Health Care Resource Management

Present and Future Challenges

Health Care Resource Management

Present and Future Challenges

Sylvia Anderson Price, PhD, RN
Professor (Retired)
College of Nursing
University of Tennessee at Memphis
Memphis, Tennessee

Marylane Wade Koch, MSN, RN, CNAA, CPHQ
Director, Community Health Outreach
Partnership for Women's and Children's Health
Methodist Health Systems/University of Tennessee
Memphis, Tennessee

Sandra Bassett, MS, RN, CPHQ, FNAHQ
Manager, Quality Management/Medical Records
Methodist Alliance Home Care Services
Memphis, Tennessee

With 23 illustrations

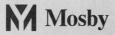 Mosby

St. Louis Baltimore Boston Carlsbad
Chicago Minneapolis New York Philadelphia Portland
London Milan Sydney Tokyo Toronto

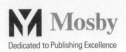
Mosby
Dedicated to Publishing Excellence

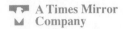
A Times Mirror
Company

Vice President and Publisher: Nancy L. Coon
Editor-In-Chief: Darlene Como
Editor: Yvonne Alexopoulos
Developmental Editor: Dana Knighten
Associate Developmental Editor: Kimberly A. Netterville
Project Manager: John Rogers
Associate Production Editor: Mary Turner
Designer: Yael Kats
Manufacturing Manager: Linda Ierardi

Printed in the United States of America
Composition by The Clarinda Company
Printing/binding by RR Donnelley & Sons Company

Mosby, Inc.
11830 Westline Industrial Drive
St. Louis, Missouri 63146

International Standard Book Number ISBN 0-8151-22985

98 99 00 01 02/9 8 7 6 5 4 3 2 1

Contributors

Sally K. Aldrich, MSN, RN, CNAA
Assistant Director
Methodist Alliance Hospice
Memphis, Tennessee

Kathy L. Beck, MSN, RN
Case Management Director
St. Joseph's Hospital
Memphis, Tennessee

Peter I. Buerhaus, PhD, RN, FAAN
Director, Harvard Nursing Research Institute,
Assistant Professor of Health Policy and Management
Harvard School of Public Health
Boston, Massachusetts

Margaret M. Calarco, PhD, RN
Director, Quality Improvement and Employee Empowerment
University of Michigan Hospitals and Health Centers
Ann Arbor, Michigan

Harriet Van Ess Coeling, PhD, RN, CNS
Associate Professor
School of Nursing
Kent State University
Kent, Ohio

Penelope Laing Cukr, DNSc, RN
Assistant Professor
School of Nursing
Kent State University
Kent, Ohio

Alice M. Davidson, MS, RN, JD
Field Representative
Joint Commission on Accreditation of Healthcare Organizations
Oakbrook Park, Illinois

Carol Dobos, PhD, RN, CNAA
Director, Children's Services,
Assistant Professor
College of Nursing
Medical University of South Carolina
Charleston, South Carolina

Deborah Esmon, MSN, RN, MBA
Director, Clinical Services
Methodist Alliance Home Care
Memphis, Tennessee

Maureen Goode, MA, RN
Clinical Nurse
Pediatric Cardiothoracic Intensive Care Unit
The Michigan Congenital Heart Center
University of Michigan Health System
Ann Arbor, Michigan

Paula R. Jaco, MSN, RN, CNAA
Vice President of Nursing Services
Marshall Regional Medical Center
Marshall, Texas

Susan R. Jacob, PhD, RN
Professor
Loewenberg School of Nursing
The University of Memphis
Memphis, Tennessee

Cheryl Slagle King, MPM, RN, CNAA
Vice President, Nursing
Allegheny General Hospital
Pittsburgh, Pennsylvania

Robert W. Koch, MSN, RN, CNA
Assistant Professor
Loewenburg School of Nursing
University of Memphis
Memphis, Tennessee

Ann E. Koliner, MBA, MHA, RN
Manager
International Services
Allegheny General Hospital
Pittsburgh, Pennsylvania

Robin Mobley, MSN, RN
Nurse Manager, ICU/BMT
St. Jude Children's Research Hospital
Memphis, Tennessee

Tommie L. Norris, MSN, RN
Instructor
Loewenberg School of Nursing
University of Memphis
Memphis, Tennessee

C. Ben Sanders, MSN, RN
Senior Consultant
Health Management Programs
Greenstone Healthcare Solutions
Kalamazoo, Michigan

Lillian M. Simms, PhD, RN, FAAN
Associate Professor of Nursing Emeritus
School of Nursing
University of Michigan
Ann Arbor, Michigan

Phyllis Skorga, PhD, RN
Senior Director
Medical Services
Southern Health Plan, Inc.
Memphis, Tennessee

Reviewers

Kathleen Duncan, PhD, RN
Assistant Professor
University of Nebraska Medical Center
Lincoln, Nebraska

Gail E. Russell, EdD, RN, CNAA
Visiting Lecturer
University of Massachusetts—Dartmouth
North Dartmouth, Massachusetts

Foreword

Resource management is the single most important skill that successful, clinically competent nurses have. Drawing from Webster's definition of management, resource management is directing, controlling, and carrying on (managing) that on which health care depends (resources). For most of a generation nurses have not directed, controlled, or carried on health care. Nurses have carried out health care and depended on nonnursing personnel to provide and allocate resources. Nursing's attention has been directed toward assessment and analysis of patient data to plan and provide care for individuals. Today those same analytical skills need to be extended to include the skillful analysis of aggregate data to secure and allocate resources to be able to provide the care that is needed. The challenge for practicing clinicians and nursing students is reclaiming this strategically significant role they have not seen fully enacted for more than a generation. Two films that portray the lost art of nursing resource management are the 1997 film *In Love and War* and the World War II film *So Proudly We Hail*. An expert nursing clinician who recently viewed one of these films commented, "I had forgotten how powerful nurses were."

Historically nurses were *the* resource managers because nurses composed the only health professional group that could envision the entire continuum of care, predict what could or would occur, and coordinate the best outcome. Human resources, equipment, health care informatics, and health care dollars are once again becoming the business of nursing because nurses are the people with the expertise to most wisely use them. As a young critical care nurse I recall with great chagrin an all-too-successful proposal to an employing hospital that "nurses needed to nurse" and business people needed to conduct the business of health care. Although I quickly learned that our young businessman with his MBA could not be taught how to manage four critical care units, nor could he be taught how to manage one without sending him to nursing school, it took some time to undo the damage that was done. Regrettably, the health care industry is still struggling with the same learning curve.

What would health care look like if every nurse clearly understood that nursing is resource management and each nurse managed resources? In hospital and home care settings professional nurses would exchange the physically arduous "doing" work of nursing that can easily be done by lesser skilled persons for the "thinking" work of nursing for which there has been no time. Professional nurses would insist on having the authority to ensure that the "doing" work was done and done well. Patients would be admitted to hospital or home care with a care path or care track that would clearly outline (1) day-to-day changes in care, (2) self-care deficits that would either be corrected or require continuing home care, (3) patient and/or caregiver education, and (4) the plan for discharge. Required variances would be analyzed to further refine predictive care models that have the best overall outcome and represent "best practices."

Practice problems would be resolved through adequate CQI procedures that are solution oriented. In hospital systems the disruptions in work flow in medical/surgical hospital units would be diminished by staffing for them via admission nurses who would fully admit patients to unit care when the entire set of admission procedures was fully completed and the plan of care in place. Perioperative time delays for the eternal search for a preoperative history and physical examination report would cease because advanced practice nurses would have performed this task.

Communication disconnects between nurses and physicians in hospital and home care would dramatically diminish through a computerized messaging system that would provide the physician with an easily obtained, brief report that includes the problems that need to be addressed. Laboratory data would be immediately linked to physician offices and would require a physician code to record the receipt of variant lab values. Using bar code technology, computer links would be established to record in all the necessary places any assessment data obtained. When vital signs, weights, intakes, and outputs were obtained, caregivers would have a bar code wand that would add this data to the proper record. With bar-coded patient wristbands medication errors would be eliminated because there would have to be a timed match between the medication and patient bar code. At the same time medications would be instantly documented.

Emergency departments would recognize that triage nurses require advanced practice skills to (1) immediately treat and discharge common and recurring problems or (2) order further diagnostic tests to be begun immediately. Much of the care that costs time in emergency departments would be dramatically reduced through the effective use of nurses across an educational continuum.

In all systems of health care, methods to produce seamless, more effective, and less costly care would be financially rewarded. When nurses once again take on the "thinking" work of nursing, they will determine that problems can be resolved. Time-wasting procedures can be eliminated. There is no other area of health care that is more deserving of study or the acquisition of expertise than the skillful management of all health care resources. The health care resources that are well managed today are the resources that are available for use tomorrow. In the words of the immortal Dr. Seuss, "Oh the places we can go and the things we can think . . . "

Toni Bargaliotti, DNSc, RN
Dean and Professor
Loewenberg School of Nursing
University of Memphis
Memphis, Tennessee

It is imperative that the nursing profession be cognizant of the limited resources and their consequences on the health care system. Resource management emphasizes using cost-effective approaches to the delivery of health care while maintaining quality nursing care. *Health Care Resource Management: Present and Future Challenges* presents an integration of the key elements of effective resource procurement and allocation and quality improvement efforts that promote quality nursing care. A proposed conceptual model for managing health care resources encompasses this process of obtaining and prudently distributing health care resources while maintaining high-quality, client-centered nursing care. Practitioners of nursing and nurse executives at all levels must lead and facilitate these endeavors.

Health care agencies are attempting to provide more services with limited resources. Gaining a competitive edge in the health care industry requires establishing resource management systems that will minimize resource consumption to maximize consumer satisfaction. Consumerism and reimbursement issues have made a significant impact on professional nursing practice. Consumers are concerned that the cost of health care is too great for the benefits received. The challenge for the nursing profession is to change this perception for consumers, reimbursers, and other health care professionals. We believe that nurses are the leaders in providing high-quality care at a reasonable cost. The nursing profession must create a culture that empowers nurses to reduce cost, as well as improve quality. Nursing has the ability and opportunity to demonstrate its worth and affect cost-effective utilization of resources within the health care delivery system.

Health Care Resource Management: Present and Future Challenges is a comprehensive analysis of the utilization of health care resources, issues relevant to nursing, and the implications for professional nursing practice. It is designed for upper-level nursing undergraduate students, registered nurses in BSN completion programs, and master's degree students. It is also a relevant reference for practicing nurses in a variety of health care settings.

We have organized this text by key issues evolving in health care. Each chapter features learning objectives and discussion questions to help the reader grasp the content of the chapter. Case studies, along with case study exercises, are presented at the end of selected chapters to reinforce the subject of the chapters. The concepts in this book are presented in four major parts:

- **Part I, Present Opportunities in Resource Management,** emphasizes that effective resource management is a primary concern for health care providers and consumers. Key concepts include managing time, human, and financial resources relative to conserving health care resources.

- **Part II, Principles and Processes Utilized in Resource Management,** explores the role of nursing in resource procurement, allocation, and conservation. Examples of research studies are presented to document cost-effectiveness of health care delivery models and the importance of time management. The importance of critical thinking skills in the leadership and decision-making roles of the professional nurse is also addressed. A comprehensive discussion and analysis of continuous quality improvement (CQI) principles presents the importance of nursing's leadership role in spearheading the quality improvement within health care organizations. The concept of work redesign and its impact on the utilization of health care resources are also explored.
- **Part III, Techniques, Strategies, and Practical Applications for Resource Management,** concerns the roles of managed care, case management, shared governance management models, and interdisciplinary collaboration in practice in conserving health care resources. Clinical pathways and quality management measurement indicators are explored as approaches to lowering health care costs. To maximize people potential in organizations through the creation of empowered environments, health care organizations must be able to adjust rapidly to change and the acceptance of innovation. The importance of research-based practice, understanding management information systems, and managing financial resources in health care and their relevance to cost containment are critically examined.
- **Part IV, Challenges of Today and Tomorrow,** focuses on a futuristic approach to managing health care resources. The theme presented is that nurses must continually pursue opportunities to nurture the growth of the profession by facilitating a learning environment that enhances the delivery of cost-effective, high-quality nursing care. The financial and economic forces responsible for the transformation of the health care industry and the implications for nursing's input and clinical resource management roles are considered relative to the economic and clinical imperatives to lower costs and improve quality. Moral principles and ethical dilemmas regarding the allocation of scarce resources are analyzed. Diversity in the workforce is addressed, stressing that health care professionals need to recognize trends affecting society today and develop strategies to address these changes. The concluding theme is that the philosophy of continuous quality improvement holds promise to both improve quality of health care and manage costs for health care products and services.

Nursing must embrace the concept of resource management to be an effective partner in health care in the twenty-first century. Our intent is to offer a futuristic book on managing health care resources that not only is informative, but also will challenge and broaden the horizons of the health care professional.

ACKNOWLEDGMENTS

Our sincere appreciation to Darlene Como, Editor-In-Chief, for her support and enthusiasm during the initial phase of the project; to Kimberly A. Netterville, Associate Developmental Editor, and Mary Turner, Associate Production Editor, for their expert editorial assistance; and to Peggy Coggins for her excellent assistance with word processing in preparing the manuscript. We also appreciate the review and suggestions on the manuscript offered by Susan Pfoutz.

Sylvia Anderson Price
Marylane Wade Koch
Sandra Bassett

Contents

5   Continuous Quality Improvement (CQI) Principles, 41

Sandra Bassett

6   Work Redesign: Rethinking Resource Utilization, 65

Robert W. Koch
Deborah Esmon

part III Techniques, Strategies, and Practical Applications for Resource Management, 75

7   Managed Care, 77

Phyllis Skorga

8   Case Management, 91

Robert W. Koch
Kathy L. Beck
Tommie L. Norris

part I

Present Opportunities in Resource Management

chapter one

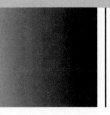

Resource Management Perspectives

Marylane Wade Koch

Learning Objectives

- Identify basic categories of resources necessary to provide a service or product in any industry and relate them to the health care industry.
- Explain key factors for change and relate them to the health care industry.
- Discuss the role of consumerism in health care resource management.
- Explore characteristics of the emerging health care system and the role of professional nurses.

Resource management is a primary concern for health care providers and consumers in today's marketplace. Health care resource management emphasizes cost-effective delivery of services and products while maintaining quality care. Consumers expect more diverse services and have higher expectations, while providers struggle with limited resources.

Nurses can take the lead in providing high-quality care at reasonable cost by effectively using health care resources. Success in demonstrating effective, quality resource management depends on knowledge, education, and skills. Understanding the dynamics of the health care environment, the role of the nurse, and the skills needed prepares the professional nurse to be a significant force in managing health care resources.

RESOURCE MANAGEMENT

Certain basic resources, usually classified as financial, physical, and human resources, are necessary to provide a product or service. Other resources include organizational systems, information systems, and technical capabilities. Management of these resources is often focused on functions of marketing, finance, research and development, operations, human resources, and information systems. How these resources are procured, allocated, and managed is critical to the success of any industry.

Marketing

Marketing links the demand by the customer to the product or service. The market position is determined by asking the question, "Who are our customers?" Through market research, industries position themselves for competitive advantage. The industries analyze trends, determine what past impact has been, and predict future impact.

Health care recognizes the importance of marketing resources as the competition for health care reimbursement dollars escalates. Consumers, the customers, will respond by purchasing and using health care products and services that are of high quality and are affordable. The industry determines who customers are and what services they desire at what price. Some health care providers may choose to develop niche markets if competition is high in primary markets.

At one time marketing was considered a small part of health care management. Competition was low, and reimbursement was plentiful. Today the reverse is true. Successful organizations know that marketing resources are critical to organizational success.

Finance

Finance is basically management of funds. The industry determines its objectives and mission and supports these through the budget process. Management of financial resources is critical to the success of an organization. Dollars must be procured and allocated to the industry's business lines to develop and offer products and services and reach the strategic objectives.

"No money, no mission" sounds harsh, but financial resource stability is necessary to achieve an organization's mission and objectives. Traditionally health care providers have been non-profit organizations that provided a mission-based service with ample reimbursement streams and support of community or religious groups. Today non-profit and for-profit organizations compete for the same limited financial resources. Community dollars and funds from churches are limited as well. Managing financial resources is critical to a health care organization's viability. In the managed care environment, health care providers constantly are challenged to do more with less.

Research and Development

An industry invests its financial resources for continued growth of product or service lines through **research and development.** With limited resources available choices among many alternatives must be determined. Human resources for research and development are costly and must be chosen carefully. Timing is critical, since a good idea developed at the wrong time for the market will result in loss of costly financial and human resources.

Research in health care may show new ways to provide services, new effective treatments, and new diagnostic possibilities. More and more research is looking at ways to provide better care for less cost with positive outcomes. The consumer wants new and/or improved products and services at an affordable cost.

Human Resources

All industries must have competent **human resources** to be successful. Jobs are matched to individuals with specific skills, aptitudes, and values. The degree to which this process is successful is reflected in job performance, employee satisfaction, and employee job absence behavior. The processes of recruitment and orientation of employees are costly in dollars, time, and energy. To maintain productivity and minimize training costs, retention of skilled workers is preferable to recruiting new ones.

Since most health care industries are labor intensive, human resource management is critical to organizational success. Quality of work life is important because individuals strive to satisfy personal needs and goals through work. Therefore employers need to consider concepts such as participative problem solving, flexible hours and work restructuring, innovative reward and incentive programs, and opportunities to be part of improvement through empowerment to improve the quality of work life for employees. People generally agree that the only long-term resource advantage for industries today is in the area of human resources.

Information Systems

Information systems are a critical resource for informed, data-driven decision making and improved productivity. Information is necessary to answer operations and strategic questions. Industries need information systems that help managers focus on critical factors for organizational success and provide high-quality, accurate data that are useful to the organization's leaders. Information systems are costly resources that can be a great strength in many areas of strategic management, such as formulation, implementation, evaluation, and control. They are also costly if poorly designed and/or ineffectively used by the organization's leaders.

Information systems play a major role in resource management in any health care system. As managed care grows, the provider of health care services must know the cost of all segments of service and product implementation. Quick access to demographics of covered lives or managed care enrollees, as well as utilization histories of health care services, makes financial decision making more accurate for organizational success. The risk-sharing opportunities in managed care make accurate data collection and analysis a must.

CUSTOMER DRIVEN CHANGE

Those living in today's information age are faced with rapidly evolving challenges. The world of work is in transformation. As change occurs some are left behind, unwilling to confront the inevitable, but most are moving to new heights of success.

Who is responsible for societal change? Consumers are more demanding in their customer requirements. They want quality services and products, at reasonable cost, provided quickly, with lots of choices. To get and keep consumer business, industry and service providers must meet these criteria and keep improving the product and the service. Purchasing power of the customers contributes to the demise of weak organizations and the success of innovative ones. In the 1930s, Joseph A. Schumpter, an economist from Czechoslovakia, termed this process "creative destruction." Industries decline as others develop. Young, aggressive companies replace weak ones that fail to adapt quickly enough through customer service development and improvement. Thus the economy basically re-creates itself (Pritchett and Pound, 1995).

KEY FACTORS FOR CHANGE

Three major factors—people, technology, and information—result in change. People are the most obvious reason for the fast rate of change. People have new ideas and, as consumers, force change. People also compete for scarce resources. As consumers demand better products and innovation improvements, business responds to these demands with change. People are both drivers and responders, producing and supporting change. The sheer number of people pushes this phenomenon. In the early 1860s the total world population was about a billion people. It took 75 years to double that number to 2 billion and only another 50 years, in 1975, to double it again to 4 billion. In the early 1990s the world population was heading toward 6 billion, with the U.S. Census Bureau predicting a world population of 10 billion by 2040 (Pritchett and Pound, 1995).

Technology is the second factor involved in forcing change. Technology is a product of human innovation, so technological trends change with population growth. Statistically, over 80% of the technological advances in our world have occurred since 1990. Since technology results in more technology, acceleration is expected to produce more change (Pritchett and Pound, 1995).

The third force that drives change is information or knowledge. More information was produced between 1965 and 1995 than in the entire period of 3000 BC to 1965. In fact, some statisticians guess that information is doubling every 5 years worldwide. This relates to another fact of people and technology: more people acquire more knowledge faster than ever through improved technology. The result? A more knowledgeable population worldwide seeking innovative improvements in products and services—change (Pritchett and Pound, 1995).

RESOURCE CHALLENGE IN THE UNITED STATES

As the population grows worldwide, competition in business to sell products and services increases. Products are cheaper to make outside the United States and offer value at a lesser price. Most Americans never hesitate to buy foreign-made products and services. Before World War II the United States was the clear leader in the world market, producing 50% of the world's manufactured goods. However, now the U.S. trade position is being challenged by aggressive competitors.

United States' economic strength was built at a time when America enjoyed rich natural resources. As Europe and Japan rebuilt their industries and the United

States lowered trade barriers and tariffs, competitors accessed the world's wealthiest customers, U.S. citizens (Pritchett and Pound, 1995).

The U.S. economic position is no longer as strong. Other countries have access to raw resources at reasonable cost. With technology, the ease of transportation, and the speed of information, competitors have gained "market share" in the global market.

CONSUMERISM: HEALTH CARE IN THE UNITED STATES

Economic change affects health care services and products, as it does in any other industry. The increasing population in the world means more need for health care resources. In the past as customers used more health care resources, demand increased and the health care market flourished. Today consumers, from individuals to insurers to government to private enterprise, desire high-quality health care services and products at reasonable costs, delivered quickly, with positive outcomes.

Consumers expect innovative health care services and state-of-the-art technology. This is often perceived as one reason for the high cost of health care in the United States: technology is expensive, and U.S. citizens consider access to health service technology a right, whether they can pay or not. The U.S. consumer is a more knowledgeable customer, raising expectations and requirements for health care products and services. This population is demanding change, and the mystique of health care healers is losing its potency (Pritchett and Pound, 1995).

Health care providers are both consumers and responders to this change. The more knowledgeable the provider, the more the expectation for valuable services at reasonable costs is accelerated. A major challenge of the U.S. health care system is similar to the economic welfare of the United States: once rich in resources, now limited in resources.

Resource management has become a major objective of health care providers. To gain a competitive edge in the current and future U.S. economy, health care providers must develop and implement effective resource management systems.

RESOURCE PRODUCTIVITY

As health care reimbursement is renegotiated in the changing world of managed care, government and other payors are seeking affordable services and products delivered within certain guidelines or regulations. Payors ask for more evidence of demonstrated quality care and customer satisfaction but offer less reimbursement for services and products. Can health care providers reach the goal of cost-efficient, quality care within reimbursement restrictions? This will be the ongoing challenge as health care organizations compete for restricted resources.

Other businesses have experienced similar situations with consumer demands and environmental regulations. Many think adding regulations or requirements raises costs. However, in the real world of dynamic competition, companies are constantly offering solutions to meet customer expectations and cover regulatory demands.

These companies are redesigning processes and looking at innovations that use resources "from raw materials to energy, to labor" (Porter and van der Linde, 1995) for enhanced **resource productivity.** Ultimately innovations actually lower costs and improve the service or product value to the customer.

An example is the Dutch flower industry, which faced strict regulations in the release of chemicals into the environment that were contaminating soil and groundwater. It developed a closed-looped system in the greenhouses that grew flowers in water and rock wood rather than soil. This process actually reduced variations in growing conditions, resulting in a better product. The net result was reduced environmental impact, lowered cost, improved-quality products, and improved competitiveness (Porter and van der Linde, 1995).

The lessons for health care providers are (1) see resource restriction and regulation as an opportunity for improvement, (2) accept that challenge, (3) review all processes and devise less costly ways to provide similar, perhaps improved, products and services, and (4) answer the questions, "Where are the wasted resources, wasted efforts, and customer dissatisfaction?" and "What can we do to provide cost-efficient quality health care services and products?"

Summary

In 1991 the Pew Health Professions Commission published a report stating that the current training and education process of health professionals was inadequate to meet the future health care needs of the American public. In a follow-up report in 1993, this group addressed the competencies needed for health care professionals in 2005. The report defined characteristics of the emerging health care systems as (1) orientation toward health, (2) population perspective, (3) intensive use of information, (4) focus on the consumer, (5) knowledge of treatment outcomes, (6) constrained resources, (7) coordination of services, (8) reconsideration of human values, (9) expectations of accountability, and (10) growing interdependence (Pew Health Professions Commission, 1993). Corresponding trends that influence nursing practice include the aging population, health promotion and disease prevention, cost-effective care, management of care, community orientation, and differentiation of practice and education (Pew Health Professions Commission, 1993). All of these have implications for health care resource management.

Nurses have the knowledge, skills, and access to effect changes in health care resource management. The changing health care environment is a constant. Nurses can choose to develop themselves and their practice value within these restrictions and seek opportunities to influence the changing profession.

Nurses can accept **stewardship** of limited health care resources to optimize and improve health care for society today. Stewardship is defined as "the conducting, supervising, or managing of something, especially the careful and responsible management of something entrusted to one's care." (*Merriam-Webster's Collegiate Dictionary,* 1993) Stewardship is a way of managing resources to create fundamental change in a system (Block, 1993). For effective stewardship, nurses must be willing to be accountable for the well-being of the health care system at large by using their skills to provide cost-efficient, quality care. In doing this, nurses help create the health care system of today and the future.

Discussion Questions

1. Why is resource management important in the health care environment of today and the future?
2. Discuss four areas of resources necessary to run a business. How do these areas relate to the health care industry?
3. Why is change occurring in the health care environment? What role do consumers play in this change?
4. What role do nurses play in health care resource management? Define stewardship and the relationship to professional nursing practice.

REFERENCES

Block P: *Stewardship,* San Francisco, 1993, Berrett-Koehler.

Merriam-Webster's Collegiate Dictionary, ed 10, Springfield, Mass, 1993, Merriam-Webster.

Pew Health Professions Commission: Healthy America: Practitioners for 2005, Durham, NC, 1991, Duke University Medical Center.

Pew Health Professions Commission: Health professions education for the future: Schools in service to the nation, San Francisco, 1993, UCSF Center for the Health Professions.

Porter ME, van der Linde C: Green and competitive: Ending the stalemate, *Harvard Business Review* 73(5):120, 1995.

Pritchett P, Pound R: *A survival guide to the stress of organization change,* Dallas, 1995, Pritchett & Associates.

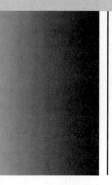

chapter two

Trends in the Health Care Environment: Managing Time, Human, and Financial Resources

Sylvia Anderson Price

Learning Objectives

- Describe the importance of time management relative to conserving health care resources.
- Analyze the effects of reimbursement mechanisms on the health care delivery system.
- Describe the health care system in the twenty-first century.

Nurse managers at all organizational levels must be committed to and personally involved in managing time, financial, and human resources. Leaders and members of thriving organizations generally set demanding goals for themselves, are more innovative, take more risks, and change at a more accelerated rate. This is relevant when you consider that the survival of health care organizations within our society depends largely on managers responding appropriately to the forces that demand effective use of resources.

TIME MANAGEMENT

Effective time management is essential for maximizing use of resources. Time management consists of the planned, organized assessment of when and how long it takes to perform an activity. Managers who use their time effectively choose their activities and decide when and how to do them. They can exercise some control over what they choose to respond to and which problems they agree to address. However, it is impossible to control all of their time because they are often interrupted and must respond to crisis situations. An administrator's time is often spent responding to requests, demands, and problems that are initiated by others. Robbins and Coulter (1996) refer to this as "response time" and treat it as uncontrollable. The portion that is under a manager's control is "discretionary time." Recommendations to improve time management apply to discretionary time, or that which is manageable.

Discretionary time tends to become available in small time slots—5 minutes here, 5 minutes there. Managers should determine what time is discretionary and then organize activities so as to accumulate this discretionary time in blocks large enough to be useful. For example, specific tasks that have priority deadlines need to be considered first. Prioritizing your activities as to how urgent they are is important—must they be done immediately, or are they important but can be done at a later time?

FINANCIAL RESOURCE MANAGEMENT

The influence of rising costs of health care, reimbursement issues, and consumerism has resulted in significant changes in health care delivery. Changes in health care are apparent as hospitals continue to downsize or "rightsize," merge and consolidate, redesign or restructure systems to survive in a highly competitive marketplace. Hospital bed capacity and occupancy rates continue to decline. To become more cost-effective and increase revenue in the present health care arena, health care providers such as hospitals and home health agencies have responded with incentives to attract more clients. For example, hospitals offer a broad range of services related to ambulatory care or outpatient services, and home health agencies are expanding their services to meet their clients' wants and needs.

Delivery Systems

An example of conserving both financial and human resources is the health care environment of managed care. **Managed care** is a delivery system that emphasizes communication and coordination of care among health care team members. The essence of this concept is that specific patient outcomes can be achieved by utilizing personnel and conserving financial resources appropriately.

Managed competition is a comprehensive use of managed care organizations in the marketplace that envisions consumer choice and selection of providers and their use of diagnostic and treatment procedures. Financial incentives promote changes in practice for providers at hospitals and in long-term care and community practice settings. Creation of health maintenance organizations (HMOs), preferred provider organizations (PPOs), and physician-hospital organizations (PHOs) facilitates closer scrutiny of financial resources through the reimbursement process. Control of costs enables service providers to compete on price.

Prospective Payment System and Capitation

The **prospective payment system (PPS),** which has been in effect since 1983, was initiated in hospitals as a way for Medicare to control expenditures by reducing length of stay yet emphasizing quality care. The health care delivery system is now moving toward a capitation system in which managed care organizations (MCOs) are paid a per capita amount for specified health services for their members or enrollees. These services are delivered either directly by the MCO or through a contract between the MCO and independent providers. Capitation tends to shift the financial risk of providing services from payors to providers and insurers. Under these contracts forces exist to use health care resources more efficiently and effectively.

Under capitation, payments are fixed for the duration of the contract and do not vary with the number of services consumed. The capitation payment rate is based on a per-member-per-month (PMPM) quantity. Grimaldi (1995a) illustrates that a capitation rate can be calculated by dividing an MCO's projected total cost by the total number of member months. For example, if projected costs are $3.6 million and 3000 members are expected to be enrolled for a total of 30,000 months, the capitation rate would equal $120 PMPM, or $3.6 million/30,000.

The MCO then divides its total costs into several categories, which include overhead and health expenses (inpatient hospital care, emergency room use, and physician office visits). Each of the services will have a projected utilization rate and the cost per unit of service the MCO expects to pay. For example, the MCO's members may average .02 day PMPM of inpatient hospital care (240 days per 1000 subscribers divided by 12 months) at a projected cost of $600 per day. The PMPM cost of inpatient hospital care would be $12, or (240/12,000) × $600.

The overhead costs are fixed expenditures that are distributed over member months. The more the portion of overhead costs remains fixed, or does not change with membership size, the greater the need for the MCO to sustain a market share (number of subscribers or enrollees) to be financially viable. If the number of members decreases, the share of the fixed cost per enrollee would increase. The capitation rate would subsequently rise, which would decrease the competitiveness of the MCO.

The monthly capitation rate can be charged by either the community rating or experience rating system. In the community rating system all members are charged the same monthly rate, which equally distributes the risk and cost of health care. In contrast, with the experience rating system, members are charged according to the group's actual utilization of services and costs of care.

Grimaldi (1995b) states, "Financial risk compels managed care organizations (MCOs) to track health costs and utilization closely, and systematically compare budgeted with actual performance." Inaccurate information may be costly, which results in avoidable losses and low quality of care. The incorrect information may also impair an MCO's ability to remedy cost problems and calculate future capitation rates.

RESOURCE ALLOCATION

Health care organizations are faced with competing pressures and demands for cost-effectiveness. Downsizing or reduction in personnel and resource allocation available for patient care services is also evident. Every health sector is affected by this reduction in health care resources. The new focus in health care is on a subscriber-based marketplace. Competition is geared toward demand, which restricts the dollars coming into the health system. The assumption is that consumers make different choices depending on their wants and needs. Through control of costs and prices, providers such as physicians and dentists compete for clients. Groups such as businesses, labor unions, and managed care organizations (MCOs) bargain with providers over prices. The assumption is that cost containment results through market forces and consumer choice.

The following example illustrates the factors that must be considered when making cost containment–related decisions. Recently Johnson & Johnson introduced a medical device known as a "stent" for cardiac patients that requires twice the hospital stay and is significantly more costly than a similar procedure. This device is a stainless steel mesh sleeve that props open blocked coronary arteries and keeps them from reclosing after an angioplasty procedure. It is predicted that 100,000 stents will be implanted in heart patients in the United States. This number could double as soon as 1997 to 50% of the estimated 400,000 patients who undergo angioplasties annually. However, some cardiologists are concerned that the rapid acceptance of the device is far ahead of the knowledge available from studies to guide its results.

"We can't take for granted that these metal sleeves will be completely innocuous and inert for years to come," states Eric J. Topol, chairman of cardiology at the Cleveland Clinic. One of the major problems is cost. The stent is priced at $1600, which is approximately four times the cost of a regular angioplasty balloon. Some patients may need more than one stent. Careful examination of reimbursement rates for the stent versus the balloon is important because of the financial impact in the hospital cardiac catheterization labs where the procedures are usually performed. The cost-benefit analysis must be carefully scrutinized as to which procedure, the balloon or the stent, would be more effective for the patient. The question is whether the device will be more cost-effective by reducing the need for repeat balloon procedures and possibly bypass surgery (Winslow, 1995).

CONSERVING RESOURCES

Legislative proposals and insurance market forces provide consumers with incentives to decrease unwarranted use of health care and to select the most cost-effective health care through managed care plans. The goal is to reduce the deductions employers can claim for medical benefits, which would encourage them to choose less costly health insurance programs. The proposals also advocate an increase in cost sharing through deductibles and copayments, which would be included in plans for the employed and also Medicare and Medicaid recipients.

Medicare home health care expenditures have risen dramatically because of increased legislative and regulatory expansions of coverage, discharging patients "quicker and sicker" from hospitals, high-tech care provided in the home, fraud and abuse in billing practices, and proliferation of home health agencies. The number of Medicare-certified agencies increased from 5700 in 1990 to 9800 in 1996. An estimated three fifths of hospitals are now operating home care agencies.

Over the past 7 years the percentage of Medicare beneficiaries using home care rose from 5.6% to 10.1%, the average number of visits per patient increased from 33 to 76, and spending rose from $3 billion to $16 billion. Costs for posthospital services such as skilled nursing and rehabilitation—with total post–acute care outlays rising from $8.3 billion to more than $30 billion—make up about one sixth of all Medicare expenses (Meyer, 1997).

The emphasis is now on reducing the costs of Medicare home health services. The Clinton administration issued a package of proposals to curb Medicare home care costs. Agencies are currently reimbursed according to their historical costs for providing services up to limits determined by national averages. By 1999 the government wants to pay a prospective rate for each episode of care, which would be adjusted for patient case mix. The cost-reduction measures proposed by the Clinton administration include setting lower limits for cost-based payments; capping average annual per-beneficiary costs at each agency; basing payment on where services are provided, not the agency's location; clarifying the definition of "homebound" for patient eligibility; and developing visit standards for each condition as a basis for making decisions on claims.

The American Hospital Association favors adopting prospective payment systems for home health and skilled nursing as soon as possible. According to Bruce Vladeck, Health Care Financing Administration's former administrator, studies indicate that the industry's preferred per-visit payment approach does not save money. Nor does its case-mix adjuster explain variation among agencies. Vladeck emphasizes that more research is needed on the adjuster and the overall prospective payment methodology to develop a system that controls cost and protects quality.

Mergers, acquisitions, alliances, and new partnerships are evident in health care. For example, Kuttner (1996) reports that conversions from non-profit to investor-owned hospitals have increased from 34 in 1994 to 58 in 1995. These mergers are a means to conserve resources or use resources more efficiently. Coordination, co-operation, and integration should prepare multihospital systems for health care reform. Communication is the essence of a successful merger. Information systems used by the facilities must interface. For example, merging with other hospitals and clinics creates an integrated network to meet changing demands in relation to health care services. Cost reduction is a critical issue, but the emphasis on quality is paramount.

Managers need to emphasize the benefits to all the agencies involved in the merger. Health care providers of varying size and ownership are attracted to the benefits, especially in shared operations arenas such as finance, purchasing, and other duplicative services. An integral part of a merger is the potential savings realized in areas such as purchasing—for example, purchasing similar products jointly from vendors so that the health care organization will get the best competitive price.

HEALTH CARE IN THE TWENTY-FIRST CENTURY

Health care is continually undergoing change. Change plays a dominant role in any enterprise. The major challenges facing nursing today and in the twenty-first century will influence the health care delivery system. Nurses must have a significant role in redesigning the health care system to effectively utilize resources and coordinate services appropriately. The survival of health care organizations in our society is dependent on their responding appropriately to the forces of change, which include changing patterns of health care delivery, advances in knowledge and technological innovations, total quality improvement, and cost-containment strategies.

The Pew Health Professions Commission (1995) stresses that most of the public and private sector demands for reform are being driven by the perception that health care is consuming too much of our nation's resources. Practitioners must be responsible for providing cost-effective and appropriate care. The system that is emerging will demand price and cost reductions, and health professionals will either participate in this process or abdicate it to non-clinicians—which would not be in the interest of the nation's health. The commission further states that health professionals must be competent and willing to manage the cost of care. The practitioner in the twenty-first century must be knowledgeable and must apply increasingly complex technologies not only in an appropriate but also a cost-effective manner to balance clinical and system demands. Health care practitioners need to recapture the tradition of a continuing commitment to lifelong learning.

Communication and information technologies are important drivers of the emerging health care system. Complex, managed, information-driven systems require health professionals who can manage and use large volumes of scientific, technological, and patient information that will enable them to deliver effective clinical care in the context of community and system needs.

The Pew commission implies that some are concerned that our enormous investment in health care is not producing the level of return that we expect. The health care industry now realizes the necessity of doing more high-quality work less expensively and more appropriately. "Using resources more efficiently will require better design, and more efficient and effective leadership and management. In a market-driven system, public accountability will have to extend to the issues of over-utilization and under-utilization." (Pew Health Professions Commission, 1995)

Summary

Can we create a health care system that has the goal of improving the health status of clients yet encouraging conservation in resource use? Health care networks and managed competition will provide more primary, preventive, and long-term care services. In initiating health promotion and primary care programs, hospitals, as well as other home health agencies, must attract clients to use such services. These primary care programs are a challenge to hospitals because these programs extend the hospital's traditional role as a provider of inpatient and emergency services. Services are extended from hospital-based, illness-related activities to a wellness emphasis. The consumer has a choice as to whether, when, and where to seek health care. These prospective clients need to be knowledgeable regarding the service or product and its desired attributes. The information disseminated must be based on what consumers need to know. Therefore practitioners should help clients participate in decisions concerning their personal health care.

The ultimate goal is to keep clients healthy while promoting high-quality care. We must provide cost-effective health care to prevent unnecessary duplication and deal directly with our clients with full responsibility and accountability for results.

Discussion Questions

1. How can nurse managers determine how effectively they manage their time?
2. Why do nurse managers need to be knowledgeable about the capitation mechanism for a managed care organization?
3. What do you envision as nurses' role in the health care system of the twenty-first century?

Case Study

After years of being financially viable, the Parker State Health Center (PSHC), a university health center, is in the "red" this fiscal year. A health center committee is deciding how to abolish 1100 jobs—amounting to 14% of the nonphysician workforce—and cut annual expenses by $100 million. Within 2 years, the PS Hospital moved from a $25 million operating profit to a $10 million loss.

Insurers, applying the cost-reduction principles of managed care, are reimbursing less and directing many clients from the health center to lower cost hospitals. Because employers have switched from traditional medical insurance plans to HMOs and PPOs, referral decisions are being made by administrators intent on reducing costs.

Managed care penetration will likely be 40% to 50% of the health care marketplace in this geographical area over the next few years. The health center's executive officer readily admits that PSHC's cost per case is more than one-third higher than that of competitors in the region, which threatens its survival. Two national networks for transplant surgery offered by Prudential and United HealthCare list several comparable health centers as providers, but not PSHC. With insurers planning more preferred provider specialty networks, if PSHC does not lower costs its patients will go elsewhere.

University health centers are a hybrid of an educational institution, research center, and business enterprise. The PSHC is staffed by more than 1100 salaried physicians and more than 700 resident physicians. This structure served Parker State well during times of plenty when insurers were reimbursing what they were billed, but not in a cost containment environment. Efforts to control costs by influencing practice patterns are hampered by independent medical faculty. The physicians, not hospital administrators or nurses, are controlling the planned $100 million spending reductions. They are the majority on the Hospital Redesign Planning Committee, which will decide on and present the downsizing recommendations to the hospital's administrators.

The financial implications for nursing at PSHC are critical. The nurse-per-patient ratio is decreasing; more critically ill patients have fewer nurses to care for them. This will inevitably affect quality nursing care.

The hospital's chief executive officer outlined ways PSHC could find $100 million in cost reductions each year for the next 3 years. Layoffs and attrition of nonphysician personnel and reduction of benefits and salary of remaining employees were given as possible cost-cutting strategies. Persuading the physicians to become more efficient by being more frugal in their prescribing and ordering patterns, another possibility, is one of the most difficult changes to achieve. The average length of stay (LOS) has actually risen over the last year. Since the hospital is reimbursed a fixed amount per admission, which is determined by diagnosis, each day represents a loss to the hospital. The average cost per case has also risen by 2% to 3%. These figures suggest that the hospital is not responding well to the current environment.

Cost-cutting scenarios such as lower staff benefits, improved purchasing, reduced capital costs, and salary concessions must occur. However, more than any other cost-cutting measure, PSHC physicians, who manage patient care, must practice medicine in ways that their competitors are already using.

Case Study cont'd

Case Study Exercise
1. Are you in agreement with the hospital administrator's recommendations for cost reductions over the next 3 years?
2. As a nurse manager at PSHC, what would you recommend as cost-cutting measures relative to the 14% reduction in the nonphysician staff?
3. How would you suggest that physicians and nurses work collaboratively in the current financial crisis?

REFERENCES

Grimaldi P: Capitation savvy a must, *Nurs Manage* 26(2):33, 1995a.

Grimaldi P: Capitation's information imperative, *Nurs Manage* 26(4):12, 1995b.

Kuttner R: Columbia/HCA and the resurgence of the for-profit hospital business, *N Engl J Med* 335(5, pt. 1):362, 1996.

Meyer H: Home (care) improvement, *Hosp Health Netw* 71(8):40, 1997.

Pew Health Professions Commission: Critical challenges: Revitalizing the health professions for the twenty-first century, San Francisco, 1995, UCSF Center for the Health Professions.

Robbins S, Coulter M: *Management,* ed 5, Upper Saddle River, NJ, 1996, Prentice Hall.

Winslow R: Simple device to prop clogged arteries open changes coronary care, *The Wall Street Journal* LXXVII(6):A1, 1995.

part II

Principles and Processes Utilized in Resource Management

chapter **three**

Role of Nursing in Resource Procurement, Allocation, and Conservation

Sylvia Anderson Price

Learning Objectives

- Explain the role of nursing in procuring, allocating, and conserving resources.
- Differentiate between a goal-driven and a resource-driven model in relation to the current nursing care delivery system.
- Analyze the impact of nursing case management on cost-effectiveness and outcomes.
- Describe the significance of time and money in the allocation and conservation of resources.

Nurses comprise the largest group of health care professionals. It is critical that all nursing personnel be able to procure, allocate, and conserve resources effectively and efficiently. All nurses need to understand the principles underlying cost containment and allocation of resources and the relationship between cost of nursing and quality outcomes. Nurses must analyze which activities are necessary and devise innovative job categories based on skill levels, using advanced nurse practitioners for more complex tasks. The issue becomes one of determining how effectively nursing is allocating its resources concerning time and competency of the staff.

A model for managing health care resources is depicted in Figure 3-1. The model represents nursing's role in managing health care resources. This role encompasses the process of obtaining (procuring) and prudently distributing (allocating and conserving) health care resources while maintaining high-quality client-centered nursing care (quality improvement). Resource procurement, allocation, and conservation will be addressed in this chapter. Refer to Chapters 5 and 21 for a comprehensive discussion of quality improvement.

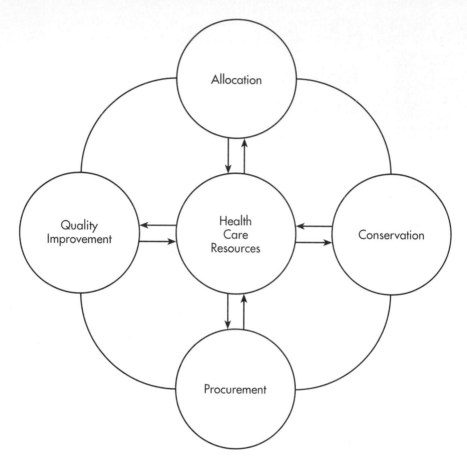

Figure 3-1   A model for managing health care resources.

RESOURCE PROCUREMENT

Barnum (1994) emphasizes that when resources are plentiful, nursing shifts to an idealized goal-driven model that is based on a single caregiver per patient viewpoint, not a task-oriented viewpoint. However, when resources are scarce it is necessary to switch to a larger group of caregivers interacting with more patients, a task-orientation or resource-driven model. Nurses take into account the environment and resources and then determine what goals can be accomplished for a patient group. A resource-driven model of care demands consideration of both quality and quantity.

The question is how much and what level of care can be given in a limited number of hours. How do nurses function in a resource-scarce environment? Barnum argues that we are once again using a task-orientation model, that is, a staff mix of different skill levels for the patient. The changes made in the restructuring of nursing practice are causing a shift toward functional nursing. Fewer staff members are needed, patient/client care is fragmented, clinical decision making is shift based, and work allocation involves the same tasks for all patients. An element of increased complexity is, however, inherent.

Barnum further emphasizes that the principle of restructured practice is one of safeguarding precious resources, namely, nursing time and expertise. Restructured nursing practice often involves fewer total staff, including registered nurses and advanced nurse practitioners. Tasks may be different depending on the health care agency. In this nursing practice someone is needed to coordinate all the necessary activities that are being done by staff with various skill levels. The case manager, who is responsible for assessing the patient care outcomes, coordinates the staff's activities. The head nurse maintains responsibility for the unit but is accountable to a case manager for patient outcomes.

NURSING CASE MANAGEMENT

The goals for nursing case management are efficient and effective nursing care delivery. Nursing case management within the hospital setting increased by 50% between 1990 and 1991 (Boston, 1993). The intent of this delivery model is to manage the utilization, quality, and cost of health care resources during the patient's illness episode. Case managers collaborate and coordinate the multidisciplinary resources needed for the patient during the episode. A **care map** is a tool of case management that is used for planning patient care. It graphs multidisciplinary staff's actions across a timeline, which is similar to a critical path with indicators for measuring quality on the same timed axis. A care map contains an outcome index in addition to descriptions of key interventions that are necessary for producing the stated outcomes. These outcome index statements are the quality descriptors (Zander, 1992). The care map analysis is recognized to be an important element in controlling resource utilization and length of stay. (See Chapter 8.)

Cohen (1991) describes an investigation assessing the cost-effectiveness of a nursing case management model in a large acute care hospital setting. The model incorporated a team nursing approach using various skill levels of nursing personnel. Patient care was monitored using critical paths and nursing care management plans. The study measured the effects of a nursing case management model on length of stay of patients hospitalized for ccsarean section. It also assessed the cost of delivering care to this patient group. A quasiexperimental design compared the experimental group (case management model) and control unit (conventional mode of patient care delivery).

RESULTS:
Length of Stay (LOS)
- Significant reduction in patient LOS on the experimental unit, which reported a mean LOS of 4.86 days, compared with 6.02 days on the control unit
- Declined by 1.16 days (19%) between the control and experimental groups

Total Direct Nursing Care Hours
- Significantly higher with the experimental group (mean of 16.84 hours), compared with the control group (mean of 12.28 hours)
  Inpatient Resources, Charges, and Expenditures
- Experimental group average charges of $5147.05 per case, compared with the control group charges of $6198.90 per case
- The average total cost per patient case was lower for the experimental compared with the control group. A savings of $930.40 per patient case was realized.

Cohen emphasizes that nursing case management provides the framework by which to collect data on the resources needed and used for delivery of patient care. This data can define the parameters and relative use of resources for patient care services in an attempt to approximate costs.

Another important area to measure is the impact of case management on preventive services, cost-effectiveness, and outcomes. An example of outcome evaluation is a study conducted by Buescher et al. (1991) of births to North Carolina women on Medicaid between 1988 and 1989. For women on Medicaid who did not receive maternity care coordinated services (case management), the incidence of low birth weight was 21% higher, that of very low birth weight was 62% higher, and the infant mortality was 23% higher than it was for those who received such services. Cost-effectiveness of case management services was also significant. It was estimated that for each $1 spent on maternity care coordination, Medicaid saved $2.02 in medical expenditures for newborns up to 60 days of age.

The effect of maternity care coordinated services, or case management, did increase participation in preventive services. Data indicate among health department patients, women who received case management during pregnancy were more likely than those who did not to enroll themselves (91% versus 67%) and their infants in the Special Supplemental Food Program for Women, Infants and Children (WIC) (77% versus 36%), to obtain a postpartum family planning examination (68% versus 39%), and to take their infants for well child care (65% versus 25%). These findings suggest that maternity care coordination can be effective in reducing low birth weight, infant mortality, and costs among babies born to low-income women.

Fields (1995) states that much of the current research that suggests that nursing case management reduces costs and maintains or improves quality does not control for extraneous variables that might influence posttest data. Thus inferences associated with causality in relation to nursing case management, reduced costs, and maintained or improved quality are weak. She investigates in the following example the effects of nursing case management on LOS and resource consumption.

Research study at a 416-bed tertiary care hospital in the mid-Atlantic region used a retrospective examination of patient records to compare pairs of similar cases, ones who had experienced case management and the comparable cases who had not. The outcome variables of LOS and costs were examined.

A sample comprised 201 case-managed patients discharged from the hospital during 1992 with selected medical-surgical diagnoses. A matched sampling was used to select non–case-managed patients. The Computerized Severity Index (CSI) was used to measure a covariate, severity of illness. Nursing intensity data were also collected. Other covariates added postmatching were ICU stay, ICU case management, and discharge destination.

RESULTS:

- Nursing case management increased LOS. The unadjusted mean difference in LOS between the two groups was 2.60 days, with the case management group having longer LOS. Differences in total costs were influenced by increased room and board costs, for which LOS serves as a good proxy. No significant differences were found in regard to ancillary charges.
- Investigation of subgroups (for example, individuals over 65 with incomes less than $25,000 who live alone) showed nursing case management had no effect.

These findings indicate that case management does not significantly reduce length of stay across a broad spectrum of patients. Further investigation into factors and services affecting cost is merited. These findings are relevant and should assist nurse administrators in decision making with regard to their choice of a care delivery system.

RESOURCE ALLOCATION AND CONSERVATION

When allocating health care resources, time and money wasted in scheduling and coordinating patient procedures are critical issues that need to be addressed. Prescott et al. (1991) specify that if more unit management responsibilities could be shifted from nurses to nonnursing personnel, approximately 48 minutes per nurse per shift could be redirected to patient care. In a hospital with 600 full-time nurses this would mean an additional 307 hours of direct patient care per day. These changes would contribute the equivalent of the work of 48 additional full-time nurses to direct patient care.

A study done by Arthur Andersen & Company reported that only 35% of a nurse's time was involved in direct patient care, which included care planning, assessment, teaching, and clinical (IVs, medications, treatments). Documentation accounted for 20% of the nurse's time (Brider, 1992).

Other studies estimate that hospital nurses spend 15% to 20% of their time documenting information concerning patients (Gwozdz and Del Tongo-Armanasco, 1992; Miller and Pastorino, 1990). The most common cause of partial shift overtime is documentation, because nurses wait until end of shift to document.

Spurck et al. (1995) emphasize that traditional communication systems such as face-to-face conversation and the use of pagers are not sufficient to cope with the increased volume and intensity of communication required among health personnel, patients, and family members. For example, nurses who are paged must leave the patient to answer the page.

A wireless telecommunication system called Spectralink was instituted on two medical-surgical units at the University Hospital in Denver, Colorado, in which nurses carried a portable (not cellular) telephone that directly interfaced with the existing phone system at the hospital. The phone has the features of call-forwarding, hold, and conferences.

Evaluation research of this system revealed significant time savings by nurses and clerical personnel. The following time savings were found:

- The time a nurse took to get to the phone decreased from 3 minutes and 25 seconds to 0 seconds, for a 100% decrease.
- The time a nurse spent waiting in the nursing station for a return page went from 52 minutes and 24 seconds to 1 minute and 46 seconds, for a 99% decrease.
- Clerical time required to locate a nurse for a phone call went from 28 minutes and 26 seconds to 20 seconds, for a 86% decrease.
- The number of incoming callers placed on hold and the length of time a caller was placed on hold both decreased by 50%.

The authors estimate that over a 1-year period the study unit could potentially save 1710 hours in lost time, which was based on calls decreasing by 50% during evening and night shifts. They state that "In addition to freeing personnel up for patient care and other productive activities, this time savings represents a significant potential cost savings for the hospital." (Spurck et al., 1995)

Quist (1992) reported on a study conducted on 42 medical/surgical, ICU, perinatal, and psychiatric nursing units in three communities and two teaching hospitals that evaluated how nurses spend their time, based on work sampling techniques.

The objectives were to verify the hours of patient care, evaluate and assess where nursing personnel were spending their time, and to compare the workload distribution of the different skill mixes. Information collected was used to determine hours per patient day (HPPD) in each of the following categories:

1. Direct care—vital signs, patient hygiene, medications, emotional support
2. Indirect care—charting, running errands, transcribing orders
3. Unit-related activities—report, checking crash carts, performing housekeeping activities
4. Personal time—meals, breaks, other "nonproductive" time

The majority of the observers were registered nurses who recorded observations every 10 or 15 minutes for two 24-hour periods on each unit. Results indicated that nursing personnel spent only 42% of their time on direct patient care, or 3.4 hours of a shift.

Approximately 24% of the direct patient care was spent on such procedures as changing dressing, ambulating, and assisting patients in breathing. Preparing and administering medications accounted for the remaining direct care time and varied from hospital to hospital. Cleaning or feeding patients averaged 4.6% of direct care activity; talking with patients, providing emotional support, or teaching consumed 3.5% of the time.

Over 16% of indirect time was spent on charting. If five nursing personnel are working a shift, this can total 7 hours per shift. Most of the units allow 30 minutes for report, however, in this study the average was 37 minutes, or 7.3% of total nursing time. If hospitals pay overtime, exploring methods for reducing this time would be advantageous.

Interestingly, in all five hospitals the nursing aides spent the most time being unproductive: 23.5%, or 2 hours per shift each. This is nearly double the expected personal time and totals $62,400 annually for five full-time equivalents (FTEs). This information would provide supportive documentation for increasing the skill mix to RNs or LPNs or changing the way a unit utilizes the various levels of personnel.

Summary

The practice of professional nursing must be responsive to limited health care resources. It is important that nurses negotiate with patients to determine their critical needs and then creatively plan for the most effective resources to meet those needs.

Pivotal to the core practice of professional nursing are the elements of accountability, responsibility, and authority for clinical decision making, which will evolve from the manager to the practitioner in partnership with the client. The nurse manager is challenged to identify and evaluate work demands and set priorities. The manager's greatest resource in this effort can be an informed and involved staff. Time, effective communication, and visibility are critical issues involved in health care resource management. Sanders, Davidson, and Price (1996) conclude that successful managerial characteristics adapt role redefinitions according to real needs. Allocation of time, support systems, and prioritizing can be adjusted for effective and efficient resource use in each of these areas.

Discussion Questions

1. Should nurse managers, in order to conserve resources, emphasize a resource-driven rather than a goal-driven model of nursing care delivery? Justify your answer.
2. What impact do delivery models such as nursing case management have on cost-effectiveness and outcomes for patient care?
3. Give some innovative examples of how nurses can conserve scarce health care resources.

REFERENCES

Barnum B: Realities in nursing practice: A strategic view, *Nurs Health Care* 15(8):400, 1994.
Boston C: Insights from the hospital personnel survey, *J Nurs Adm* 23(2):11, 1993.
Brider P: The move to patient-focused care, *Am J Nurs* 92(9):27, 1992.

Buescher P et al.: An evaluation of the impact of maternity care coordination on Medicaid birth outcomes in North Carolina, *Am J Public Health* 81(12):1625, 1991.

Cohen E: Nursing case management: Does it pay? *J Nurs Adm* 21(4):20, 1991.

Fields B: The effect of nursing case management on length of stay and resource consumption. Poster presentation at the Sixth National Conference on Nursing Administration Research, St Paul, Oct 27, 1995.

Gwozdz D, Del Togno-Armanasco V: Streamlining patient care documentation, *J Nurs Adm* 22(5):35, 1992.

Miller P, Pastorino C: Daily nursing documentation can be quick and thorough! *Nurs Manage* 21(11):47, 1990.

Prescott P et al.: Changing how nurses spend their time, *Image J Nurs Sch* 23(1):23, 1991.

Quist B: Work sampling nursing units, *Nurs Manage* 23(9):50, 1992.

Sanders B, Davidson A, Price S: The unit nurse executive: A changing perspective, *Nurs Manage* 27(1):42, 1996.

Spurck P et al.: The impact of a wireless telecommunication system on time efficiency, *J Nurs Adm* 25(6):21, 1995.

Zander K: Quantifying, managing and improving quality: How CareMaps link CQI to the patient, *The New Definition* 7(2):1, 1992.

chapter **four**

Critical Thinking

Sally K. Aldrich

Learning Objectives

- Define the term *critical thinking.*
- Discuss the process of reasoning and the various steps to follow.
- Discuss different practice methods that help promote intellectual discipline.
- Discuss how to incorporate "socratic" questioning into didactic sessions.
- Define the role of critical thinking as it relates to resource management.

Demands for insightful problem solving, long-range planning, vision, creativity, and analytical thinking have made critical thinking skills a crucial element for success in the pivotal leadership role of today's professional nurse. Yet at this stage of increasing complexity and rapid change in health care, many nurses feel inadequate to meet the challenges that require clear, insightful thinking. Many feel increasing pressure to handle problems they don't think they can manage because no one has given them any answers or told them where to look. Often nurses are heard to say, "No one ever taught me this in school" or "I wish I had known it would be like this." Many believe something is missing from the purely traditional education most nurses have received. In addition, their management training and professional experience seem only to add to their sense of unease with the climate that surrounds them. Nurses often express that they think they do not have the strength or ability to handle the multiple issues and problems their patients face, be they in the acute care, community, or long-term care setting. Managed care has also brought about new pressures of streamlining, increasing patient populations, and limited resources. Nursing can no longer afford to waste its efforts, people, or time, all of which are now considered precious commodities.

Where is the source of this unease? Could it be that, in the rush to inculcate nurses with as much technical information as they need for safe practice in today's high-tech hospital environment, nurses have forgotten how to think? All too often the phrase "cookbook nursing" arises in discussions about what is missing. Students are given a mass of information to memorize, and instructors expect them to learn it all for the upcoming exam. Little processing is involved; they simply have too much to learn in a short period of time, and multiple-choice exams have become the way to test. Memorize it today, forget it tomorrow—after the exam.

Practicing nurses are caught in a similar bind; they are given a list of things to do when certain conditions arise, but all too often patients refuse to fit the prescribed mold and nurses are at a loss as to how to proceed without rules to follow. The skills of observation, reflection, and informed decision making seem to get pushed aside in the rush to get multiple tasks done with few resources and within a constrained period of time. It is a complex problem with few simple answers. One place to begin is to look at our educational and clinical practice settings to see where the concept of critical thinking can fit.

LITERATURE REVIEW

The literature on critical thinking and its role in nursing reveals an abundance of opinion articles but is very limited in research studies. In an overview of those discussions, the authors are in agreement that critical thinking is a valuable and necessary asset for effective nursing practice and leadership in the current health care environment. For nurses to develop critical thinking skills, the process must begin early in their nursing education and practice; however, authors generally agree that this is not occurring (Harbison, 1991; Miller and Malcolm, 1990; Pond, Bradshaw, and Turner, 1991; Schank, 1990; Watson and Glaser, 1980).

CRITICAL THINKING DEFINED

Critical thinking can be defined as "intellectual discipline." Dr. Richard Paul of the Center for Critical Thinking at Sonoma State University, Rohnert Park, California, (1993) describes the development of a "fit" mind:

- Clearly and concisely define the problem or question.
- Identify what information is needed and know where to get it.
- Comprehend the significance of the information and reach a point of understanding.

Critical thinking is defined by Schumacher and Severson (1996) as a "formal reasoning process which appreciates context within the attitude of inquiry."

The Reasoning Process

Using the reasoning process, nurses learn to think in a purposeful manner and nurture the solid reasoning skills of precision, relevance, depth, accuracy, and sufficiency. The key is to literally "think about what you are thinking" and improve on it. **Reasoning** is the process of figuring things out, and it contains several fundamental steps (Paul, 1993).

1. **Purpose**—What is the goal, purpose, or need that must be met? Is the goal unrealistic, in conflict with other goals, or confused?
2. **Problem**—What is the question at issue, the problem to be solved? Is the question clear, relevant, and solvable?
3. **Point of view**—What is our frame of reference? Is it too narrow? Does it contain contradictions, or is it clear and consistently adhered to?
4. **Information**—What evidence is presented? Are the data clear and relevant?
5. **Concepts**—What theories, principles, or rules are being used? Are they clear and relevant?
6. **Assumptions**—All reasoning begins somewhere, and one must take some things for granted. Are the assumptions clear, justifiable, and consistent?
7. **Implications**—What are the consequences of a specific line of reasoning? Are they precise and realistic?
8. **Inferences**—"Because this is so, that is also so." Are the conclusions drawn deep or superficial? Are they consistent?

Studies and discussions of the humanities have been shown to be one form of inquiry to help nurture the sharper vision and quality of mind essential to critical thinking. Discussion of value questions, ethics, and multifaceted ideas as seen in liberal arts programs can help participants add to their traditional education and thus promote the more independent, sophisticated skills so necessary for survival and action. Nurses filled with technical knowledge need to learn how to use that knowledge; they need to be able to analyze clearly and make informed decisions. To achieve balance between information and intellectual strength requires the nurturance of thinking skills, thus the phrase "critical thinking." (Paul, 1993)

DEVELOPING CRITICAL THINKING THROUGH CASE STUDIES

One experimental program that was developed to help nurture critical thinking occurred between a large health system in the southeastern United States and a small, distinguished liberal arts university in the community. The overall goal was to merge the traditional educational background of the nursing participants with the strong humanities focus of the college and to foster a larger repertory of perspectives while developing expanded critical thinking skills. The health system's foundation agreed to help fund the program as part of its dedication to promoting nursing continuing education.

A 6-week curriculum was designed by the college in collaboration with the coordinator for nursing management resources, with readings and discussions centered around literature, ethics, history, and philosophy. Nurses were encouraged to apply for the program, and 20 were selected to participate. The class was kept small to preserve the trust and intimacy of the group.

The program was first conducted in 1992 and repeated in 1993, again with 20 participants. The format for both sessions included six weekly classes, the first one designed as an evening program so participants could get acquainted with each other and the group leaders. The five classroom sessions met each Wednesday morning for 3 hours and required 2 to 3 hours of reading before class. The directed discussion was led by faculty members of the college. Discussion topics included historical and cultural perspectives, ethical decision making, dealing with change, women's ways of knowing and leading, and enlarging personal perspectives. Specific readings were assigned before each session with the purpose of challenging students' frame of reference and stereotypical thinking.

Before the first session, a search began for a tool to measure what, if any, progress had been made in the development of critical thinking skills and if the humanities program had any effect. The Watson-Glaser Critical Thinking Appraisal tool (WGCTA), developed by the Psychological Corporation in San Antonio, Texas, was selected for its demonstrated validity and reliability, ease of use, and minimal cost (Howenstein et al., 1996; Maynard, 1996; White et al., 1990). The tool contains 80 questions divided into five subsets: (1) inference, (2) recognition of assumptions, (3) deductions, (4) interpretation, and (5) evaluation of arguments (Watson and Glaser, 1980). A sample question from one of the subsets is as follows:

Should all young men in the United States go to college?
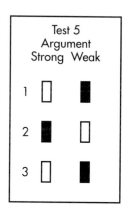

1. Yes: College provides an opportunity for them to learn school songs and cheers. (This is a silly reason for spending years in college)
2. No: A large percent of young men do not have much ability to derive any benefits from college training. (If this is true, as the directions require us to assume, it is a weighty argument against all young men going to college)
3. No: Excessive studying permanently warps an individual's personality. (This argument, although of great general importance when accepted as true, is not directly related to the question, because attendance at college does not necessarily require excessive studying)

A local norm group had to be established, involving at least 100 nurses. This control group was selected from practicing nurses in the community, while the experimental group comprised those attending the college program. The WGCTA was administered to both groups, with the experimental group taking the test again 6 months after participating in the humanities course.

The overall mean for the entire nursing norm group was 61.6 (N = 106). For just the nurses who attended the humanities program, the preprogram raw scores showed a mean of 58.8 (N = 12), and postprogram scores showed a mean of 62.8 (N = 9). The highest score attainable on the tool is 80. With such small control and experimental groups, the statistical significance was not determined. Greater numbers are needed for comparison across the country (Howenstein et al., 1996).

While the WGCTA tool has received some criticism for its lack of applicability to nursing process, it continues as one of the main measurements broadly in use (Schumacher and Severson, 1996).

From a qualitative perspective, 6 weeks of discussion once a week with a group of already practicing nurses seems to be insufficient time to create dramatic improvements in critical thinking. Cost constraints on the part of the hospital system and time constraints on the part of the nurses are realities that must be incorporated into any educational effort. Perhaps a more efficient and permanent hope for developing intellectual discipline lies within the drive for learning and growth each individual possesses.

How did the participants feel about the program? In a feedback session conducted by the college, comments were overwhelmingly positive. Nurses were challenged in an atmosphere that was conducive to sharing and learning. They believed they had been opened to new perspectives and ways of thinking. An additional benefit not previously anticipated was the feeling of trust and closeness that was generated within the group. Nurses often do not get time in the busy setting of work to get to know one another well. The course helped to solidify a sense of camaraderie that they had not experienced since their nursing school days.

SOLUTIONS

Where are the answers for nursing? Where can the spark of creativity that will promote critical thinking in nursing practice be enhanced? All too often our own educational structure creates bad intellectual habits such as passivity, fear of being corrected and ridiculed, poor reading and writing skills, poor speaking and listening skills, few reasoning skills, and a limited view of what education has to offer. We, as educators, have created some of the problems because our teaching often becomes rote, unimaginative, and unchallenging. Students come to class just to collect the information they need to memorize in order to pass the test; the information is not retained because its usefulness has never been demonstrated and embraced.

How can this trend be changed? One step to take is to challenge the notion that nurses can be made to think; instead, what we must focus on is creating an environment where they *want* to think. Spoon-feeding information is a method for gaining knowledge quickly, but retaining it long term is difficult. Although we recognize that learning and thinking are not passive endeavors, we know they also involve hard work and tremendous effort on the part of the professional nurse and the manager to make them a part of our everyday workplace. Some tactics, however, can work.

Begin by putting the emphasis on reasoning and not simply memorizing. Didactic material can be incorporated into the clinical setting; exercises and information should be given in short increments, with specific examples presented to help illustrate key concepts and make the new information "real" to the nurse. Group discussions and case studies are crucial to helping managers and nurses learn to think out loud, to critique reasoning skills, and to analyze situations (Schumacher and Severson, 1996). Having nurses question each other instead of always looking to the manager for the answer helps to increase reasoning skills as well as self-confidence.

Creating an atmosphere where mistakes are permissible but passivity is not tolerated is necessary if independence and autonomy are to develop. Making mistakes together in a group setting, manager and nurse alike, creates trust and allows participants to take risks. Intellectual courage can be gained when sharing, inquiry, and energy are allowed (Paul, 1993).

A method of guided discussion described by Dr. Richard Paul (1993) is that of **socratic questioning,** by which managers and nurses listen to each other, challenge assumptions, probe to follow the steps of reasoning, and draw conclusions. One person plays the role of questioner, and a question is posed to the group as a whole. The group tries to figure out the answer and discusses it; the questioner verbally analyzes what was said and asks further questions of the group. An appointed monitor observes the thinking of the nurses and plays the intellectual "conscience," challenging the direction the group and/or questioner is taking. Eventually, the group does get somewhere; something is figured out and, often more important, participants come to know what they *don't* know.

A similar tactic is that of debate, in which an established position is taken on an issue with "pro" and "con" arguments presented. Ethical issues lend themselves to this type of discussion format, and this is an excellent way for a group to analyze reasoning skills. It provides an active, participative component to the alternative of the passive, one-way communication process (Degazon and Lunney, 1995).

Writing needs to be promoted more because it forces nurses to think about what they are thinking about. Multiple-choice tests, so common in nursing school, force a response and a decision. Narrative writing can help nurses struggle with questions and concepts through the very process of description itself; they can work through their confusion, defend a line of thinking, and draw conclusions through essay construction.

As an aside, writing promotes proper grammar and can increase vocabulary, two components necessary for good verbal communication with fellow members of the health care team.

When nurses write narratively, the responsibility of the manager then becomes to provide staff with specific intellectual standards, against which their writing will be judged. This can help the manager and the nurses assess development of composition skills; intellectual growth then becomes a personal, as well as a managerial, responsibility (Paul, 1993).

Keeping a journal is another helpful way to encourage nurses toward self-assessment. Have staff describe a situation they have experienced. How did they feel? How did they react at the time? What was their thinking? Did they trust their judgment? Have them go on to analyze their reaction critically and then discuss the implications of their actions. What conclusions can be drawn? Whereas many of them function at the feeling/reacting level, those with sound critical thinking skills will function at the higher level of analysis and consequences (Degazon and Lunney, 1995; Paul, 1993).

The method of **critical reading** is an excellent professional exercise. The nurse reads a case study/ethical dilemma out loud, and the group discusses what they do and do not understand. The staff is engaged in the discussion, and thoughts are exchanged; this encourages "close" reading—really examining what is being said, what inconsistencies have been uncovered, what inferences are drawn. This can also help nurses feel more comfortable handling the concept of debate, as well as speaking in front of a group (Paul, 1993).

Use the reasoning process of purpose, problem, point of view, information, concepts, assumptions, implications, and inferences to help everyone in the group develop intellectual discipline. Sound reasoning depends on it. The manager must challenge those nurses who rely on saying, "It's my opinion." How did they get to that opinion? What was their thought process? How did they come to that judgment?

Distinguishing among knowledge, opinion, and judgment is important. Knowledge is the right answer when only one answer to a specific question is acceptable. Opinion is an individual's subjective preference when no specific answer is required. Judgment is required when multiple competing answers exist and one must give evidence of reasoning; this is where the phrase "good and better answers" comes into play (Paul, 1993).

In 1993 the Department of Education mandated critical thinking enhancement for our country's college graduates. The National League of Nursing (NLN) has taken a leadership position in promoting critical thinking measurement through use of sophisticated multiple choice and short essay testing in the classroom setting, along with case study presentations. It has been innovative in creating connections between critical thinking, clinical judgment, and development of nursing knowledge in school curriculums. A result is the emergence of creative, challenging approaches to nursing education that will promote the development of "expert judgment." (Facione, 1995)

RESOURCE MANAGEMENT

The skill of critical thinking becomes even more important in the realm of resource management. The challenge managed care has placed before nursing and the entire health care system is how to provide "more with less." See more patients at less cost but with higher quality of effort. The demand for high quality coupled with decreasing reimbursement drives the market of today, and nursing is being pressured to develop new solutions to the old problems of how to handle the increased demand. The old adage of "work smarter, not harder" has never been more appropriate, and no longer can nursing afford the traditional "FTE (full-time equivalent) fix" of adding more staff nurses to do the work. The resources of people, time, and dollars must be utilized in the most efficient manner possible, with the target of high-quality care being ever at the center.

Does that sound impossible? It does not have to be, if the principles of critical thinking are applied with diligence. The skill of observation helps promote proper problem definition, and reflection can help answer the questions of how to use the professional's time more efficiently and streamline effort. Using groups of nurses to challenge each other to arrive at creative solutions can promote whole new modes of thought, entire new systems of work, efficient division of labor, and futuristic planning. Nurses then arrive at informed decision making, and a new course of action can be plotted; nurses can literally rethink how they can deliver patient care better, instead of allowing those outside the field to dictate. New methods can be developed in a rational, thoughtful manner rather than by emotional reaction. The idea is to increase creativity and arrive at new processes, not to add more people and expense to an already burdened system. Other questions to be asked are: What do nurses really *do?* What does nursing *affect?* What outcomes does nursing *promote?* When nursing can articulate the answers to these questions to the managed care world, then the profession has added value to its practice.

Summary

The challenge of building a mind possessed of strong intellectual inquiry is a daunting one, but it is essential for survival and progress in today's rapidly paced world. As information becomes overwhelming, the ability to sift, absorb, and discard it and arrive at sensible conclusions seems all that much more important. It is no different in the world of health care and certainly no different for nurses. In a way, it is more important in the world of health care, since it is often the nurse who remains the only true patient advocate, the only one who has access to the individual, family, home setting, medical plan, goals, choices, and decisions to be made. If the nurse can demonstrate sound reasoning skills when deciding to do what is "right" for the patient in any given circumstance, the results of efficient, effective care and patient satisfaction become evident.

Critical thinking skills must be promoted and developed at all levels of nursing, from nursing management and school curriculums to the individual professional (Facione, 1995). All nurses can be continually challenged to expand their ongoing education, develop their intellectual capabilities, and articulate the vision for nursing. Managers can help staff deal with reality in their everyday lives and do so honestly; to take charge of their own minds is to take responsibility for their own lives. It involves self-discipline, and this discipline can produce the intellectually "fit."

The ability of nurses to make such intelligent, informed, encompassing decisions in the field of health care today will enable them to take the leadership positions necessary in an ever-changing environment tomorrow. Nurses who are able to articulate what makes them essential to health care will be effective providers. Without such ability, nurses may forever be put in the more passive roles of following treatment plans, being viewed as blue-collar workers, and finding themselves in an ever-shrinking market. Nonlicensed hospital workers may continue to be trained to perform patient care "tasks," and the RN may be seen as a high-priced worker of little value to the institution, agency, or health care setting.

Our opportunities become clear; we all can become more aware of how we educate ourselves and our students, families, and children. How we educate and develop ourselves and our profession will determine our gifts and successes in the future. Strength lies in knowledge and the ability to use it wisely.

Discussion Questions

1. What was your education like? Do you believe you were taught to think or taught to take tests?
2. What is the most important aspect of education for nurses? What makes a professional a professional?
3. What types of learning do you find most beneficial? Most stimulating? What helps you retain knowledge the best? Conversely, what is the worst?
4. What areas do you think you need to develop in order to become a more disciplined thinker? What will give you confidence that you can do so?
5. Where do you think the challenge will lie in the future? What are the threats and the opportunities for nurses? How can critical thinking help/hinder?
6. What do nurses *do?* What makes them different from other health care workers?

REFERENCES

Degazon C, Lunney M: Clinical tool: A tool to foster critical thinking for advanced level of competence, *Clin Nurse Specialist* 9(5):270, 1995.

Facione NC: Critical thinking and clinical judgment: Goals 2000 for nursing science. Paper presented at annual meeting of the Western Institute of Nursing, San Diego, 1995.

Harbison J: Clinical decision making in nursing, *J Adv Nurs* 16:404, 1991.

Howenstein M et al.: Factors associated with critical thinking among nurses, *J Continuing Educ Nurs* 27(3):100, 1996.

Maynard C: Relationship of critical thinking ability to professional nursing competence, *J Nurs Educ* 35(1):12, 1996.

Miller MA, Malcolm NS: Critical thinking in the nursing curriculum, *Nurs Health Care* 11:67, 1990.

Paul R, Center for Critical Thinking, Sonoma State University, Rohnert Park, Calif: Personal communication, 1993.

Pond EF, Bradshaw MJ, Turner SL: Teaching strategies for critical thinking, *Nurse Educator* 16:18, 1991.

Schank MJ: Wanted: Nurses with critical thinking skills, *J Continuing Educ Nurs* 21:86, 1990.

Schumacher J, Severson A: Building bridges for future practice: An innovative approach to foster critical thinking, *J Nurs Educ* 35(1):31, 1996.

Watson G, Glaser E: *Watson-Glaser critical thinking appraisal manual,* San Antonio, Tex, 1980, The Psychological Corp.

White NE et al.: Promoting critical thinking skills, *Nurse Educator* 15:16, 1990.

chapter five

Continuous Quality Improvement (CQI) Principles

Sandra Bassett

Learning Objectives

- Describe the origins of the health care and industrial models of quality.
- Understand the basic principles of continuous quality improvement (CQI)/total quality management (TQM).
- Describe at least one statistical tool and one nonstatistical tool for quality improvement.
- Identify steps in the improvement process.
- Describe the components of an effective team.
- Discuss the quality improvement implications for nursing.

Many nurses have questioned whether or not they can affect cost or quality. The professional nurse plays an integral role in quality and resource management. Controlling costs and improving quality of patient care are interwoven into the nurse's everyday activities.

Commitment to quality reduces expenditures. Research on cost of quality repeatedly shows that 20% to 30% of a typical organization's expenses are the result of redundancy of effort, reworking, error, inefficiency, recurrent problems, untrained personnel, and cumbersome systems. On the other side of the quotient, 10% of loss revenue is attributable to problems in maintaining quality (Leebov, 1991). As a member of the health care team, the professional nurse can indeed affect quality and cost of patient care. Background information relating to quality helps the nurse move forward.

HISTORY OF THE HEALTH CARE MODEL OF QUALITY

The concept of quality measurement in health care began in the mid 1850s. During the Crimean War Florence Nightingale focused on improving nursing practice through problem identification and resolution. As a result of Dr. A.E. Codman's work in 1916, the American College of Surgeons (ACS) was formed in 1918 to oversee peer review among its members. In addition, the group developed and implemented standards of care and provided education to physicians. The Joint Commission on Accreditation of Healthcare Organizations (JCAHO) was formed in 1951 to conduct voluntary surveys of hospitals. This non-profit organization replaced the function of the ACS. With passage of the Medicare bill in 1965, the JCAHO standards were considered the benchmark of quality.

In an attempt to encourage hospitals to follow Codman's lead, the JCAHO required hospitals to conduct peer review activities. This was achieved by auditing physicians' practice and identifying problems, with the desired outcome of improvement in patient care. Very little was accomplished by this endeavor. In regard to accredited hospitals, physicians and hospitals went through the motions. Physicians viewed this as punitive and hesitated to address the outcomes of the audits.

The underlying goal or focus of the JCAHO has always been to improve the quality of patient care. In keeping with this goal the first standards relating to quality (quality assurance) were implemented in 1980. The question, "How can you ensure quality?" was impossible to answer. Quality assurance programs, an inspection model, focused on outliers, or "bad apples" in care. Many employees believed they were being threatened and became defensive. The standards only related to select departments within the hospital setting. The programs were commonly the responsibility of one individual with very little leadership support. In many cases increased quality activities were evident just before an accreditation survey. Movement from quality assurance to monitoring and evaluation to quality assessment failed to meet the goal of improving patient care.

The Joint Commission reorganized its approach to focus on improving organizational performance. The philosophy, which combined theories of clinical and industrial quality improvement, is commonly referred to as total quality management (TQM) or **continuous quality improvement (CQI).** Although the Joint Commission does not mandate a particular model or approach, the expectation of improving patient care must be attained through attention to processes that are interdepartmental and interdisciplinary. The components of the standard "Improving Organizational Performance" are plan, design, measure, assess, and improve. Performance is defined as doing the right thing and doing the right thing well. The Joint Commission has identified dimensions of performance as efficacy, appropriateness, availability, timeliness, effectiveness, continuity, safety, efficiency, and respect and caring (JCAHO, 1997-98).

In addition, state and federal regulations, for example, those involving licensure, Medicaid, Medicare, Crippled Children, Hill Burton, PSRO, and PRO, establish various standards of care. The Agency for Health Care Policy and Research (AHCPR, 1992-1996) published guidelines relating to pain management in 1992.

Since that time the AHCPR has published guidelines relating to 19 different diagnoses, with the latest in 1996 entitled, "Alzheimer's Disease and Related Dementia." The National Committee for Quality Assurance (NCQA) released the first national standards in April 1996 for managed behavioral health care organizations. In 1994 the American Medical Association published its strategies for patient management in its *Directory of practice parameters*. The American College of Physicians published the *Clinical efficacy assessment project* in 1994, which is divided into eight anatomical systems.

THE INDUSTRIAL MODEL OF QUALITY

Walter Shewhart, an engineer at Bell Laboratories, recognized that some variations result in small, normal change, and others come from abnormal causes. The changes are commonly referred to as "common cause" and "special cause," respectively. Common cause relates to issues dealing with usual occurrences within a given process, and special cause relates to unusual occurrences such as equipment malfunction. Although a special cause variation could be costly, it is usually something that does not occur frequently. Shewhart's techniques, known as statistical quality control (SQC), graphically differentiated common cause from special cause variations. During this era this responsibility was assigned to technical specialists and was not considered a role of managers (Schmele, 1996).

At the end of World War II little competition for products contributed to industries losing site of assessing and improving the quality of products. During the 1950s quality measurement advanced. In addition, experts in the field, such as Dr. W. Edward Deming and Joseph Juran, supported the philosophy that quality is everyone's responsibility.

Japan viewed quality improvement in a different manner from the United States. Japan wanted to rebuild factories, improve production, and improve the quality of life of its people. Japanese leaders quickly determined that this could be accomplished through quality improvement (Walton, 1986). Although Deming was not received well in the United States, the leaders of Japan supported the commitment to their people through major quality improvement training initiatives led by him.

Deming combined Shewhart's statistical control techniques with his own emphasis on adopting a systematic approach to problem solving and the attention to process or how things are done (Garvin, 1988). Deming utilized Shewhart's approach, called the Plan-Do-Check-Act cycle. The involvement of all employees and meeting customer expectations are central to this concept (Ishikawa, 1985). Deming's philosophy (1982) is demonstrated by his 14 principles:

1. Create a constancy of purpose for service improvement.
2. Adopt a new philosophy.
3. Cease dependence on mass inspection.
4. End practice of awarding business on price alone.
5. Find problems. Constantly improve every process for planning, production, and service.

6. Institute training on the job.
7. Institute leadership for system improvement.
8. Drive out fear for effective environment.
9. Break down barriers between staff areas and departments.
10. Eliminate slogans, posters, and numerical goals asking for improved productivity without providing methods.
11. Eliminate numerical quotas for workforce.
12. Remove barriers to pride of workmanship.
13. Institute a vigorous program of education and self-improvement for everyone.
14. Create a structure in top management that will push every day for the above.

In addition to Deming, Joseph Juran led many seminars for Japanese executives. Juran influenced the progression toward total organizational involvement in quality improvement. He recognized that quality does not just happen. It occurs through careful planning. He defines two aspects of quality, with the first being freedom from deficiencies. Reduced reworking, need for inspection, and customer dissatisfaction would result in lower cost. The second aspect is product features or attributes such as value and customer expectations (Juran, 1989). Juran states that product features make products appealing to customers, increase competitiveness, and increase sales, thereby decreasing costs. Juran defines seven steps, by which management can improve quality (Vasilash, 1988):

1. Awareness of the competitive challenges and your own competitive position
2. Understanding of the new definition of quality and of the role of quality in the success of your company
3. Vision of how good your company can really be
4. Plan for action. Clearly define the steps you need to take to achieve your vision
5. Train your people to provide the knowledge, skills, and tools they need to make your plan happen
6. Support to ensure changes are made, problem causes are eliminated, and gains are held
7. Reward and recognize to make sure that successes spread throughout the company and become part of the business plan

Phillip Crosby, another leader in the quality arena, believed that all the results in a company are made by people. He emphasized the importance of improving all levels of the system and utilizing statistical quality control to help employees identify when things are going wrong. In his book *Quality Without Tears* Crosby (1984) identifies four absolutes of quality management:

1. The definition of quality is conformance to requirements. Quality improvement is built on getting everyone to do it right the first time. The key is conveying requirements so that they are clearly understood by everyone and making it possible for people to comply with the requirements.
2. The system of quality is prevention. Checking or inspecting only identifies errors which have already occurred. This process is expensive and unreliable in making sure things are right.

3. The performance standard is zero defects. Management must embrace and enforce this philosophy. Otherwise, the workforce will continue with the concept of allowable errors.
4. The measurement of quality is the price of nonconformance. The price of nonconformance includes all expenses of doing things wrong. Crosby estimates nonconformance represents 20% or more of sales in manufacturing companies and 35% of operating costs in service companies. Conversely, the price of conformance deals with all the things required in doing things right. It usually represents about 3% to 4% of sales in a well-run company.

Crosby states the way to make money is to give customers what they were promised and eliminate the hassle for the employee. Doing it right the first time is the key to quality. He defines "it" as requirements or expectations of the customer.

BASIC CQI/TQM PRINCIPLES

Health care has learned much from the industrial gurus. Several principles are basic to continuous improvement.

1. *Leaders play a key role.* Leaders must set the stage by initiating a different culture for the employees. The entire organization must embrace the vision, mission, and strategic direction. Measurable objectives are developed to coincide with the vision, mission, and direction. Management must commit money and support for training, including additional resources to cover for those in training. Leaders set the priorities for the organization. With this in place, individual team members know their boundaries and expectations. Leaders must be patient. Continuous quality improvement takes time.
2. *Customer requirements are identified.* Customer requirements are central to continuous improvement. Customers (for example, patients, families, physicians, and staff) are both internal and external to any given process. Each customer becomes a supplier at any point in the process. A customer is one who receives a service from another, whereas a supplier gives a service to another. For example, the pharmacist (supplier) provides the correct medication to the nurse (customer). The nurse (supplier) gives the medication to the patient (customer). In this example the customer requirements of the nurse include receiving the medication with the correct label, strength, and stability, as requested. The patient expects to receive the correct medication in a safe manner.
3. *Majority of problems are related to process.* According to Dr. Deming, 85% of the problems relate to process or system rather than special causes such as individual or equipment. As stated earlier, the process of focusing on 15% of the problem, or outliers, causes staff to become skeptical about continuous improvement. The old process of inspecting something after the fact does not prevent the problem. By being proactive, the staff can identify a defect in the process as it occurs or, even better, prevent it from occurring.
4. *Cross-functional approach is imperative.* A process seldom stands alone. Processes

normally cross function(s) within an area of a department or multiple areas or departments. The focus is on the organization as a whole. Therefore every department and every person are involved in continuous improvement. The "old turf" orientation becomes a thing of the past. The organization of today is viewed as a structure without walls.

5. *Processes are improved and stability maintained.* A process is made up of a sequence of steps or activities that are dependent on each other. Every process has suppliers and customers. To improve and maintain stability of the process, the customer and supplier expectations are addressed. Problem identification is usually one of the easier steps in continuous improvement. Consistent and reliable data are the basis for measuring improvement. Because of the attention a problem or issue receives, one would expect improvement early in the process. The key is to maintain the improvement over time by continually measuring the effectiveness of the change.

QUALITY IMPROVEMENT TOOLS

Quality improvement tools are divided into two broad categories, statistical and nonstatistical. **Statistical tools** are used in describing quantitative data, that is, data expressed as numbers. The tools include run chart, histogram, control chart, scatter diagram, and pareto chart. Conversely, **nonstatistical tools** are used to describe qualitative data, that is, data expressed as occurrences or conditions. Examples of this type of tool are process flow diagram, cause and effect diagram, and survey.

Tools used in continuous improvement activities are designed for different purposes. The following tools are discussed in order of usage in the improvement process.

1. Listing and Prioritizing Improvement Opportunities

- *Brainstorming.* Brainstorming is used to generate ideas related to a specific topic or problem. This tool can be used at any step in the quality improvement process to identify potential opportunities, data collection techniques, or potential solutions. The group members should be considerate of each other during this process to allow everyone's participation. Remember there is never a "dumb" idea or suggestion. The ideas are documented on a flip chart that can be taped to the wall for everyone to view.
- *Nominal group technique.* This technique requires each person on the team to offer one suggestion at a time. If the member does not have a suggestion, the member passes until next time. The process continues until all members have exhausted potential ideas. Likewise, the ideas are documented on a flip chart and taped to the wall for viewing.
- *Affinity diagram.* This process is used if a large number of ideas or suggestions need to be organized into related groups. This allows for manageable discussion. One easy way of displaying them is to write ideas or suggestions on Post-it notes. The notes can be moved under identified categories, thus eliminating having to rewrite each item. Figure 5-1 is an example using an affinity diagram for visit information.

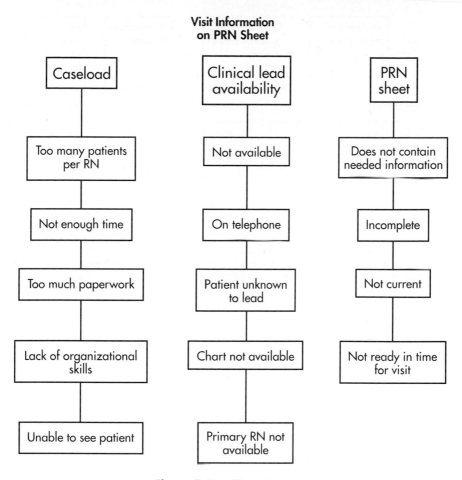

Figure 5-1   Affinity diagram.

- *Selection matrix.* The selection matrix is used to compare and evaluate each of the improvement ideas or suggestions to identify the order of priority. The ideas or suggestions are listed in the left column, with evaluation criteria listed across the top. Examples of criteria are, "Does it support organizational objectives?" "Is it of value to the customer?" "Can it be implemented?" "Does it have a deadline?", and "What are the estimated costs/savings to the organization?"

2. Defining Customer Requirements

- *Process flow diagram.* This tool portrays in a sequential manner the flow of the process. It paints a picture. All parties involved in a particular process must be present to adequately complete the task. Since any one individual usually does not know the entire process, team members gain understanding through shared knowledge. The process identifies inefficiency, redundancy, and areas that work well. The following symbols are used in the process: a circle indicates either starting or stopping the process, a rectangle reflects a single step in

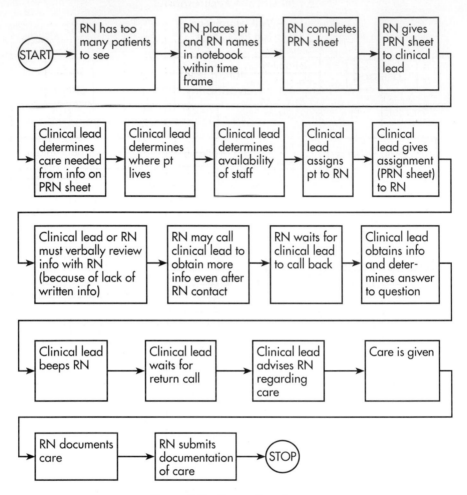

Figure 5-2 Process flow diagram.

the process, a half oval shape signifies a delay or waiting period, a diamond documents a decision point, and arrows between symbols indicate the direction of flow of steps. The symbols are helpful in the analysis phase. For example, the decision symbols could be evaluated to determine whether adequate criteria were used in decision making. Likewise, one could evaluate whether the waiting periods were appropriate. Figure 5-2 is an example of a process flow diagram.

3. Measuring Tools

- *Checksheet or log.* This tool is used to record individual occurrences as they happen over a period of time. (See Figure 5-3.) Checksheet or log is constructed by identifying the required item that is expected to occur. Each item must be clear, concise, and easily understood by all who will collect the data. The items are normally listed in the left column, with the time, day, etc., listed

Customer Requirements

REQUIREMENT	DIMENSION	YES	NO	IMPORTANCE
1. Patient Name	Courtesy	P/K		5
2. MR Number	Reliability	P/K		5
3. Medications	Performance	K	P	5
4. Diagnosis	Reliability	K	P	5
5. Date of Birth	Courtesy	K	P	3
6. Race	Courtesy	K	P	3
7. Allergies	Performance	K	P	5
8. Pharmacy #	Reliability	K	P	4
9. Medicare #	Reliability	K	P	5
10. Recert Date	Reliability	K	P	3
11. Emergency Contact	Reliability		K/P	5
12. Start of Care	Reliability	K	P	2
13. Diet	Performance	P	K	4
14. PRN Visits per Cert	Reliability		K/P	2
15. Map Page w/Directions	Security	P/K		5
16. Date & Time Visits	Security	P	K	5
17. HHA Sup Visits	Performance	K	P	4
18. Lab Tests	Performance	P/K		4
19. Doctor	Reliability	P/K		5
20. Supplies	Performance		P/K	5
21. Visit Instructions	Performance	P	K	5
22. Foley Cath (Yes or No)	Performance	P/K		3
23. Wound Care	Performance	P/K		5
24. Type of Visit	Features		P/K	4
25. IVs	Performance	P/K		5
26. Dressing Changes	Performance	P/K		5
27. Type of Line	Performance		P/K	5
28. Telephone #	Reliability	K	P	5
29. Discipline Frequency	Features	K	P	5

Requirement — Customer Requirements
Dimension — Requirement Dimensions
P — PRN Form
K — Kardex
Importance — How Important Is it to the RN?
        Ranked from 1 to 5 with 5 being most important

Figure 5-3 Checksheet.

The "PT/ST Only" Admission Process Team requests your assistance in evaluating the current admission process for patients with PT or ST only. Your input will be greatly appreciated. Circle either "most of the time," "sometimes," "rarely," or "never" in response to the following questions.

1. How often do you talk to your patients about medications, including side effects?	most of the time	sometimes	rarely	never
2. How often do you talk to your patients about their diet?	most of the time	sometimes	rarely	never
3. How often do you talk to your patients about food and drug interactions?	most of the time	sometimes	rarely	never
4. How often does your patient ask you about medication?	most of the time	sometimes	rarely	never
5. How often does your patient ask you about diet?	most of the time	sometimes	rarely	never
6. How often does your patient ask you about drug/food interactions?	most of the time	sometimes	rarely	never
7. I feel comfortable completing the "PT/ST Only" evaluation.	most of the time	sometimes	rarely	never
8. I feel confident that the "PT/ST Only" evaluation process provides quality patient care.	most of the time	sometimes	rarely	never

Comments/ideas for improvement: _____

_____

_____

Figure 5-4   Survey.

across the top. Considerations for identifying the items for collection are to focus on essential information, measure what is in your control, focus measurement on the activity, and involve others in the process.

- *Surveys.* Surveys are tools to collect information directly from individuals. (See Figure 5-4.) Survey questions fall into two categories—open-ended and closed-ended questions. Open-ended questions offer an unlimited number of responses, whereas closed-ended ones have a limited number of responses. Most closed-ended questions include multiple-choice, yes/no, or a ranking sys-

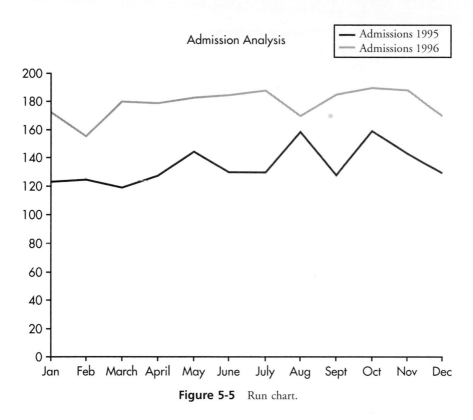

Figure 5-5   Run chart.

tem. Surveys can be obtained through mail-out questionnaire or through personal or telephone interview format. Both types of surveys, however, have potential problems. Personal interview is time consuming, and varied responses for the same questions are received if different people are administering the tool. Mail-out questionnaires may elicit varied responses because of individual interpretation of the questions. Return of the surveys is always a problem. Therefore more surveys may be required to have an adequate response rate.

4. Displaying Data

- *Run chart.* A run chart is used to display changes within a process over time. (See Figure 5-5.) This tool can be used before solutions are implemented to document baseline information. In addition, a run chart can demonstrate the effect of a solution on the process. The chart can identify trends, fluctuations, or unusual occurrences. Usually, the horizontal (X) axis represents time, whereas the vertical (Y) axis documents the values of measurement or frequency at which an event occurs.
- *Histogram.* A histogram is a bar graph that displays the distribution or variation of data points. (See Figure 5-6.) A histogram is useful in displaying many data points. Large amounts of data are difficult to understand. Grouping data

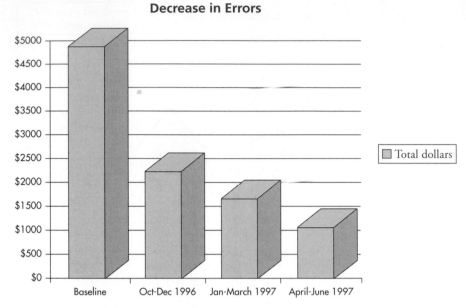

Figure 5-6   Histogram.

together at specific, equal intervals displays data in a manageable form. The overall patterns provide information relative to performance of the process and the level of variation. The horizontal (X) axis indicates what is being displayed and the unit of measure. The vertical (Y) axis depicts what is being measured and the intervals of measurement.

- *Double bar chart.* A double bar chart is useful when comparing two or more items relative to several different categories. For example, in Figure 5-7 last year's referrals are compared with the current year's referrals.
- *Control chart.* A control chart is a run chart with established upper and lower control limits. (See Figure 5-8.) The control limits are commonly three standard deviations from the average. The control chart is helpful in differentiating between common cause and special cause variations. The data points within the upper and lower control lines are said to be the result of common cause variation, whereas those points outside the upper and lower control lines are the result of special cause variation. To affect common cause variation, the process itself must be changed.
- *Pie chart.* A pie chart displays the amount each part represents out of the whole amount of data collected. (See Figure 5-9.) Usually the data are displayed in terms of percentages.
- *Scatter diagram.* A scatter diagram depicts the relationship (if any) between two variables. (See Figure 5-10.) The purpose of this tool is to determine if the relationship has a positive or negative effect on the variables. When the points resemble a straight line, the relationship is said to be tight. If the line demon-

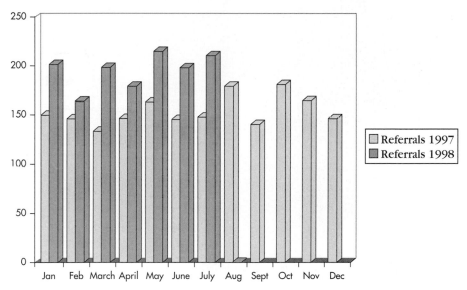

Figure 5-7 Double bar chart.

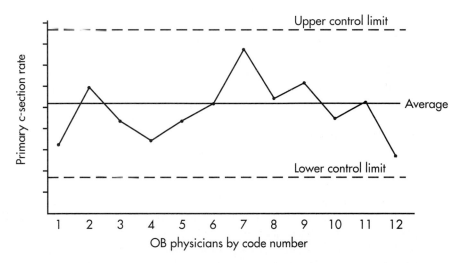

Figure 5-8 Control chart.

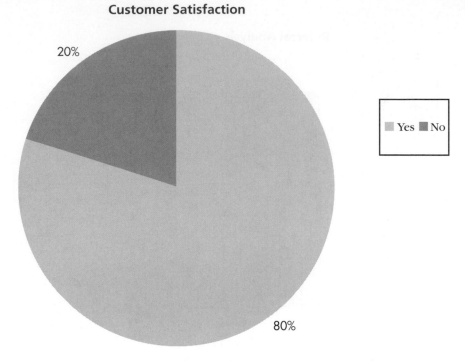

Figure 5-9   Pie chart.

strates upward movement, the relationship is positive, whereas a downward line represents a negative relationship.

5.   Analyzing Data

- *Fishbone diagram.* The fishbone diagram is also known as the cause and effect diagram. Named for its resemblance to a fish, the tool is used to collect and organize information and identify potential root causes. The effect, opportunity, or desired outcome is documented at the "head" of the fish. The causes, which are divided into four basic categories, are displayed on the major spines. Often referred to as the "4 M's," the groups are man, method, material, and machine. Other categories can be added to the fishbone. In Figure 5-11 man refers to everyone involved in the process. Method relates to how the process is accomplished, for example, procedures, systems, policies, standards, and other practices relative to the process. Supplies, forms, and manuals are examples of things that make up the material category, whereas machines involve things like computers, printers, or equipment. Each spine can have sub-spines. The point is to identify all areas that are related to the process.
- *Pareto chart.* The pareto chart is a way of displaying data identified through the fishbone diagram. The chart is based on the 80/20 rule, which states that

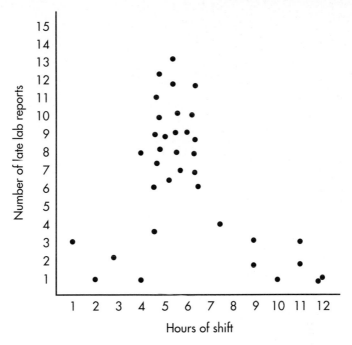

Figure 5-10   Scatter diagram.

80% of problems or effects come from 20% of the causes. Data are collected relative to frequency of occurrence. The left vertical axis is labeled by frequency. The horizontal axis is labeled by categories, ranking from largest tosmallest. The right vertical axis denotes percentage—0 to 100. Each category is designated by a bar on the graph. Ranking and determining the percentage of each category focuses on the areas that need immediate attention.

6. Generating Potential and Selecting Best Solutions

- *Force field analysis.* The force field analysis technique is used to identify potential solutions to resolve root causes of a problem. (See Figure 5-12.) To construct the tool, draw a horizontal line in the center of the page/flip chart. At the end of the line, document the cause and enclose it in a box. Label the section above the line as restraining forces and the section below the line as driving forces. Brainstorming is used to generate as many restraining forces related to the cause of the problem. For each restraining force, using brainstorming, identify at least one driving force. Many times more than one can be identified. Change occurs when one force overpowers another force. Performance declines when the restraining force dominates the driving force. Conversely, performance improves when the driving force emerges over the restraining force.
- *Solution selection matrix.* The solution selection matrix is used to select the best opportunity or solution for the problem. It resembles the selection matrix

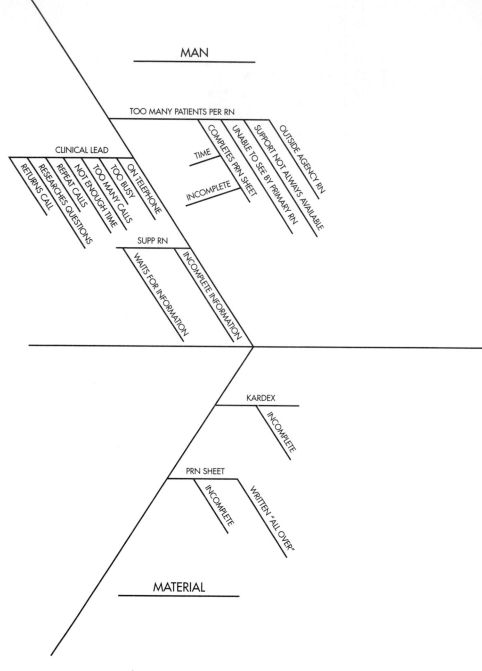

Figure 5-11 Fishbone diagram.

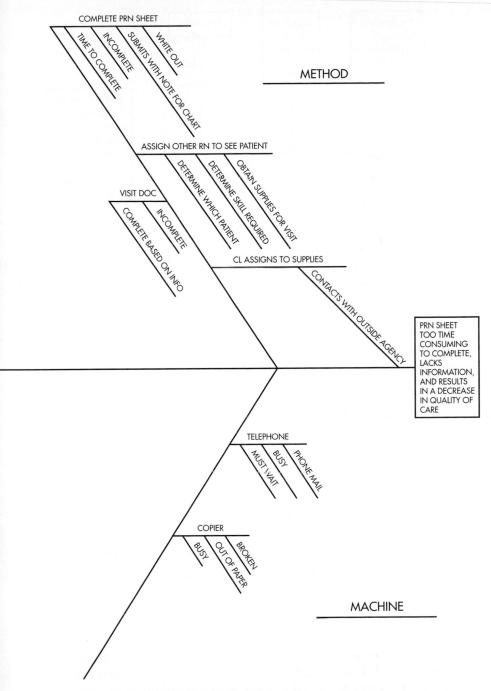

Figure 5-11, cont'd Fishbone diagram.

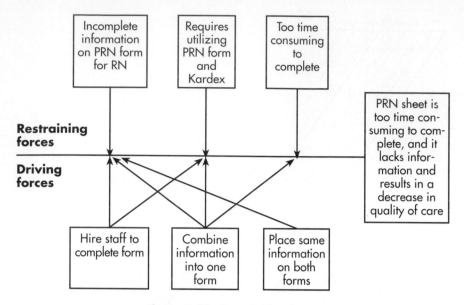

Figure 5-12 Force field analysis.

Possible Solution	Cost to Implement	Savings & Gains	Chance of Success	Percentage of Root Causes Removed
Hire staff to complete form	HIGH	LOW	LOW	LOW
Combine information into one form	LOW	MED	HIGH	HIGH
Place same information on both forms	HIGH	LOW	LOW	LOW

Figure 5-13 Solution selection matrix.

in construction. (See Figure 5-13.) The matrix utilizes the potential solutions identified in the force field analysis process. The tool helps in visualizing the advantages and disadvantages of each possible solution, as well as determining other data needs. Down the left side of the chart, document the potential solutions, and identify the criteria that will be used to evaluate them across the top. Examples of criteria are estimated cost of implementation, estimated savings and gains, chance of success, percentage of root causes removed, or effec-

Average RN Time

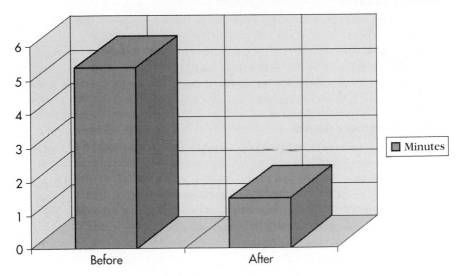

Figure 5-14   Tracking effectiveness.

tiveness of solution, and correlation to organizational mission and goals. The team determines the mechanism for scoring the solutions and criteria, for example, low to high or 1 to 5.

7. Implementing the Solution and Evaluating and Tracking Effectiveness

- *Implementation plan.* The implementation plan is critical to the success of a new or adjusted process. The following issues must be addressed: what needs to be done, who will do it, when it will be done, and how it will be monitored and the progress or effectiveness will be tracked. A simple worksheet can address each of the questions.
- *Gantt chart.* A Gantt chart is used to visually display projected start and completion dates of each activity. The team can easily refer to the chart and track actual progress against the plan. The tasks or activities are listed down the left side in the order of start dates. The time increments, for example, days, weeks, or months, are listed across the bottom. The estimated start and end dates for each task are indicated by a line.
- *Tracking effectiveness.* Effectiveness can be demonstrated by using the tools previously discussed, such as run chart, control chart, bar chart or histogram, and double bar chart. Figure 5-14 provides an example for tracking effectiveness. A major decision is what, when, and how to track. Responsibility in data collection and reporting back to the team in a timely manner is imperative.

WORK GROUPS AND TEAMS

Team Purpose

For the purpose of this discussion, work groups and teams are viewed as the same. In *Quality Without Tears*, Crosby describes the purpose of a team as guiding the process and helping it along. He states that it is not to clear each action beforehand, to be the all-wise oracle, or to hold things back. The purpose is to coordinate and support the team members. The professional nurse has historically been a part of the medical team. Therefore, the team concept is not new to the nursing profession.

Team Member Skills

The basic requirements or skills of team members are listening, giving and receiving feedback, asking questions, clarifying statements and questions, and valuing and respecting each other. In addition, the team needs the ability to establish and live by ground rules, to exhibit sound decision making, and participate in collaborative problem solving. The team members maintain focus on the issue at hand and respect the interdependence of diversity. The group demonstrates a synergistic effect, in that the whole is greater than any one of its parts. The team consists of a leader, facilitator, and members.

Team leader

The team leader guides the team to achieve the desired outcomes and goals. The leader is responsible for providing direction and support for the team members. In addition, this individual can share in the work of the team and has voting powers. All decisions, however, are not made by the leader.

Team facilitator

The team facilitator's responsibility is to promote group effectiveness and positive group dynamics within the team structure. The facilitator is not considered a team member; this person is seen as a coach or consultant. In smaller settings the leader of the team also serves as the facilitator without a vote. The most effective facilitator is one who has no vested interest in the opportunity or problem. This decreases the potential for the facilitator to lead or sway the team.

Team members

The responsibility of the member is to share knowledge and information about the particular process under review. The members share the responsibilities of staying focused on the given objectives; collecting, organizing, and interpreting data; maintaining effective group dynamics; making decisions; keeping on target; and sharing in the success of the team.

Team Size

The size of the team is driven by the issue and direction of the team. The size, usually five to eight people, should be manageable; it should not compromise the purpose. If the number of team players is too large, the team should consider a subteam or the idea of invited guests. In both cases the individuals would not necessarily become a part of the core team.

Effective Teams

Each member of an effective team demonstrates participation, individually and collectively. Honest, open discussions are imperative to form a working relationship. Each member has unique talents and knowledge that enhance the progress toward meeting the objectives of the team and its outcomes. Quality improvement tools are utilized throughout the process. In most cases the leaders and facilitators have been trained relative to teams, group dynamics, and tools. The members receive "just-in-time" training as needed. Since members do not continually serve on teams, the individuals lose the techniques required for team participation after being removed from the team setting.

BENCHMARKING

Benchmarking, initially used in industry, is identifying and adapting best practices to improve work processes. It is not a comparison of indicators of same processes between similar companies. Benchmarking requires people to meticulously study work processes in other organizations and apply those processes in their own company. The question is, "What do other organizations do to get better results?" Organizations are more open today and are highly recognized for their efforts in benchmarking. A by-product of winning the Malcolm Baldridge Award is the organization's responsibility to share its successes with others in the industry.

IMPLICATIONS FOR THE PROFESSIONAL NURSE

Leaders must spearhead the quality improvement movement within the organization. The nursing professional can take a leadership role, officially or unofficially. Many of the quality improvement techniques have been learned during the years of education and preparation. The nursing process, including patient education, utilizes some of the same techniques as improvement processes. In nursing research many of the improvement tools are the same, as well. The professional nurse can influence other staff members relative to collaborative practice and team approach. They can learn the importance of synergy. Responding to needs of staff and patients demonstrates customer requirements and expectations, thereby leading to customer satisfaction. Changes in health care delivery necessitate major change in roles of nursing. Nurses must respond to the change in positive ways by being a mentor, teacher, leader, facilitator, and team member.

Summary

Quality improvement in health care has evolved through the years. The health care and industrial models have helped shape the improvement process as it is known today. Dr. A.E. Codman, an early pioneer, focused on improving patient care. The American College of Surgeons formalized the process, and the Joint Commission on Accreditation of Healthcare Organizations established the first documented standards relating to quality. In addition, state, federal, and other organizations have developed standards and/or guidelines for the purpose of improving health care in the United States. In the industrial arena Deming combined Shewhart's statistical control techniques with his own ideas to develop a systematic approach to problem solving. Joseph Juran focused on total organizational involvement in quality improvement. Phillip Crosby believed that all results are made by the people. He focused on helping employees identify when things go wrong so that improvement in processes could occur. Health care has developed basic CQI/TQM principles with the basic knowledge learned from the industrial gurus.

Quality improvement tools are divided into two broad categories, statistical and nonstatistical. Whereas statistical tools describe quantitative data, nonstatistical tools describe qualitative data. Tools used in continuous improvement activities are designed for different purposes.

Depending on the selected model of improvement process, the steps vary in name and number. An important point to remember is that improving a process should be approached in a systematic method. The key to success is data. Without baseline data, the employees will not know where they have been, where they are going, or when they get there. The organization has to select a particular model of improvement process and educate its members on the steps of the model. When possible, benchmarking should be employed in continuous improvement. Benchmarking goes a step beyond comparing internal or to like organizations. Benchmarking compares the best of a similar or same process.

Likewise, organizations teach the employees how work groups or teams function. The key components are the purpose of the team; skills required of team members; leaders, and facilitators; responsibilities of each member and leader; the size of the team; and the concepts of an effective team.

The professional nurse is prepared through education to make a difference in patient care. The nursing process utilizes some of the basic concepts and tools of quality improvement. Changes in health care delivery necessitate major changes in roles of the professional nurse. More and more opportunities are available outside the acute care setting. Nurses must regard the changes in a positive manner.

Discussion Questions

1. What implications did the health care model and the industrial model have on the development of quality improvement in health care as it is known today?
2. What roles if any do statistical and nonstatistical tools have on the quality improvement process?
3. Why is it important to educate staff and managers at all levels regarding quality improvement principles, methodology, and tools?
4. What is the significance of benchmarking?
5. What are the implications of continuous quality improvement for the professional nurse?

Case Study

Historically, patients who are admitted to home care for only physical therapy services have been admitted by the registered nurse. The charge for the initial admission by the RN has been administrative because of the lack of an order for skilled nursing services. Because of increasing caseload and a need to control resources, the administration determined that a physical therapist could complete the admission. The therapist has concerns regarding basic knowledge about requirements of admission and scope of practice. A team was formed consisting of two physical therapists, rehab manager, rehab coordinator, two RNs, and an educator.

Case Study Exercise
1. Who should lead the team?
2. What type of education should the team members receive before working on the issue?
3. Does this type of concern warrant a quality improvement process team?
4. What type of data should be collected?

REFERENCES

Agency for Health Care Policy and Research, Public Health Service: Pain management, Rockville, Md, 1992.

Agency for Health Care Policy and Research, Public Health Service: Alzheimer's disease and related dementia, Rockville, Md, 1996.

American College of Physicians: *Clinical efficacy assessment project,* Chicago, 1994, The College.

American Medical Association: *Directory of practice parameters,* Chicago, 1994, The Association.

Crosby PB: *Quality without tears,* New York, 1984, A Plume Book.

Deming WE: *Quality, productivity, and competitive position,* Cambridge, Mass, 1982, Institute of Technology Center for Advanced Engineering Study.

Garvin D: *Managing quality: The strategic and competitive edge,* New York, 1988, The Free Press.

Ishikawa K: *What is total quality control? The Japanese way,* Englewood Cliffs, NJ, 1985, Prentice-Hall.

Joint Commission on Accreditation of Healthcare Organizations: *JCAHO comprehensive accreditation manual for home care,* Chicago, 1997-98, The Commission.

Juran JM: *Juran on leadership for quality,* New York, 1989, The Free Press.

Leebov W, Ersoz CJ: *The health care manager's guide to continuous quality improvement,* 1991, American Hospital Publishing.

Schmele JA: *Quality management in nursing and health care,* New York, 1996, Delmar.

Standards for managed behavioral healthcare organizations, Washington, DC, 1996, National Committee for Quality Assurance.

Vasilash GS: Buried treasures and other benefits of quality, *The Juran Report* 9:30, 1988.

Walton M: *The Deming management method,* New York, 1986, Perigee Books.

chapter six

Work Redesign: Rethinking Resource Utilization

Robert W. Koch
Deborah Esmon

Learning Objectives

- Define societal forces that prompt health care facilities to consider work redesign options.
- Identify central goals and desired outcomes in work redesign programs.
- Identify changes that occur in the workplace and workforce secondary to work redesign.
- Discuss the American Nurses Association (ANA) position statement on work redesign.
- Discuss the impact that work redesign has on utilization of health care resources.

Imagine yourself in a world that has no health care system, where medicine and nursing do not exist—a place where care for the sick and injured has never been organized. What type of health care system would you create? How would this system look? How would you make the system effective? What resources would be needed to create the perfect system?

This is the kind of thinking required in the process called *work redesign*. Work redesign is one of the hottest trends in health care today and is unlikely to go away. The focus of work redesign is a re-creation of systems to improve performance and outcome. Nursing can play a significant role in the creation of this new system. But first we must understand the principles and concepts involved in work redesign.

The process of work redesign is centered on starting over from scratch. Work redesign is not about fixing the existing problematic environment. The work redesign process is truly "health care reform," manifesting itself at the bedside (Blanchett and Flarey, 1995).

Work redesign is quickly becoming a major force shaping the health care future. With the current emphasis on reform, health care facilities are closely evaluating the processes used in delivering care. However, because health care facilities are reexamining how and by whom care is accomplished, there is no one right way to redesign. Therefore those involved have many questions concerning the best way to redesign. Two factors to be considered in any attempt to redesign the health care work area are (1) health care must be cost-effective and (2) health care must maintain quality outcomes (Greenberg, 1994).

WORK REDESIGN DEFINED

Work redesign is both a concept and a process. As a concept, work redesign is a powerful tool for meeting current challenges because it focuses on the total organizational system rather than on separate components. As a process, redesign recreates the entire health care facility rather than "fixing" separate components of the system (Kerfoot and Green, 1993). Work redesign is a process of change occurring in the work environment that begins with a clean slate, examining all procedures, activities, and structural components, and evaluating their contribution to the overall goal. Irrelevant components of the work process are eliminated, and more efficient ones are redesigned.

A SHIFTING PARADIGM

The term *paradigm* has been used in a variety of ways. In fact, it may be one of the most over-used terms to come along in the last 10 to 20 years. Thomas Kuhn (1962) was the first to use the term to describe and explain scientific progress. In his writings the concept of paradigm referred to an encompassing world view that included a set of assumptions about the nature of the world used to develop a theory to explain and predict natural phenomena. Since Kuhn's use, paradigm has taken on additional meanings. Paradigms may also be related to cultures or shared knowledge about what is and/or what ought to be (Lenze, 1992).

When people live or work within a given paradigm, they cannot imagine any other way to behave. The prevailing paradigm is viewed as the accepted way of doing things. Looking back at history, one can identify a number of paradigms that have determined the behavior of people. Consider the prevailing paradigm in medicine before the germ theory was established. Before the germ theory, sanitary conditions were poor compared with today's standard. Yet to the people who lived in those times, considering another way to live was not possible.

Paradigm shift occurs when the accepted beliefs about the way things should be change. However, a paradigm shift is not comfortable. Persons who operate within a paradigm become uneasy or downright reactive when others challenge the status quo or suggest a new way of thinking and behaving. When the status quo is challenged, it is often a time of upheaval, conflict, reaction, and resistance to change (Lenze, 1992).

Currently, a major paradigm shift is occurring in the delivery of health care. A variety of factors have precipitated the shift. These factors include changes in population demographic trends, such as (1) aging of the baby boom generation, (2) increasing racial and ethnic diversity, and (3) a demanding, better-educated consumer. Other influential factors include increased competition for scarce resources and the resulting need to contain cost, as well as a view that today's health care system is not working well and needs major revisions. These factors have created a considerable amount of pressure to monitor both cost and quality in the health care arena. A rethinking of how the business of health care is delivered is presently a very important issue.

The paradigm shift that has been occurring within the corporate world for some time now has spread to the health care industry. There is, as a consequence, more concern with the perceptions of the customer and more attention to the service that the customer receives (Druker, 1991). Instead of health care facilities operating essentially for the convenience of the employees, the radical idea of focusing on the convenience of the customer is the mind-set of today.

Understandably, nurses may be apprehensive about redesign efforts. They may even fear that change may affect their professional roles. However, the opportunity for nursing can be tremendous. The involvement of nursing can make an enormous difference in establishing a well-planned redesign that will benefit everyone, including patients, nurses, and the health care facility.

Nurses need to be knowledgeable about work redesign in order to voice opinions that are informed and credible. It is when nurses cannot articulate their concerns or offer feasible solutions to problems that everyone suffers. In the following discussion the essential issues important to nursing in work redesign projects will be considered.

UNDERSTANDING PURPOSE, GOALS, AND PHILOSOPHY IN WORK REDESIGN

In work redesign clearly defined goals have to be established. Redesign is frequently a long and sometimes difficult process, and in order to achieve success all members of the organization need to understand the desired outcome.

The overall goals of most redesign projects include improving efficiency, cost-effectiveness, and customer satisfaction. Of utmost importance is maintaining a balance between productivity and quality patient care. Some health care facilities identify more specific objectives such as decreasing length of patient stay or achieving quicker return of laboratory or x-ray reports. Others focus on decreasing the number of personnel with whom the patient interacts during hospitalization (Mang, 1995).

In the establishment of goals for this type of re-creation, it has become obvious to health care executives that they cannot achieve the changes that are necessary in work redesign without involvement of the people actually providing the care or service. The work redesign movement has made it clear that workers (those closest to the patient) have the greatest impact and play the most important role in representing the organization.

Many of the old processes and procedures of the organization, which have evolved through time or have become the traditional way of doing things, have actually hindered the effectiveness of most health care organizations. It is only when these antiquated processes that do not directly support the patient/provider relationship are removed that the goal of work redesign can be effective (Porter-O'Grady, 1996).

Many organizations have adopted continuous quality improvement (CQI) as a framework for implementing the changes resulting from work redesign efforts. One major principle of CQI is active participation of the workers or staff. Frequently staff members can offer valuable insights into setting goals. It is often the front-line worker who can identify barriers and strengthen the implementation that will enhance quality of care. The likelihood of meeting goals of a redesign project frequently depends on continuous staff commitment (Blanchett and Flarey, 1995).

The organization's philosophy should be representative of a culture that supports the redesign movement. The culture of the institution—that is, the underlying values—should provide ways workers can be recognized as having a strong effect on the quality of care. Health care facilities that promote a unity of purpose among administrators and health care providers will provide everyone with a sense of collective ownership. A philosophy that enhances work redesign should enable the institution to be supportive and to offer a challenging work environment. Workers should be empowered to make commitments and to take risks that enhance the quality of patient care. Communication must be open and honest. Secrets between management and staff should not exist. For work redesign to be successful, everyone must become a stakeholder in the organization and have the right to know what is really going on. It is vital that the organization embrace this type of philosophical commitment in order to successfully implement the kind of changes necessary for work redesign (Miller, 1995).

REDESIGNING: THE ROLES

Currently, the trend in many redesign efforts has been to bring services to the patient rather than sending the patient to the services. Traditionally, health care facilities such as hospitals have been organized around departments rather than around the patient. In work redesign, the patient becomes the center of the organization. This can be accomplished in many ways.

One method commonly used is development of **multi-skilled workers** and cross-training. In health care a multi-skilled worker is an individual who has been taught to assume multiple roles in the institution. Examples include having one individual who can perform ECGs, phlebotomy, respiratory care procedures, and certain aspects of direct patient care that are usually considered nursing duties.

The main objective in cross-training is to create a core team of multi-skilled care providers who provide multiple services at bedside. The team concept decreases the number of people who interact with patients during their stay in the health care facility. This is not a totally new concept; many nurses trained during the height of "team nursing" will recognize an old concept recycled. In theory, proponents of the redesign concept believe that this team model enhances continuity of care by having one group of individuals who are responsible for all aspects of the individual's care.

Patient care provider duties and roles are reexamined as part of the work redesign project. In many instances, efforts to redesign the workplace have included massive cross-training efforts. One of the most common concerns in redesigning roles and cross-training is the competency of the providers. One development in the redesign movement that has been controversial has been the role of unlicensed assistive personnel.

The team approach with cross-training may sound like the answer to all problems. However, today and in the past, there have been concerns associated with revamping health care provider duties, roles, and/or responsibilities. Ensuring the competency of providers is an important issue. Competency in health care can be thought of as the degree of knowledge/proficiency needed to successfully accomplish a task, duty, or responsibility. In defining roles, some institutions use the categories of professional, technical, and service provider. In accordance with this categorization of roles, an additional role has been added—unlicensed assistive personnel (UAP).

There is a great deal of confusion, as well as concern, regarding UAPs and their role in patient care. Some health care organizations have dramatically increased their utilization of UAPs in areas in which only RNs or LPNs would have been acceptable in the past.

One of the major problems that exists with the UAP role is that there are no mandated federal or state guidelines related to training. Programs designed for UAPs in acute or subacute care settings vary tremendously in both content and length. However, this is not true in long-term care, for which specific guidelines have been established since the passing of the Omnibus Reconciliation Act (OBRA) of 1987. This federal mandate precisely identifies curriculum and program length for certified nursing assistants employed in a nursing home setting.

The regulations of the Joint Commission on Accreditation of Healthcare Organizations (JCAHO) require that UAPs demonstrate "competence" and that the health care facility employing UAPs validate their competence in the desired specific skill. But the problem remains: what criteria will be used to establish competence in a given area?

One central issue of the health care provider debate is regulation of UAPs. Some providers believe that regulation of UAPs will help to ensure safe care through standardization training and utilization. However, others oppose the regulation of UAPs because they feel the regulation will create another "legitimate occupation" that can be more readily substituted for the RN.

There is insufficient research to clearly demonstrate that patient care is compromised by the increased use of UAPs. However, numerous anecdotal reports indicate that a decrease in professional nursing and an increase in unlicensed persons providing care are detrimental to the patient (Shoffner, 1997).

Health care facilities considering the addition or implementation of another level of patient care provider should weigh many factors before taking this action. When resource allocation is a central concern, individuals involved in a work redesign program should explore all options concerning the acquisition and retention of nurses and other licensed caretakers. If nursing duties are to be delegated, the competence of unlicensed personnel must be ensured. When human and fiscal resources are scarce, as in the health care arena, the utilization of an unlicensed person may be a viable option. Many unanswered questions related to quality outcomes and the use of UAPs need to be settled.

REDESIGNING: THE WORK

Ask any nurse why something is done a certain way or at a certain time and you most likely will be given the answer "because it's always been done that way." Other times the response may be that the work environment is set up to function a certain way. Yet alternative methods of "getting the work done" may be more beneficial to the patient. Work redesigners are finding that in many health care facilities the established "way of doing things" exists only to support the department, unit, or facility. The process of work redesign calls for a break in traditions, rules, or routines, especially if these fail to consider patient welfare first.

The process of work redesign eliminates fundamental assumptions that are outdated and that have dictated the operation of the organization for years. Work redesign calls for a fresh approach, one that is creative and innovative. Work redesign requires that all processes be focused on the product, which, in this case, is delivery of health care to the patient (Murphy et al., 1994).

Task simplification is one of the key elements in work redesign. It involves restructuring and redesigning every aspect of giving care and making the process more efficient. In some cases the tasks required to perform patient care are simplified by moving the activity closer to the patient. Also in redesign, it is necessary to look closely at how and by whom tasks are completed. An example will clarify this point.

In hospital X, after work redesign, one person may perform housekeeping services, serve the patient meals, assist with patient transport, and fill the patient's water pitcher. Before work redesign, these tasks required the services of at least three people. There are definite advantages to compressing several jobs into one.

One advantage of combining job functions is that health care facilities have decreased the number of workers with which the patient must interact and increase the customer's overall level of satisfaction. Stress, fatigue, and frustration appear to be only a few of the side effects patients suffer when forced to deal with a multitude of health care workers. The redesign method does not necessarily demand a loss of jobs or a reduced number of employees, although this sometimes happens.

REDESIGNING: THE ENVIRONMENT

Changing the physical environment is not mandated in redesigning the workplace. However, the physical plant of an institution may hinder redesign efforts. Many health care agencies undergoing work redesign have made conscious efforts to decentralize the workplace.

Decentralization brings services closer to the patient and aids in creating self-standing entities within the institution. The process of decentralization allows the nursing unit to become an independent care center, reducing dependency on central departments. In some work redesign efforts, decentralization is evident by the deletion of traditional centralized departments such as admissions, laboratory, pharmacy, and dietary. Although these services are still essential to the operation of the organization, they are brought closer to the area of patient care.

Obviously, decentralization is costly but may well be worth the effort in the overall plan of work redesign. One benefit to decentralizing is that it minimizes the amount of scheduling, paperwork, and distance a patient has to travel through a hospital because it provides proximity of patient service. It also reduces the number of "process steps" required to get a job done quickly—a very important factor that profoundly affects patient length of stay and the economic status of the facility.

Other redesigned facilities have focused on optimizing the patient environment. To optimize patient care, supplies and equipment may be decentralized or routinely stocked in the patient's room to accommodate a particular patient's needs, thereby decreasing unnecessary steps required by the health care worker. Reducing personnel travel time to obtain items necessary for patient care not only increases worker and patient satisfaction but also saves dollars for the facility. Generally speaking, efforts to decentralize as much as possible reduce lengthy process steps, wasteful delays, and lost information, and improve overall efficiency (Mang, 1995).

BEWARE: ALL THAT SPARKLES . . .

Lately, the term *work redesign* has acquired bad publicity because many health care workers have become victims of unsuccessful work redesign projects. Negative attitudes have developed because the concept of work redesign has been poorly understood by those attempting to bring about change. One word of warning to health care professionals—not all change occurring in a health care organization entitled "work redesign" is actually work redesign in its truest form.

In some situations work redesign has been nothing more than organizational restructuring, workforce reductions, environmental remodeling, marketing tactics, or automating. These efforts are work redesign in name only and are attempts at a quick solution to long-standing problems. In most cases work redesign is a dismal failure when the underlying principles of paradigm shift, quality care, worker empowerment, and departmental decentralization are ignored or poorly understood. Work redesign will be successful only when all these elements are considered.

NURSING'S POSITION ON WORK REDESIGN

Various professional nursing organizations have established policy statements regarding work redesign and the role of registered nurses. One of the most notable positions has been taken by the American Nurses Association (ANA). This organization has been very active in identifying and assisting with nursing issues related to work redesign programs.

ANA opposes any work redesign programs that delegate professional nursing re-

---

| **Box 6-1** |

The ANA Position on Work Redesign

The ANA Supports:

1. Registered nurses participation as full partners in workplace redesign decisions.
2. Promotion of the role of registered nurses to educate corporate management that registered nurses are skilled, cost effective practitioners of safe, quality patient care.
3. Additional education for registered nurses to apply their skills to new or enhanced patient care environments.
4. Collaboration with SNAs to vigorously resist work redesign models to the detriment of patient safety.
5. Public information campaigns to raise consumer awareness about quality and patient outcomes.
6. Collaboration with nursing organizations, agencies, and private sector to address key issues to strengthen local and state collective action toward common goals of safe quality care.

(American Nurses Association: ANA position statement on restructuring, work redesign, and the job and career security of registered nurses, *Tenn Nurse* 59(1):17, 1996.)

---

sponsibilities to UAPs and other nonregistered nursing personnel. The ANA strongly believes such substitutions will lead to decline in the quality of patient care. The ANA also believes that work redesign programs that downsize RN staffing levels or lower RN skill mix will prove to be detrimental to patient safety.

Therefore when work redesign decisions affecting RN practice are made by health care facilities, ANA advocates that RNs be involved as full participants in the decision-making process. Box 6-1 is an excerpt taken from the ANA position statement on work redesign and the job and career security of RNs.

THE OUTCOME: MEASURE OF SUCCESS

Have institutions participating in work redesign efforts been effective? Many examples in the literature have illustrated effective programs of redesigning the workplace for health care workers. Determined by the use of standardized surveys and instruments, many variables related to quality in health care settings have shown improvement.

Murphy et al. (1994) in their study reported a 13% increase in staff satisfaction after the implementation of a newly redesigned workplace. Staff turnover decreased by 11%, and unplanned single-day absenteeism of staff dropped by 66%. Physicians and community members expressed satisfaction with improved quality of care after the work redesign was initiated.

One West Coast hospital reported saving up to $200,000 per year on their 34-bed medical/surgical unit after a successful redesign project (Farley, 1994). Other quality indicators cited in the literature include a decrease in length of patient stay, improvement in speed of discharge and in patient teaching, decreased readmission rates, and increased patient and family involvement in care (Farley, 1994).

Summary

We are living in a time of ever-present change; consequently, the health care delivery system that once existed has disappeared. The health care traditions that have been universally accepted are being challenged, abandoned, or reconsidered. Nurses are facing a new paradigm through work redesign, a process that offers multiple opportunities for the professional growth of nurses.

Redesign can be exciting, with great potential for positive outcomes in patient care. Redesign requires adapting to change and working together to design new systems that will improve quality and optimize resource utilization. Today nurses have the unique advantage of being able to use their creativity and innovative skills to help shape the future of health care delivery.

Discussion Questions

1. How have the following factors prompted a paradigm shift in today's health care system? Baby boomers, racial and ethnic diversity, demanding, educated consumers.
2. Discuss the statement, "Today's health care system is not working well." Do you agree or disagree? Give examples to support your belief.
3. What does the term *organization culture* mean? How does it affect work redesign efforts?
4. Discuss the pros and cons of decentralization in a health care facility.
5. Develop a process chart of various activities that you have observed on a typical nursing unit (for example, laboratory tests, dietary orders, and requisitions for equipment). How many people are involved? How many procedural steps are needed to get the job done? Can any steps be eliminated? Discuss how this job could be redesigned.

Case Study

A nurse working on a general medical/surgical floor for a number of years is concerned with recent talk about redesign activities being planned in the agency in which she is employed.

Case Study Exercise
Discuss what actions and alternatives are available to the nurse as the redesign is being planned.

REFERENCES

American Nurses Association: ANA position statement on restructuring, work redesign, and the job and career security of registered nurses, *Tenn Nurse* 59(1):17, 1996.

Blanchett SS, Flarey DL: *Reengineering nursing and health care,* Gaithersburg, Md, 1995, Aspen.

Druker P: The new productivity challenge, *Harvard Business Review* 69(6):69, 1991.

Farley E: How we survived a redesign, *Am J Nurs* March 1994, p 43.

Greenberg L: Work redesign: An overview, *J Emerg Nurs* 20(3):28A, 1994.

Kerfoot K, Green S: Redesign vs "fix-it-up": The case for reengineering, *Cap Com Nurs Leadership Manage* 1(4):1, 1993.

Kuhn T: *The structure of scientific revolution,* Chicago, 1962, University of Chicago Press.

Lenze ER: Paradigm shifts, changing context, and graduate nursing education. Paper presented to the Southern Council on Collegiate Education for Nursing, New Orleans, 1992.

Mang AL: Implementing strategies of patient-focused care, *Hosp Health Serv Adm* 40(3):426, 1995.

Miller K: The next wave of care delivery re-engineering, *J Healthcare Res* 8(7):1, 1995.

Murphy R et al.: Work redesign: A return to basics, *Nurs Manage* 25(2):37, 1994.

Porter-O'Grady T: The seven basic rules for successful redesign, *J Nurs Adm* 26(1):46, 1996.

Shoffner D: Who's behind the mask? UAP unveiled, *Tenn Nurse* 60(2):13, 1997.

part III

Techniques, Strategies, and Practical Applications for Resource Management

chapter seven

Managed Care

Phyllis Skorga

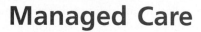

Learning Objectives

- Describe the role of managed care in relation to demand for health services and mechanisms of cost containment.
- Explain differences among the types of managed care organizations.
- Identify the nursing components of utilization and quality management.
- Analyze national accreditation programs for managed care organizations.
- Evaluate present and future implications of managed care in resource allocation.

A national health care transformation has materialized over the past several decades as health care costs have escalated. With the cost of health care spiraling, managed care has been espoused by employers, insurers, providers (hospitals and physicians), and subscribers (members or customers) as a means of resource allocation and resultant cost containment. The issue of quality care delivery has attained parallel importance.

This chapter will examine the impact of trends in health insurance—that is, managed care—on the demand for health care. From an economic perspective, the concern is efficient allocation of health care resources. The efficient allocation of resources occurs when the cost of bringing the health care services/products to market equals the value in the market to the client buying the services. Insurance can lead to increased expenditures on health services and increased benefits to the consumer through reduction of financial risk. Health insurance protects the consumer against risk by preventing potential and substantial loss (Folland, Goodman, and Stano, 1993). Managed care as a form of prepaid health insurance is the current guardian against misallocation of resources in health care.

DEFINITION OF MANAGED CARE

Although managed care is the principal form of health care delivery in the United States today, a universal definition of managed care does not exist. Most consider managed care to be a system of health care delivery that uses financial incentives and management controls to direct members to efficient providers of health services (both physicians and hospitals) while promoting appropriate medical care in efficient treatment settings. Effectively managed health care systems control quality and utilization of services, as well as medical costs and administrative expenses.

Trends in Managed Care

Employer demands to decrease the rate of employee medical expenses propels the momentum toward managed care. According to health care analyst Kenneth Abramovitz, increasingly sophisticated and expensive technology, an aging population, massive excess capacity of providers, and increased demand for services caused by patient insensitivity to cost drives health care costs up (Abramovitz, 1993). To control costs, managed care links health care service use with associated costs. Managed care organizations control use and cost by providing incentives to patients and providers to consider treatment alternatives and to promote economical use of health care resources (Stano, 1996).

The future development and direction of managed care depends on responsible and equitable sharing of health care risks and rewards. To date, research in the field, although limited in scope, indicates that managed care has achieved cost savings primarily by avoiding unnecessary care, reducing hospital admissions, and decreasing lengths of hospital stay. Current research findings suggest that 15% to 40% of major procedures such as hip replacements, coronary artery bypass graft surgery, etc., appear to be unnecessary (Wennberg and Gittelsohn, 1982). Research studies also indicate that physician recommendations for follow-up, laboratory testing, and x-rays can be directly linked to the number of competing physicians in the area (Rossiter and Wilensky, 1983). The practice of medicine is tied to economic and payment factors.

Ongoing assessment of managed care efforts indicates that access to medical care has not been compromised within the managed care environment. Managed care members achieve comparable or higher levels of satisfaction than their fee-for-service counterparts (Winslow, 1994). As managed care organizations mature, the focus of research moves to outcomes management and demonstration of the quality of clinical care and service delivery.

However, a backlash effort is directed at the managed care movement's attempt to reform health care delivery. The media are very attentive to this subject, and bad publicity abounds. In addition, several national and state legislative efforts are directed at curbing the extent of reform. The fact that managed care has slowed the growth of medical spending is often lost in the criticism and debate. A better understanding of managed care can help to resolve this issue.

TYPES AND CHARACTERISTICS OF MANAGED CARE ORGANIZATIONS

Managed health care has evolved over the last 10 to 20 years to become a hybrid industry. Historically the health maintenance organization (HMO) was the model of managed health care delivery. This traditional indemnity-style insurance product then added management controls and specialized contracting to become the preferred provider organization (PPO). A new derivative that blurs the distinctions between these two types is the point of service (POS) option. Each of these types of managed care is explained in greater detail in the following discussion.

Health Maintenance Organizations

Health maintenance organizations (HMOs) have grown incredibly from enrolling 2 million people in the United States in 1970 to 20 million in 1985 to 51 million in 1995 (Findlay, 1995). They provide health care services to patients with the philosophy that maintenance and promotion of health will result in savings. HMOs attempt to control unnecessary medical services through peer review and various forms of provider risk sharing. One premise of provider risk sharing is to encourage the prescription of appropriate and necessary services by paying providers a fixed payment per patient for comprehensive health services, no matter what the cost of treatment. This form of risk sharing tends to reverse the incentive for higher utilization inherent in the fee-for-service payment mechanism.

Payment can be in the form of a salary or a capitated fee. With capitation, physicians are paid a set per-member-per-month payment to deliver specified care over a set period of time for a defined patient population. Physician risk is high, but it varies depending on how many services the capitation rate covers. In addition, a portion of the payment to physicians may be withheld until the end of the year to create an incentive for efficient care. If physicians exceed utilization norms, they may not receive the payment that was withheld.

There are four main varieties of HMOs identified by their financial and organizational arrangements with the physicians who provide services.

IPA model

The largest and fastest growing of the HMO types is the **independent practice association (IPA),** with 65% of the HMO market share in 1994 (*HMO-PPO Digest,* 1995). The IPA model of HMO contracts with individual physicians who practice in their own offices or with associated independent groups of doctors in private practice. Physicians in the IPA model provide care for private pay patients, as well as HMO members.

Staff model

The **staff model** HMO is the so-called traditional type of HMO with hired staffs of physicians on salary. Traditionally, physicians in this model have few if any fee-for-service patients, and the HMO may be called a closed panel. This type of HMO structure is able to exert tight utilization controls and has shown the most cost-efficiency.

Group model

The **group model** HMO is a third type that contracts with a group of physicians that practice in a group setting. The group is usually paid a set amount per patient to provide a specified range of services. The group of physicians then decides individual salaries, often sharing profits.

Network model

The **network model** is an extension of the group type and is identified by contracts with more than one group of solo practice physicians, multi-specialty groups, or independent group practice physicians. Each of the contracted groups provides care for HMO patients, as well as fee-for-service patients, in the group offices (Lopez, 1995).

Membership

The largest of the managed care organizations ranked by total enrollment are the Blue Cross and Blue Shield Association with 7.3 million members, followed by Kaiser Foundation with 6.6 million members, United HealthCare Corporation with 3.7 million members, and Prudential Health Care Plan with 2.2 million members (Data Watch, 1995). The lines separating the various model types have blurred with the impact of mergers, mega-mergers, and acquisitions. As managed care expands, the number of HMOs shrinks and fewer companies control a majority of managed care enrollees. The pace of integration and consolidation has also increased. In the managed care sector there is increased understanding that the greatest potential for economy lies in effectively using manpower and systems, promotion, and capitation. The challenge continues to be ensuring that the managed care product is evaluated on quality rather than solely on price.

Preferred Provider Organizations

Preferred provider organizations (PPOs) are sponsored by insurers, employers, providers, and independent agents. In 1995, 79 million workers were covered by 802 PPOs in the United States (Dimmitt, 1996). The sponsoring groups contract with physicians to provide services for a discount on customary charges in return for higher volume. Volume is achieved by sending patients to a panel of preferred providers. Provider charges are usually 10% to 20% below customary fees. Physicians do not assume risk and are paid a fee for service. This is the dominant method of payment for PPOs. This payment method favors providing more care to more patients.

PPO members can receive health services at a non-participating provider site, but the rate of insurance coverage is reduced. PPOs have been endorsed as an alternative to the strict utilization parameters and risk contracts of HMOs. However, employers have indicated that PPOs are less capable of controlling costs than was projected originally, and this weakness may be related to less stringent utilization review practices (*HMO-PPO Digest,* 1995).

Point of Service Options

The **point of service (POS)** plan has shown tremendous growth in the last few years. Once considered to be an interim measure, smoothing the road to more restrictive, in-network only HMOs, it now appears that POS is here to stay. The POS option allows the member the choice at the time of service delivery to use a non-member physician or health care provider in return for reduced reimbursement. The POS plan has multiplied rapidly as employees have demanded the choice of providers that it offers.

INSTITUTIONAL REIMBURSEMENT

In the past, hospitals received full-cost reimbursement for all of their billed services. Currently, most are paid one of the following ways: discounted charges, per diem, per case, and/or capitation.

Discounted Charges

With **discounted charges,** the hospital receives specific fees, based on its own rates and discounted by a contracted percentage. Most risk is carried by the payor, but the hospital could lose if its rates do not reflect true costs. Incentives in this system favor additional admissions, longer lengths of stay, and more services.

Per Diem

The **per diem** method allows a set payment per day for each case. The hospital is at risk if the cost of care exceeds the per diem. The payor retains risk for the number of admissions and patient days. Incentives favor efficient utilization but encourage longer hospital stays.

Per Case

The **per case** payment allows a global set amount to provide all care necessary for the patient, based on a schedule developed for various types of cases or by diagnosis. The hospital is at risk if treatment exceeds the set payment. Incentives favor utilization efficiency and shorter admissions. Medicare uses this system with diagnosis-related groups, as do many HMOs.

Capitation

Capitation provides a set payment to the hospital or physician per member per month whether or not hospital services are needed or used. As a buffer against extraordinary costs, or for a year-end bonus to the hospital, partial payment may be withheld in a risk pool. A **risk pool** is an account of payment dollars set aside and not paid to the service provider until the predetermined criteria (for example, overall efficiency and/or effectiveness of services) have been analyzed. At that time the pool of payment dollars is allocated. Hence the risk involves sharing financial exposure for specified outcomes. The hospital retains risk for the expense and number of cases because it has a fixed amount of incoming revenue. The larger the number of capitated cases, the lower the risk from individual catastrophic cases. Incentives favor efficient utilization, reduced lengths of hospital stay, and decreased admissions (Milstein, Bergthold, and Selbovitz, 1993).

Ancillary Services

Providers of ancillary health care services (physical therapy, home health services, hospice, etc.) are afforded the same method of payments. Use and volume of services often depends on the payment scheme. The payment method reflects the strictness of the managed care organization in terms of model type and philosophy of management.

Pharmacy

The pharmaceutical arena also is evolving in response to revenue changes resulting from managed care. Prescription drug sales are now more often covered under managed care and are therefore subject to direct and indirect controls such as formularies that restrict or discourage prescription of selected drugs, discounted fees for pharmacy services, volume discounts, rebates, and generic substitution.

UTILIZATION MANAGEMENT

The major activity used to control health costs has been utilization management of unnecessary health care services. **Utilization management** includes a deliberate action to evaluate treatment options to determine medical necessity and appropriateness of treatment setting without sacrificing health outcomes. Utilization management includes effective selection of both hospital and physician providers. Properly credentialed providers who have demonstrated efficient practice profiles are preferentially selected. Both HMOs and PPOs rely on this method of utilization control.

Utilization Management Controls

The main focus of utilization management is the use of independent professionals, usually registered nurses, to scrutinize and control unnecessary health services, typically before they are provided. **Utilization review** is intended to ensure the highest standard of quality while discouraging inappropriate and unnecessary use of services. Utilization management activities include pre-service, concurrent, and retrospective review; second opinion consultation; and case management (Skorga, 1989; Terry, 1995).

Pre-service review

Pre-service review indicates that a registered nurse, as a first-level reviewer, analyze the proposed health care service—whether it be an inpatient hospitalization, outpatient procedure, ambulatory surgery, or same-day surgical admission. The analysis includes comparison to standard written screening criteria that contain rigorous utilization data. If the first-level reviewer questions the medical necessity or appropriateness of a planned service, a second-level reviewer, a physician, is consulted. The physician reviewer provides expert opinion, in terms of knowledge of the procedure or service requested and support in the face of potential attending physician resistance to change or to acceptance of the decision of the review team. The physician reviewer should demonstrate diplomacy and discretion in defending the utilization management program.

The pre-service review component also includes review of home health services, home infusion therapy, prosthetic and orthotic services, and out-of-network services such as chiropractic services.

Concurrent review

Concurrent review involves professional evaluation by first-level reviewers of documented service delivery and continued hospital stays. The review may be by telephone or on site in the particular hospital. As in pre-service review, the intent of concurrent review is to determine medical necessity and appropriateness of setting for the services ordered or anticipated. Services documented in the medical record are compared by diagnosis and procedure. Unnecessary and inappropriate services are further evaluated by the managed care organization's physician reviewer.

Retrospective review

If utilization management does not occur before service, **retrospective review** can be conducted; this is done by first-level and/or second-level reviewers. In this scenario, the same criteria and reasons for analysis are employed, but after the delivery of health care services. In many circumstances the review occurs in collaboration with individual claims review. Manual claims review is often aided by software-based screens of medical algorithms to determine medical need and appropriateness.

Second opinion consultation

At any point in the review process a third-level review from a **second opinion** consulting care physician or specialty physician can be requested. The purpose of this review is to obtain independent analysis of the anticipated health care service and to determine medical necessity and appropriateness of care and setting. This level of medical peer review is used in selected appeals and to improve the reliability of decision making.

Case management

Case management is the focus of current utilization management activities and involves an effort to maximize care and cost-efficiency. Case management includes discharge planning and appropriate utilization of home health services and medical equipment. Case management is often directed at high-cost cases and chronic and/or catastrophic situations. Alternative health care settings are explored and, when appropriate, are recommended for use in lieu of traditional inpatient hospitalization. Disease management programs that target selected conditions for intensive education, risk assessment, and case management are employed as adjunctive methods for controlling utilization and costs (Feldstein, 1988). Case management is further explored as a means of resource allocation in Chapter 8.

Utilization management programs that have incorporated the medical services identified in this section have been studied for effectiveness in reducing hospital use and decreasing overall medical expenditures (Congressional Budget Office, 1993; Feldstein, Wickizer, and Wheeler, 1988). In these studies utilization management has been found to reduce admissions by 13%, inpatient days by 11%, hospital room and board expenditures by 7%, hospital ancillary service expenditures by 9%, and total medical expenditures by 6%. Studies were controlled for a number of potentially confounding variables and naturally occurring trends toward lower utilization. Results support the belief in managed care cost controls as an effective means of resource allocation (Skorga, 1989; Terry, 1995). According to the Congressional Budget Office, current managed care systems reduce the use of services by 7% compared with unmanaged care and 4% compared with fee-for-service plans (Dimmitt, 1995).

MANAGED CARE ACCREDITATION

As managed care has evolved, accreditation has been spearheaded by employers, who see it as a safety measure to explain to employees that standards are being met as health care costs are lowered. Accreditation indicates that an independent third party completely external to the managed care organization has applied a set of accepted standards to the policies, procedures, and initiatives of the managed care organization and has determined a score or rank for the organization. The most prominent accrediting bodies for managed care entities are the National Committee for Quality Assurance (NCQA), Joint Commission on Accreditation of Healthcare Organizations (JCAHO), and the Utilization Review Accreditation Commission (URAC).

All three of these accrediting bodies share a strong bond requiring quality improvement to achieve accreditation. Although the programs have unique features, they share many of the same objectives and standards.

National Committee for Quality Assurance

The National Committee for Quality Assurance (NCQA) was established in 1990. The NCQA, based in Washington, D.C., typically accredits HMOs, PPOs, and POS plans. To be accredited, organizations must have provided comprehensive inpatient and outpatient care through an organized delivery system for at least 18 months and must have defined administrative processes in place.

Standards and sub-standards for NCQA address the areas of quality improvement, utilization management, provider credentialing, member rights and responsibilities, preventive health services, and medical records.

In documenting quality improvement for NCQA, health plans must produce a plan for assessing the quality of care given to members, as well as the coordination of parts of the plan. Health plans are asked to demonstrate that patients have access to care in a reasonable period of time and that improvements have been made in patient care and services. There is a requirement for a written quality improvement program, with specific conditions for oversight and accountability of the quality improvement committee. Quality improvement actions and the results of these actions must be documented. Provider contracts must obligate the physicians to participate in a quality management and improvement process within the health plan. Members with chronic or high-risk illnesses must be identified, educated, and appropriately managed through disease management programs.

For physician credentialing, health plans must have written policies for credentialing, recredentialing, and reappointment. Health plans must keep track of physicians' performance and use that information in periodic evaluations. The network must have evidence that it requests information on practitioners from recognized monitoring organizations, and it must make site visits to ensure conformance with standards. The managed care organization must have procedures for disciplinary action against providers. Other entities such as hospitals, laboratories, and nursing homes must have accreditation from a recognized accrediting body or have developed standards of participation with assessment of the organization based on standards.

NCQA examines the process for deciding what health services are appropriate and for responding to member and physician appeals when payment for services is denied. A physician must review all clinical services denied. A written protocol for utilization management must be in place along with a mechanism to evaluate the utilization management program using member and provider satisfaction data. A protocol for evaluating new medical technologies must also be in place. In terms of member rights and responsibilities, health plans must inform members how to access providers and choose and change physicians. This section must include complaint mechanisms and use of member satisfaction data as evaluation material.

Health plans must offer preventive services and have practice guidelines for the use of services. Specific screening and preventive programs must be in place for selected conditions such as childhood and adult immunizations, prenatal care, cholesterol, cancer, and hypertension. For medical records the standards call for consistency and verification of compliance within established guidelines (Graham, 1996; McQuire, 1996). In addition, NCQA publishes national comparison of health plans and has developed the Health Plan Employer Data and Information Set (HEDIS). HEDIS is a measurement system that quantifies health plan processes and outcomes of quality, enrollment, utilization, and other data (Edlen, 1996; Pallarito and Morrisey, 1996).

Joint Commission on Accreditation of Healthcare Organizations

The Joint Commission on Accreditation of Healthcare Organizations (JCAHO) was established in 1951. JCAHO, based in Chicago, Illinois, accredits hospital and health care networks that deliver integrated health services to a defined population, offer specialty services, and have a central structure. An option for early survey can be obtained for organizations with less than 6 months' experience or those that are not yet ready for a complete survey.

JCAHO standards address rights, responsibilities, and ethics; the continuum of care; education and communication; health promotion and disease prevention;

leadership; management of human resources; management of information; and improvement of network performance.

Standards require a written code of ethics that protects the integrity of clinical decision making regardless of how the network compensates practitioners. For JCAHO, the code contains information regarding how treatment decisions are made and deals with privacy and confidentiality of medical records, as well as a process for addressing complaints and grievances. Health plans must demonstrate that services are integrated into a seamless continuum of care. The code also requires that members be informed of services and how to access services. Communication includes information on fees, out-of-network benefits, and education on self-care and disease prevention. For health promotion and disease prevention, a requirement exists for documentation of appropriate services for the population served.

Networks must demonstrate effective leadership in terms of planning, directing, and coordinating the provision and improvement of health care services that are cost-effective and responsive to member and community needs. The number and qualifications of providers must also be consistent with the needs of members. Data must show evaluation and actions to improve practice patterns. JCAHO standards evaluate the adequacy of information systems with protocols to protect confidentiality and integrity of data. Networks must demonstrate a continuing effort to improve performance by measuring and assessing performance standards continually (Graham, 1996; McQuire, 1996).

Utilization Review Accreditation Commission

The Utilization Review Accreditation Commission (URAC) was established in 1990. Now known as American Accreditation Healthcare Commission/URAC (AAHC/URAC), it is based in Washington, D.C., and accredits utilization review organizations, both freestanding and within managed care organizations. URAC focuses on the policies and procedures of utilization review and is an operational requirement in certain states. The following discussion explains external review in greater detail (Berger, 1996).

URAC strives to improve the quality of utilization review organizations by evaluating network participation and management standards; quality, utilization, and provider credentialing standards; member protection and participation; confidentiality of patient information; and marketing and sales standards.

According to URAC, to participate as a network, written criteria must exist for physicians, inpatient and outpatient facilities, and outsourced components. These criteria must include standards for quality of care and service, access, and out-of-network needs. Networks must establish provider relations programs to maintain the panel through recruitment and training. Physicians must be involved with network management through boards, peer review committees, etc. URAC requires a written agreement with providers that mandates established responsibilities, dispute resolution, and reimbursement methods.

To monitor quality, URAC requires statistical studies, screenings, treatment outcome studies, and treatment protocols on quality of care and service. For utilization review, standards are most rigorous and include training and credentialing of first-, second-, and third-level reviewers and a documented process for appeals. In addition, written policies governing all aspects of utilization management are included. Credentialing standards are very similar to those of NCQA and include a credentialing committee and a written plan with criteria for evaluation and verification. For member protection, a process for complaints and grievances must be used with a mechanism to educate members on their rights. Practitioners are expected to sign confidentiality and conflict of interest agreements.

URAC has developed a unique area of focus in their standards to prevent misrepresentation of benefits. Networks must inform plan members of exclusions, limitations, benefit reductions, utilization management requirements, provider networks, and satisfaction statistics (Graham, 1996; McQuire, 1996).

FUTURE IMPLICATIONS FOR MANAGED CARE

As managed care helps to shape the future of health care in the United States, many believe that a majority of hospitals and insurers will move to for-profit status, that a majority of Americans will be covered by some form of managed care, and that all parties will strive to allocate resources in a best-care scenario for a large aged population. The future will also include a continuum of health care with long-term care as a necessity. The most important site for health care will move from the hospital to the home. It is also believed that the drive for medical data will be commonplace; data from all avenues will be provided on-line (Smith, Wong, and Eichert, 1996). The next generation of health care services will include health plan administrators, providers, patients, and payors as partners in developing incentives and risk-sharing arrangements designed to achieve health care objectives. The future will include managed care companies and payors reinvesting the savings gained from utilization management in activities designed to improve the overall health of patients and to contain health care costs over the long term.

Summary

This chapter has explored the importance of managed care in terms of resource allocation for current health care delivery. The dominant types of managed care have been explained along with reimbursement methods driving the process. Activities to monitor and manage utilization and disease states have been identified. Finally, standards of external oversight agencies have been explained because the quest for quality initiatives dictates accreditation results. Predictions regarding health care in the future include greater penetration of managed care as a means of resource allocation in health care.

Discussion Questions

1. How does managed care promote effective and efficient health care services?
2. Compare and contrast types of managed care organizations.
3. Explain utilization management techniques used to control costs.
4. What are the similarities among the standards of NCQA, JCAHO, and URAC?
5. Explain methods of resource allocation attributed to managed care operations in providing health care services.

Case Study

Dr. Saber's office nurse called the HMO pre-service review hotline to provide medical information supporting insurance benefits' approval for an inpatient admission. The member was described as a 41-year-old white female who was experiencing acute depression. The member had been referred to an in-network psychiatrist by her primary care physician and had been receiving outpatient therapy without success. Her diagnosis was listed as depressive disorder, and hospital admission was planned to provide intensive therapy and medication adjustment. Hospital services were reviewed by a concurrent review nurse, and length of stay was monitored against national averages for the diagnostic grouping. During hospitalization and treatment the patient's diagnosis was altered to reflect thorough assessment and analysis. Her primary diagnosis was changed to schizoaffective disorder, and treatment was appropriately defined. At discharge the patient was recommended for an alternative form of therapy. The HMO continued case management and approved benefits coverage for partial hospitalization treatment. The nurse case manager monitored treatment and, with physician concurrence, recommended a step down to regular outpatient treatment. The episode of care demonstrated appropriate assessment, diagnosis, intervention, and analysis while reducing hospital length of stay and utilizing alternative less expensive but equally effective forms of treatment. The member continued to make progress with her psychiatrist, and the primary care physician coordinated ongoing care as needed.

Case Study Exercise

1. What utilization management controls were applied to this case?
2. Why was case management recommended for this patient?
3. How was hospitalization minimized?

REFERENCES

Abramovitz K: Changing trends in health care delivery. In Boland P, editor: *Making managed health care work,* Gaithersburg, Md, 1993, Aspen.

Berger D: Playing the accreditation game: Strategies for networks, *Health Care Innovations* 6(2):8, 1996.

Congressional Budget Office: *Managed competition and its potential to reduce health care spending,* Washington, DC, 1993, U.S. Government Printing Office.

Data watch, *Bus Health* 13(1):22, 1995.

Dimmitt B: Accreditation: What's the big deal? *Bus Health* 13(12):38, 1995.

Dimmitt B: Follow the money, *State Health Care Am:*6, 1996.

Edlen M: Define your health plan value with reporting, *Health Manage Technol* 17(8):11, 1996.

Feldstein P, Wickizer T, Wheeler J: The effects of utilization review programs on health care use and expenditures, *N Engl J Med* 318(20):1310, 1988.

Findlay S: Will big HMOs stamp out competition? *Bus Health* 13(10):52, 1995.

Folland S, Goodman A, Stano M: *Insurance, the economics of health and health care,* New York, 1993, MacMillan.

Graham J: The rise of the health care consumer, *State Health Care Am:*49, 1996.

HMO-PPO digest, Kansas City, Mo, 1995, Hoescht Marion Roussel.

Lopez L: Choosing the best HMO, *Bus Health* 13(1):22, 1995.

McQuire D: NCQA unveils draft version, *Manage Care Outlook* 9(15):n5, 1996.

Milstein A, Bergthold L, Selbovitz L: Utilization review techniques. In Boland P, editor: *Making managed health care work,* Gaithersburg, Md, 1993, Aspen.

Pallarito K, Morrisey J: The future, *Modern Healthcare* 26(35):932, 1996.

Rossiter L, Wilensky G: An examination of the use of physicians' services: The role of physician initiated demand, *Inquiry* 20:162, 1983.

Skorga P: Evolving trends in managed care, *Office Nurse* 2(6):26, 1989.

Smith D, Wong H, Eichert J: The third generation of managed care, *Am J Manage Care* 6(7):821, 1996.

Stano M: An alternative framework for evaluating the efficiency of managed care, *Am J Manage Care* 2(6):639, 1996.

Terry K: Disease management, *Bus Health* 13(4):65, 1995.

Wennberg J, Gittelsohn A: Variations in medical care among small areas, *Sci Am* 246:120, 1982.

Winslow R: Performance of HMOs is rated higher than fee for service plans in study, *Wall Street Journal* B7, June 23, 1994.

chapter **eight**

Case Management

Robert W. Koch
Kathy L. Beck
Tommie L. Norris

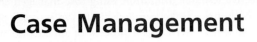

Learning Objectives

- Discuss the historical perspective of case management.
- Identify various models of case management.
- Discuss the role of case management in community care, acute care, and disease management.
- Identify the advantages of case management in health care resource management.

Case management, although not a new concept, is a good way to manage scarce health care resources in today's cost-conscious environment. As early as the 1970s the literature describes studies of case management research in behavioral health, social work, and health services (Chamberlain and Rapp, 1991). In the 1980s case management in long-term care developed. The process of case management improves the quality of care and manages costs associated with adults and children at high risk for health problems and social complications (Capitman, Haskins, and Bernstein, 1986). Many social health maintenance organizations (SHMOs) use case management techniques to care for acute and long-term care Medicare clients (Abrahams et al., 1989).

Given the increased emphasis on managed care and cost containment, nursing has become a leader in developing new and innovative models of case management. The current models of case management originate from community health nursing. Although the literature on nursing case management is essentially descriptive, nurse case managers historically (1) have worked with populations at high risk for adverse health outcomes, (2) have been held responsible for utilizing nursing process to improve quality and cost outcomes, and (3) have maintained an in-depth knowledge of the continuum of health care services available to the client (Lamb, 1992).

THE ISSUE OF RESOURCE MANAGEMENT

Case management has been implemented to address quality and cost in health care. The process of effective resource utilization using case management principles can often be complex. McKenzie, Torkelson, and Holt (1989, p. 30) define **case management** as a "set of logical steps and a process of interaction with service networks." The steps or processes are frequently identified through the use of various types of tools; one such tool is the critical path. A **critical path** is an interdisciplinary plan of key processes and expected outcomes to be completed in a specified span of time (Zander, 1988). The case manager in most situations is responsible for monitoring the critical path, investigating deviations, recommending care alternatives, and defining outcomes.

Multiple studies indicate that case management is an effective method of maximizing critical resources. In one exploration of case management, McKenzie, Torkelson, and Holt (1989) describe 84 patients following coronary bypass surgery who received case management services. In comparison to control groups, the researchers found shorter lengths of hospital stay and decreased pharmacy, laboratory, and radiology costs among those patients followed by a nurse case manager. Mahn (1993) reported a similar study, and again the results showed decreased length of stay and costs, along with fewer hospital readmissions.

In 1991 Chamberlain and Rapp compared hospital expenses involving "case-managed" women who had had cesarean sections and women who were not "case managed." Given the use of critical paths and an increased emphasis on teaching and discharge planning, with case management there were fewer hospital days and lower hospital costs.

A growing number of studies support the positive impact of nurse case management on managing scarce health care resources. Many reports also reveal a higher level of satisfaction by patients whose care is case managed by nurses. Further research is necessary to document the advantages of nurse case management in health care resource decision making.

MODELS OF CASE MANAGEMENT

All definitions of case management involve an individual who is skilled in public relations and health care issues and who coordinates all aspects of a client's care in a cost-effective, efficient, and culturally sensitive manner (Rogers, Riordan, and Swindle, 1991; Stanhope and Lancaster, 1996).

The American Nurses Association (1991) categorized models of case management into three groups: reimbursement, agency, and social welfare. (See Box 8-1.) The case manager in the reimbursement category assesses needs and justifies health care services while ensuring quality care is rendered in a cost-effective manner. Case management with an agency focus is based on diagnostic-related groups (DRGs) for a specific health problem and coordinates care along an established "norm" for the problem. Case management based on the social welfare category matches resources with client needs (Molloy, 1994).

Box 8-1	

ANA Case Management Categories

Model Category	Function
Reimbursement	Justifies health care services
	Ensures quality care in a cost-effective manner
Agency	Based on diagnostic-related groups (DRGs)
	Coordinates care along an established "norm"
Social welfare	Matches resources with client needs

Esposito (1994) also described various models of case management. The collaborative practice model ensures a cooperative practice involving the physician and the case manager, in which a mutually acceptable plan of care is developed that meets the needs of the client and caregivers. Other members of the health care team, such as the medical social worker and physical or speech therapist, also contribute to the plan of care.

The family caregiver model consists of competencies that promote self-help. Orem's theory of self-care is the basis for the model. This model identifies several major competencies required for successful case management. One of the fundamental competencies includes a strong and trusting relationship between the client and the health care team. Another includes the ability to detect barriers that impede efficient health care. The model also addresses availability, mobilization, and collaboration to obtain needed resources or acceptable alternatives. Other competencies include problem solving, crises management, and conflict resolution.

The multisystem model, as the name implies, embraces all elements of case management plus having the nurse perform a multisystem assessment. In this model the case manager assesses the client in seven domains; these domains are environmental, psychosocial, physiological, health behaviors, therapeutic regimen, noncompliance, and technical procedures. The formulation of goals is based on the client's formal and informal support systems. The case manager reviews the plan of care to ensure that the client's needs are being satisfactorily met.

Box 8-2 describes characteristics of each of Esposito's models of case management.

Molloy (1994) has identified one problem in defining the case management role. Definition of case management may be difficult because of numerous meanings assigned to the term and common misuse of the term. This confusion exists within agencies, such as insurance companies, that hire nurses for the primary purpose of utilization review and then call these individual "case managers." Also case management can be performed by a wide variety of individuals with differing educational backgrounds and titles, thereby adding to the confusion.

Case managers, in fact, may perform utilization review functions. However, if an individual focuses only retrospectively on resources that were used in patient care or

---

Box 8-2

Esposito: Models of Case Management

Model	Characteristics
Collaborative practice model	Cooperative practice involving the physician and the case manager
	Mutually acceptable plan of care
	Other members of the health care team contribute to the plan of care
Family caregiver model	Competencies that promote self-help
	Model based on Orem's theory of self-care
Multisystem model	Seven assessment domains: environmental, psychosocial, physiological, health behaviors, therapeutic regimen, noncompliance, and technical procedures

---

authorizes hospitalization and outpatient treatments, the role is something other than case management. Universal concepts of case management include integration of health care services and evaluation of the care provided, both essential to the role definition.

CASE MANAGEMENT SETTINGS

Case Management in Community Health Care

Various case management programs can be found in several areas of community health nursing. Case management is an effective management strategy for community-based and public health care. Public health nurses are a vital link to the health care system for clients and their informal caregivers. Case management in the community setting began during the late 1960s with the deinstitutionalization of mentally ill individuals. Frequently these clients needed follow-up and monitoring of their health care needs (Lyon, 1993).

Rogers, Riordan, and Swindle (1991) describe the multiple benefits of nursing case management in the community setting. Case management allows the community client easier access to a health care system that is often complicated, fragmented, and confusing. Another advantage includes providing nurses in the community setting with increased authority over their practice. Also case management provides health care administrators with a mechanism for financial savings.

Community-based case managers work with a wide variety of clients who often have complex problems. Both urban and rural dwellers are confronted with many barriers to health care. Oftentimes, the client is unable to seek needed medical care because of functional, financial, or geographical limitations.

In the rural setting clients may postpone seeking medical care for a variety of reasons. Rural workers may not be eligible for sick leave or may fear losing their jobs because of illness-related absence. Also the time and expense required for lengthy transportation to a health care provider may add additional difficulties. At times, simple essentials that are often taken for granted are not available to the rural client. Running water, indoor plumbing, telephone services, and desirable living environments are issues that the community-based case manager may face.

Although urban dwellers may have less of a distance to travel to obtain health care, they are also faced with obstacles. Difficulties may include economic barriers or a lack of knowledge about how to access the health care system. Case managers may also work with the homeless population, transient workers, or immigrants. Typically these individuals are without health insurance and have no regular health care provider.

Community-based case managers develop a plan of care for the specific and unique needs of the client. By assessing the available community resources and having a working knowledge of the health care system, including reimbursement and financial aid, the case manager can effectively coordinate the client's health care.

Educating the public is another important role for the community-based case manager because prevention may decrease the ever-escalating cost of health care. Case managers dealing with child health may coordinate care by addressing obstacles such as poverty, abuse, lack of knowledge by the caregiver, economic limitations, and peer pressure. Additional assignments for case managers in the community setting may include coordinating care for children with special needs, dealing with women's health care issues, or representing the elderly population, who have unique needs involving the potential for fraud, dementia, or the inability to independently continue activities of daily living.

Three levels of prevention must be utilized by the case manager in the community setting (Swanson and Albrecht, 1993). Primary prevention is directed toward the prevention of disease. Secondary prevention is aimed at early screening and discovery of diseases already present in the individual. Tertiary prevention is focused on abbreviating the adverse consequences of disease and preventing the spread of communicable diseases to a susceptible population. Such public health nursing issues frequently provide an area where case management techniques are employed. In such settings, the case manager may focus on the aggregate health care needs of an entire population.

Case Management in Home Care

Home health care is another area in which case management is commonly used. By providing care in the home, visiting home health care nurses can manage chronic diseases and assess barriers that interfere with successful patient recovery. In most cases the home care nurse coordinates care with the client's physician who initiates the orders. Referrals to physical therapy, occupational therapy, speech therapy, medical social work, respiratory therapy, nursing assistants/homemakers, the pharmacist, equipment companies, and even dietary consultation may be a part of home health care case management.

One major advantage of case management in the home is that the nurse case manager is able to assess a client's knowledge deficit in carrying out health-related instructions for therapy and medication. The case manager can also assess the client's formal and informal resources and can evaluate "caretaker burnout" in the client's family or among significant others. Last, because of multiple issues that face the terminally ill, many clients benefit from home hospice care, which is frequently coordinated by the case manager.

Case Management in Acute Care

With the advent of increased competition and health care costs, health care providers in the acute care setting must begin to pursue avenues to achieve the major goal of increased quality at a decreased cost. Case management has been used in other environments to effectively meet this goal.

In many facilities, case management techniques have been modified for use in the acute care setting. However, the emphasis remains on increased quality at a decreased cost, as well as enhanced patient outcomes, patient satisfaction, and professional satisfaction (Van Dongen and Jambunathan, 1992). Frequently acute care case management is referred to as "episodic case management."

In the acute care environment several roles may be combined with case management—for instance, utilization review, quality improvement, outcomes management, discharge planning, and social services. The goals of acute care case management are to ensure cost containment and efficient use of resources, coordinate alternate forms of care, increase access to care, coordinate services, improve the patient's functional status, ensure early discharge with an appropriate length of stay, promote expected patient outcomes, promote collaboration among members of the health care team, and promote professional satisfaction of the health care team (Easterling et al., 1995).

Acute care case management focuses on coordination of the patient's care from pre-admission to post-discharge. However, some programs coordinate the patient's care beyond inpatient admission to the continuum of including preventive services, self-care services, and acute care services. The coordination of acute care services includes managing cost-effective use of resources, planning for care after discharge, decreasing hospital stay, increasing communication between patient and health care providers, and decreasing fragmentation of care by collaborative practice.

The process

Before admission, the case manager may contact the patient to begin teaching, assist with self-care, coordinate preadmission testing, coordinate scheduling of outpatient procedures or appointments, and prevent unnecessary emergency room admissions. These contacts may be in person, by telephone, or through home health referrals. Part of the preadmission testing is related to what case management is—how it can assist patients and how their care will progress. Also the case manager will answer any questions patients may have.

Once the patient is admitted, various tools are used to guide patient care. These tools include clinical pathways (also called care maps and care paths), guidelines, and protocols. These items are used to standardize care and thus decrease trial-and-error techniques. Clinical pathways serve as outlines for expected needs of the patient. They also serve as valuable tools for teaching less experienced staff and as guides for all staff members. Often these pathways are shared with the patient to assist with education regarding expectations, service and treatments provided and patient goals to be achieved (Flynn and Kilgallen, 1993; Rudisill, Phillips, and Payne, 1994).

Case managers use the pathways to micro-manage the care provided to patients covered under these guidelines. Frequently, meetings are held with the health care team. The case manager also coordinates care among consultants, checking for redundancies and communicating patient information to the health care team (Perry, 1996). Variances to the norm or deviations from the pathway are reported and analyzed to improve quality and performance as needed. Interdisciplinary teams are used to monitor, evaluate, and make improvements as needed in the pathway.

Many acute care case managers also manage patients after discharge. Patients who are managed after discharge are contacted periodically by phone, scheduled for follow-up appointments, scheduled for outpatient educational sessions, and/or are seen by home health nurses. Preparation for discharge includes evaluation of need for financial resources, support systems, durable medical equipment, transportation, community linkages, counseling, and education, to name a few. Patients are followed closely to prevent readmission to the acute care setting, a particular concern as the norm for length of stay in the acute care arena continues to shrink.

Case management models for acute care

Various staffing models have been used for acute care case management, ranging from RN case managers, case managers with any clinical specialty, social worker case managers, and teams with combinations of these (Borland, McRae, and Lycan, 1989; Goering et al., 1988). In addition, RN case managers have ranged from staff nurses, clinical nurse specialists, advanced practice nurses, to nurse practitioners.

The caseload of case managers varies greatly, depending on the severity of illness of the patient population, the type of service being provided, or the coverage of patients (acute care only or across the continuum of care). Case managers are assigned to particular nursing units, diagnostic-related groups (DRGs), disease categories, or combinations of any of these. Coverage of patients may be based on the patient's risk level, particular disease, DRG, clinical pathway, or the type of reimbursement (for instance, Medicare) (Lamb, 1995).

In some models the case manager provides direct patient care (Lyon, 1993). The advantage of this model is intimate knowledge of the patient and day-to-day activities. However, disadvantages can occur because, if staffing is short, this vital role is neglected in favor of the pressing clinical needs of the patient.

Despite the wide range of staffing models and coverage models, acute care case management has three predominate staffing models: the New England model, the discharge planner and arbitrator case management model, and the geriatric clinical nurse specialist model (Lyon, 1993). Box 8-3 gives characteristics of each predominate acute care case management model.

Box 8-3

Predominate Acute Care Case Management Models

Model	Characteristics
New England model	Based on primary nursing
	Responsible for the clinical care of the patient, as well as the financial implications, clinical pathway, and discharge planning
	Manages the patient according to the clinical pathway
Discharge planner and arbitrator case management model	Case managed by staff nurse providing direct patient care
	The RN, who serves as the discharge planner, also performs quality improvement/utilization review
	Quality improvement/utilization review activities are also performed in the traditional manner by a separate department
Geriatric clinical nurse specialist model	Focused on the geriatric population
	Case management is performed by a master's-prepared geriatric clinical nurse specialist
	Patients are typically followed at least 2 weeks postdischarge
	Geriatric clinical nurse specialist performs quality improvement/utilization review

The first, the New England model, is based on primary nursing. A primary nurse is assigned a group of patients to provide primary care, as well as manage their cases and to another group of patients for which she/he is not the primary care provider. The nurse as primary care provider is responsible for the clinical care of the patient, as well as for financial implications, clinical pathway, and discharge planning. Instead of using a nursing plan of care, the nurse manages the patient according to the clinical pathway, which consists of an interdisciplinary plan of care. In this model the primary nurse does not manage the patient before or after admission, except for one follow-up telephone call.

The second model, the discharge planner and arbitrator case management model, is also managed by a staff nurse providing direct patient care. The RN, who serves as the discharge planner, also performs quality improvement/utilization review activities. In this model, however, the bulk of the quality improvement/utilization review activities are performed in the traditional manner by a separate department.

The last model, the geriatric clinical nurse specialist model, is focused on the geriatric population with case management performed by a master's-prepared geriatric clinical nurse specialist. Comprehensive discharge protocols are used by the geriatric clinical nurse specialist. Geriatric patients are typically followed for at least 2 weeks post-discharge via telephone or home visits. The geriatric clinical nurse specialist performs quality improvement/utilization review activities and manages the financial, as well as clinical, outcomes of the patient.

Regardless of the staffing model used, the primary goals of case management are to decrease cost and increase or maintain quality. Case managers must coordinate care across departments, serve as a communication link among members of the health care team, evaluate discharge planning needs, assess the financial impact of illness on the patient and family, guide the patient toward support agencies or resources, coordinate patient education, monitor patient outcomes, evaluate quality of care, and ensure effective use of resources.

NURSES' ROLE IN DISEASE CASE MANAGEMENT

With increasing costs of chronic disease management and the growth of numbers in an aging America, resource allocation is a primary focus for the future of health care. The illness-driven model is no longer affordable and is ineffective in managing quality or costs. The nurse case manager can provide education, planning, and administration of care to ensure optimal use of resources in a disease-management model.

Disease management refers to the "application of systems necessary to minimize health care expenditures." (Stolte, 1996) Another way to describe this approach is that it is

> . . . a systematic proactive case management model that uses an organized approach to provide early intervention along a continuum of care, and that includes active patient self-care participation in maintaining their optimum state of health (Lee, 1996).

Disease management is usually population based and must have proactive patient involvement, as well as an integrated health care delivery system. Patients must have knowledge of disease and the resources necessary to maintain an achievable level of health (Stolte, 1996). Zitter (1994) describes five principles necessary to manage the disease process:

1. Understanding the course of the particular disease process and typical costs associated with it
2. Diagnosis and treatment provided for the disease process without influence of reimbursement available for the therapy
3. Education and compliance programs for management of chronic disease
4. Care for the patient in a continuum across all care settings
5. Allocation of necessary resources to provide the most powerful and cost-effective treatment available

The nurse case manager in the disease management model can demonstrate management of care for those most likely to consume valuable health care resources and dollars. This may delay or actually help avoid acute exacerbation of the disease process and may decrease costs. Education and patient compliance programs are critical to success. Using a systems approach, the nurse case manager can decrease the overall costs of health care resource consumption by identifying and educating the patient to avoid secondary complications, by tailoring education to the patient level, and by initiating early treatment for chronic disease populations (Stolte, 1996). This process helps the patient learn self-management and achieve long-term optimal health.

Summary

Case management is one tool for conserving health care resources while providing satisfying quality care for patients in all settings from community care to acute care. Evolving variations of case management are proving effective in care management. Disease case management is an example of this as nurses move to proactive prevention and management of chronic disease. The patient is an active partner in this process, with education and self-care being key. Using the case management approach, nurses can make a major impact in providing cost-efficient, quality care.

Discussion Questions

1. List the attributes and personal characteristics needed to become a successful case manager. How can people prepare themselves to assume this role?
2. Identify universal concepts inherent in all models of case management. Discuss how these concepts affect resource utilization.
3. Identify the advantages and disadvantages of implementing case management in a health care facility.

Case Study

Jill is a 35-year-old divorced woman with four school-age children. While at work, she suffered a severe burn over 25% of her body, including both arms and part of her torso. She has recently been admitted to an acute care facility but is past the acute phase of her recovery.

Case Study Exercise
1. Develop a case management plan of care for this client in both the acute care setting and the community setting.
2. What services and resources should be used?

REFERENCES

Abrahams R et al.: Variations in care planning practice in the social/HMO: An exploratory study, *Gerontologist* 29:725, 1989.

American Nurses Association: *Standard of Community Health Nursing Practice,* Kansas City, Mo, 1991, The Association.

Borland A, McRae J, Lycan C: Outcomes of five years of continuous intensive case management, *Hosp Community Psychiatry* 40:369, 1989.

Capitman JA, Haskins B, Bernstein J: Case management approaches in coordinated community-oriented long-term care demonstrations, *Gerontologist* 26:398, 1986.

Chamberlain R, Rapp CA: A decade of case management: A methodological review of outcome research, *Community Ment Health J* 27:171, 1991.

Easterling A et al.: *The case manager's guide: Acquiring the skills for success,* Chicago, 1995, American Hospital Publishing.

Esposito L: Home health case management, *Home Healthcare Nurse* 12(3):38, 1994.

Flynn AM, Kilgallen ME: Case management: A multidisciplinary approach to the evaluation of cost and quality standards, *J Nurs Care Qual* 8(1):58, 1993.

Goering PN et al.: Improved functioning for case management clients, *Psychosoc Rehab J* 12(1):3, 1988.

Lamb GS: Conceptual and methodological issues in nurse case management research, *ANS Adv Nurs Sci* 15(2):16, 1992.

Lamb GS: Case management. In Fitzpatrick JJ, Stevenson JS, editors: *Annual review of nursing research,* New York, 1995, Springer.

Lee S: New trends in disease management, *Contin Care* 4:32, 1996.

Lyon JC: Models of nursing care delivery and case management: Clarification of term, *Nurs Econ* 11(3):163, 1993.

Mahn V: Clinical nurse case management: A service line approach, *Nurs Manage* 24(9):48, 1993.

McKenzie CB, Torkelson NG, Holt MA: Care and cost: Nursing case management improves both, *Nurs Manage* 20(10):30, 1989.

Molloy SP: Defining case management, *Home Healthcare Nurse* 12(3):51, 1994.

Perry LE: Case managers eliminate "parallel play" in health care, FAX Bulletin (excerpts from the First Annual Hospital Case Management Conference) April 4, 1996, American Health Consultants.

Rogers M, Riordan J, Swindle D: Community-based nursing case management pays off, *Nurs Manage* 22(3):30, 1991.

Rudisill PT, Phillips M, Payne CM: Clinical paths for cardiac surgery patients: A multidisciplinary approach to quality improvement outcomes, *J Nurs Care Qual* 8(3):27, 1994.

Stanhope M, Lancaster J: *Community health nursing: Promoting health of aggregates, families, and individuals,* ed 4, St. Louis, 1996, Mosby.

Stolte CM: Nurses' role in disease case management, *Healthcare Res* 15(10):21, 1996.

Swanson JM, Albrecht M: *Community health nursing: Promoting the health of aggregates,* Philadelphia, 1993, WB Saunders.

Van Dongen CJ, Jambunathan J: Pilot study results: The psychiatric RN case manager, *J Psychosoc Nurs Ment Health Serv* 30(11):11, 1992.

Zander K: Nursing case management: Strategic management of cost and quality outcomes, *J Nurs Adm* 18(5):23, 1988.

Zitter M: *Special report: Disease management,* San Francisco, 1994, The Zimmer Group.

chapter nine

Clinical Pathways

Sandra Bassett

- Discuss key benefits for implementing clinical pathways.
- Identify at least three questions organizational leaders must address before a critical pathway initiative is begun.
- Define system-, patient-, and clinical-related variances.
- Differentiate between negative and positive variances.

The rising cost of health care is forcing organizations to rethink the way care is delivered. The focus is on controlling cost by decreasing resource utilization and length of stay. Resources may include staff, diagnostic and therapeutic processes and procedures, and pharmaceuticals. Third party payors and managed care companies are asking for improved results. Outcome information relates not only to clinical outcomes, but also to cost savings. For example, if Health Care Organization A can demonstrate that it can provide cost-effective care without negative impact to the patient, as compared with Health Care Organization B, Health Care Organization A will in most cases receive the contract. With all things equal, the contracting companies focus on cost.

One approach to lowering cost is clinical pathways, also referred to as guidelines, critical pathways, maps, paths, protocols, or algorithms. **Clinical pathways** or guidelines are developed around a specific diagnosis or procedure, such as congestive heart failure or total hip replacement. A pathway includes key functions or events of care processes; it is one of many case management tools or models. The development and use of pathways reduce variations by defining the most common or preferred courses of treatment. Variations from these courses may represent improved treatment, uncontrollable or unrecognized patient variables, or poor care (Hopkins, 1993). Pathway templates organize, sequence, and specify timelines for interventions by each discipline. Pathways establish specific goals and outcomes for the patient. One or more disciplines may be involved in the process.

In addition to controlling cost, pathways encourage consistent practice patterns within a discipline. Variation occurs among disciplines, geographical locations, and places of employment. The professional nurse combines education and experience

Box 9-1
Clinical Pathway Process
Planning phase Current practice phase Designing phase Testing phase Variance phase Evaluation phase

to formulate a particular practice pattern. Since staff members do not share the same education and experience, various practice patterns emerge for similar or the same diagnosis or procedure. Identification of best practices is the goal in developing effective pathways. Therefore resource consumption varies among staff and patients.

Patients appear to achieve goals faster when clinical pathways are used. Goals, interventions, time frames, and expected outcomes based on best practices are shared with the patient at the entry level of the pathway. At this point expectations are established between the patient and care team. Flexibility within the pathway allows for variances among patients, if needed.

Pathways are excellent communication tools. Each day or encounter, the nurse documents the patient's relationship to the pathway. At any point the nurse relays information to the physician, managed care professional, or case manager. The physician can alter the intervention at any time, as determined by the patient's needs. The pathway can serve as the basis of a teaching tool for patients and physicians and other members of the care team.

CLINICAL PATHWAY PROCESS

How does an organization begin? The decision is made to adopt a pathway available for purchase or to develop one internally. Either way, the pathway must meet the organizational goals, mission, and strategies. The leaders establish how the success of the pathway will be measured. Accountability for the process is assigned. The phases of the clinical pathway process are listed in Box 9-1.

Planning Phase

First, leaders must identify high-volume, recurring diagnoses or procedures. In most cases developing and implementing a pathway for a small population are not cost-effective. The following questions must also be addressed. How prevalent is the diagnosis or procedure within the community or referral base? Does the organization have experienced staff relating to the anticipated pathway? What is the required investment by the organization? Although the focus is on controlling costs, developing, implementing, and tracking a pathway are costly.

What is the projected target for the pathway? The target usually relates to reduction in cost or a reduction in length of stay or number of visits. Are the data available, accurate, and in a format that is easily understood by staff? Who will collect the data, and how will they be used? Can the data be derived via computer software or must they be obtained manually?

Current Practice Phase

The next phase involves identifying and understanding current practice among the care team members by performing medical record review of patients with the diagnosis or procedure. Depending on the total number of cases, a sample size, usually at least 25 and not more than 50, is determined. Each intervention, contact with the patient, and outcome of care is documented on a worksheet. The care provider is recorded by intervention. After data collection is complete, summaries of interventions by day or visit are composed. Converting the data into meaningful information can be difficult and confusing; determining what is and is not important is a challenge. The outcome of this process will allow the team to identify best practices by care provider.

Designing Phase

The pathway is designed around best practices of care. During the designing process developers should anticipate response to and from payors. The design is based on goals, interventions, and outcomes in a day-to-day or visit-by-visit sequence. Goals are specific, measurable, and patient oriented. Interventions are bound by time, for example, day 1, day 2, week 1, week 2, visit 1, or visit 2.

The pathway can be developed to include all disciplines, or separate pathways can be written for each discipline to use for the same diagnosis. Documentation may be incorporated in the actual pathway tool or in nurses' notes. The patient's and care provider's responsibilities are specified. Patient education material is one way to address the patient's/caregiver's role in the pathway. The pathway has designated outcomes that are also bound by time. A survey tool may be one approach to ascertain the patient's/caregiver's perception of the success of the clinical pathway. Before implementation, the type of patient as it relates to the pathway is defined. Appendixes 9-1 through 9-4 at the end of this chapter present examples of clinical pathways.

The components of the pathway often include specific information regarding the disease process surrounding the diagnosis or procedure, nutrition, fluid and electrolytes, functional activity, and community resources. In addition, education is an important part, since the goal is to assist the patient in becoming independent in a shorter period of time. Education centers around understanding medication regimen, purpose, and side effects and procedures or other interventions. Discharge planning is included from the entry point of the pathway and continues until discharge. Other data included in the pathway are name of patient, diagnosis or procedure with corresponding ICD-9 codes, age, race, sex, date of entry into pathway, and date of discharge from pathway. The key components of a pathway are listed in Box 9-2.

Testing Phase

The involved physicians and other care team members must embrace the entire process, including the trial testing phase, which is imperative for success. Input

---

Box 9-2

Components of Pathway

Disease process
Nutrition
Fluid and electrolytes
Functional activity
Community resources
Education
Discharge planning

---

should be consistent and ongoing. The components of the pathway must be adjusted as needed. During implementation the team starts small, with a few patients and selected team members. Constant surveillance during the testing phase is a must. Only those patients who meet the definition will be admitted into the pathway. Caution should be taken not to admit other patients.

Variance Phase

The term *variance* is being used to mean the difference between what is planned and what actually happens. (See Appendix 9-1C.) During testing and implementation, variances among care team members, patients, and physicians occur. Some variances are in our control, whereas others are not. The variances should be examined to determine which components of the pathway need adjustments, if possible.

To clarify differences among types of variations the variances should be categorized into, at least, system-, patient-, and clinical-related variances. System variances are related to supplies, equipment, or services that are not available when needed. Patient-controlled situations such as their being too ill to participate in or comply with the intervention and unavailability, are examples of patient-related variances. Clinical variances relate to areas such as a care team member's not advancing parenteral fluids to oral fluids when the patient can tolerate oral feedings, not consulting physician when indicated, or failure to perform an intervention as outlined on the pathway.

Variances are further categorized as positive or negative. Positive variances refer to the patient's meeting the goal in the specified time frame and at a cost equal to or less than anticipated. Conversely, negative variances relate to the patient's not meeting the goal within the time frame at a cost equal to or greater than anticipated. Communication of all types of variances should be timely and in a format that staff can understand.

Evaluation Phase

After successful development and implementation are complete, the next step in the pathway process is the evaluation phase. This process addresses both quality and cost. Outcomes can be defined in terms of the patient's physiological progression or functionality or in terms of systems outcomes (Strassner, 1996). The goals that were established during the planning phase are applied to the pathway. For example, has a reduction in cost or decrease in length of stay or number of visits occurred? Did patient and family satisfaction change? The satisfaction of the patient and family can be measured with a patient interview survey. (See Appendix 9-1D.)

Critical pathways will not be successful in regard to quality or cost for each and every patient. Because of the complex nature of the patient and the patient's environment, some patients are not suited for a pathway; this is one reason to carefully define which patients will enter the pathway before implementation. Other issues that may result in negative outcomes include lack of collaboration of care team members and lack of consensus of professional staff regarding practice. Lack of feedback from staff or staff's perception that leaders are not supportive can decrease momentum. In addition, pathways with no demonstrated added value to the patient may be ineffective.

EDUCATION

Education of all care team members is essential for success. Overview of current and future trends in health care support the need for a new, creative approach to the delivery of health care. A brief summary of the pathway from beginning to end should be included in team members' education. A detailed orientation of the pathway, including goals, interventions, outcomes, and definition of patient types should also be covered. An explanation of variances regarding definition of types should be included. The care team must embrace the pathway process. Leadership must strive to gain support for it. Ongoing feedback about both negative and positive variances must be given to staff. Members can learn from each other, and leaders can respond to variances as needed and make necessary adjustments.

BENEFITS OF PATHWAYS

Developing and implementing pathways benefit those involved in many ways. The most obvious goals are to improve quality of patient care and reduce overall costs. Some other results of the process that are just as important are listed in Box 9-3.

Summary

The rising cost of health care is forcing organizations to reevaluate how care is delivered. Payors want more care delivered at a lower cost without jeopardizing quality. Companies negotiating contracts ask for outcomes, and health care organizations have the ability to define them. The clinical pathway is just one model of managing care in today's health care environment. The components of pathways are goals, interventions, and outcomes that are bound by time and resources. A few of the benefits of developing and implementing clinical pathways are enhanced collaborative practice, established baselines relative to standards of care for clinical competency, and identified outcomes of care.

> **Box 9-3**
>
> **Benefits of Clinical Pathways**
>
> Methodical approach to care increases patient and family satisfaction.
> Communication among care team members and patients increases.
> Baselines for standards of care are established for clinical competency.
> Responsibilities of care team members and patients are clarified.
> Quality improvement endeavors are enhanced.
> Orientation process of new staff members encourages consistent practice from the start of employment; pathways reduce inconsistencies in care.
> The pathway process identifies outcomes that can be utilized for benchmarking with other organizations.
> Collaborative practice among professional and nonprofessional staff is encouraged.
> Clinical pathway process provides for a holistic approach to care, as opposed to the traditional model.
> Outcomes of pathways can serve as a negotiating tool when discussing coverage of services with payors.
> The concept of team is demonstrated through implementation of the pathway.

Discussion Questions

1. Why should an organization start developing and implementing clinical pathways?
2. What questions should organizational leaders address before clinical pathway initiatives are begun?
3. What are system-, patient-, and clinical-related variances?
4. What are the differences between and similarities of negative and positive variances?

Case Study

Comfort Hospice Services is interested in implementing clinical pathways. The hospice staff is interested in learning more about ovarian cancer and would like to start a pathway in this area.

The admission data for the past 2 months indicate the following:

End-stage cardiac disease	5 patients
End-stage renal disease	3 patients
Ovarian carcinoma	4 patients
Lung carcinoma	7 patients
Metastatic carcinoma	25 patients

Case Study Exercise

1. Discuss the pros and cons of the staff's selection. Who should make the determination relative to selection of diagnosis?
2. What steps should the staff follow?
3. Which components would you include in the pathway?

REFERENCES

Hopkins TL: Avoiding the pathway potholes, *QRC Advisor* 9(3):1, 1993.
Strassner L: Evaluating critical pathways, *Contin Care* 15(4):24, 1996.

Appendix 9-1 Critical Path for Congestive Heart Failure

9-1A: Critical Path: DRG 127-Congestive Heart Failure
9-1B: Congestive Heart Failure Clinical Path
9-1C: CHF Critical Path Compliance Study
9-1D: CHF Patient Interview Survey (Post D/C Call)
9-1E: CHF Patient and Family Clinical Path Letter

Appendix 9-2 Critical Path for Skilled Nursing

9-2A: Critical Path: Skilled Nursing
9-2B: Critical Path: Skilled Nursing
9-2C: Critical Path: Skilled Nursing

Appendix 9-3 Clinical Pathway for CVA/TIA

Appendix 9-4 Clinical Pathway for COPD

9-4A: Clinical Pathway for COPD, Nursing
9-4B: Clinical Pathway for COPD, Physical Therapy

Latest revision date: 7/97

	Admission Day	**Post-Admission Day 1**	

Tests	EKG
	CXR-PA
	CBC with Diff
	Card. Profile
	Chem Profile
	Dig Level
	O$_2$ Sat
		Echocardiogram (if more than year
		   since previous one or at MD discre-
		   tion)
		Card. Profile (if applicable)
		Chem 7	

Assessments & Interventions	Admission Weight Strict I&O Telemetry VS Q 2-4 hours Breath Sounds q shift O$_2$ Protocol (if indicated) KVO IV (or heplock)	Daily Weight I&O Telemetry VS Q 4 hours Breath Sounds q shift O$_2$ Protocol KVO IV (or heplock)	
Activity	Elevate HOB BR/BSC	Elevate HOB BR/BSC	
Diet	Low Na per order Fluid Restriction (per MD order) No Caffeine	Low Na per order No Caffeine	
Medications	Diuretic K+ Supplement Lanoxin ACE Inhibitor	Per MD order	
Education and Continuum of Care Planning	Notify CardPulm Rehab Notify Dietitian Assess Educational needs Provide patient with copy of "Patient CHF path"	Initiate CHF teaching CardPulm Rehab Dietitian CM evaluation	
Outcomes	Hemodynamically stable; Diuresis	5-10 lb weight loss; Improved Resp. Status; Decreasing edema; VSS	

IMPORTANT NOTE: This critical path is a guideline and is not intended to create a standard of care. The pathway can be modified based on individual patient need.

(Courtesy NorthCrest Medical Center, Springfield, Tennessee.)

Post-Admission Day 2	Post-Admission Day 3	Discharge Day
		Lytes and BUN
		Dig Level (if newly started on Dig)
Daily Weight I&O D/C Telemetry if stable VS Q 4 hours Breath Sounds q shift O$_2$ Protocol (if still applicable) KVO IV (or heplock)	Daily Weight I&O VS QID Breath Sounds QD D/C IV (or heplock)	Discharge Weight AM VS Discharge Breath Sounds
Ambulate in room	Ambulate in hall	
Low Na per order No Caffeine	Low Na per order No Caffeine	Low Na per order No Caffeine
Per MD	Per MD	Per MD: Home prescriptions given
Continue teaching and counseling	Continue teaching and counseling	Finalize teaching and continuum of care planning; Affirm patient/family understanding prior to discharge
Continues improvement in respiratory status—off O$_2$ or plans for home O$_2$ in progress; No weight increases; Advancing through CHF education plan	Tolerates ambulation of short distances; I&O values approximate; Continues to advance through teaching plan	Stable for discharge with outpatient, Home Health or Nursing home management

Latest revision date: 7/97

	The first 1-2 days of your hospital stay	
Your Medical Care	The doctors and hospital staff will want to check the function of your heart and lungs: • The nurse will check your vital signs (pulse, blood pressure, and breathing rate) every few hours. • You will be weighed. • Doctors, nurses, and other staff may listen to the sounds made when you breathe. • Someone will examine your neck veins and look at your feet to detect swelling. • The fluids you drink and urine you expel will be measured (I&O). • You will have lab work and other tests as ordered by your doctor. • You may have an IV (tube in your vein) and a catheter (tube in your bladder). • You may be given some oxygen to ease your breathing.	
Activity	Rest is very important since we are trying to ease the workload on your heart. You will be confined to bed. The head of your bed will probably be raised. If your condition permits, your doctor may let you out of bed to use a bedside commode, but **YOU MUST NOT GET UP WITHOUT YOUR NURSE.** Call your nurse if you need to use the bathroom. **NO SMOKING!!!!**	
Diet	You will be served a diet low in salt (sodium). Salt causes your body to hold fluids, making it harder for your heart to work. Caffeine will not be allowed because it can add stress to your heart. You should continue to avoid adding salt and caffeine to your diet after discharge. The Nutrition Services Hostess will give you the brochure "To Our Guests." Fill it out if you have special food likes and dislikes.	
Medica-tions	Tell the nurse what medications you currently take at home and what medications you have taken today. Depending on your history and current condition, your doctor may prescribe new medications to treat your congestive heart failure. Your nurse, doctor, or a hospital pharmacist will explain any new drugs to you.	
Education & Planning for Discharge	Our hospital has a team of individuals that will help you understand and manage your disease. Your disease will be discussed with you and you will be given a booklet. A case manager will be assigned to help you with special discharge planning needs.	
Feeling Better	Within a few hours of arrival, you should begin to breathe easier and feel better. You will probably produce a lot of urine which is a sign that your body is getting rid of extra fluid.	

(Courtesy NorthCrest Medical Center, Springfield, Tennessee.)

The next 1-2 days of your stay	Discharge day
• You will be weighed every day. • You will have your intake and output measured. • As you begin to feel better, your IV and catheter will be removed. • Your oxygen will be discontinued when you no longer require it.	Your doctor has determined that you are ready for discharge. Remember to weigh daily after you go home. Weight gain of more than 3 pounds in a day, swelling, and increased shortness of breath are indications that your congestive heart failure may be worsening. Call your doctor or seek medical care immediately.
As you improve, you will be allowed to get up in your room and walk in the hall—BUT ONLY WITH ASSISTANCE. Do not get out of bed by yourself. Assist with your bath as you feel able.	Take it easy today. You will undergo a lot of activity in preparing for discharge. Don't forget to continue "pacing yourself" after discharge. Remember that too much stress on your heart makes your disease worse. Avoid tobacco and alcohol as these will aggravate your condition. Ask a health care professional if you need information about smoking cessation.
Rest before and after your meal and eat as much as you are able. A dietitian or nurse has information for you about your special dietary needs.	If you have any questions about what you should or should not eat after going home, please be sure to tell your nurse. If necessary, she can make arrangements for you to meet with the dietitian either before or after discharge.
Learn about your medications so that you can manage your condition after you leave the hospital.	Your doctor will give you discharge prescriptions. Be sure to take your medicines as directed. Notify your doctor if you have any problems related to your medicines.
Review your "CHF" booklet and any other material the hospital staff has shared with you. Ask questions!	Tell your nurse or doctor if you have questions. Don't hesitate to call the doctor or hospital if you find you have questions later.
Your clinical condition is stabilizing. You must focus on learning how to best manage your disease.	You are ready for discharge but will need close management by your doctor and other health providers.

	Y	N
1. New diagnosis?	○	○
2. Was this a readmission within 31 days (related to CHF)?	○	○
3. Cardiac Consult?	○	○

4. LOS

    ○ 1 day   ○ 2 days   ○ 3 days   ○ 4 days   ○ 5 days   ○ 6 days

    ○ 7 days   ○ 8 days   ○ 9 days   ○ Over 9 days

5. Discharge status

    ○ Home   ○ Home Health

    ○ ECF   ○ Expired

    ○ Other _____

6. Adherence to path

    ○ Strong variation from ○ Moderate variation from ○ Generally followed
       path   path   path

7. Ejection Fraction

    ○ <20   ○ <30   ○ <40   ○ >40   ○ Not noted

	Y	N
8. Daily weights	○	○
9. Intake and Output	○	○
10. Cardiopulmonary rehab visited?	○	○
11. Patient education (including life-style modification) noted?	○	○
12. Diuretics administered?	○	○
13. ACE Inhibitors administered?	○	○
14. Dig. administered?	○	○
15. Documented medication usage education?	○	○

Comments

```



```

_____
(Courtesy NorthCrest Medical Center, Springfield, Tennessee.)

Did you (the patient) receive instructions about the following?

	Y	N
1. Congestive Heart Failure	○	○
2. Low salt diet	○	○
3. Limiting use of alcohol and tobacco	○	○
4. Weighing yourself daily	○	○
5. Adapting your activity so you can conserve your energy	○	○
6. Your medications	○	○
7. When to call your doctor	○	○

Patient Satisfaction

	Y	N
8. Overall, were you satisfied with your care and treatment at NorthCrest?	○	○
9. Were the instructions we provided useful?	○	○

Patient Outcomes

	Y	N
10. Are you weighing yourself daily or every other day?	○	○
11. Have you had any trouble with increased swelling, cough, weight gain or shortness of breath?	○	○

12. If yes, have you notified your physician of the problem?

　○ Yes　　○ No　　○ Not applicable

13. Are you able to carry out simple activities such as walking, brushing your hair and bathing?

　○ Yes　　○ No　　○ Not applicable

Do you have any comments, questions, or suggestions for us?

Surveyor comments (name of nurse placing call, date of call, observations/actions)

(Courtesy NorthCrest Medical Center, Springfield, Tennessee.)

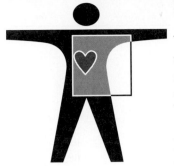

Dear Patient and Family:

You will receive information about **Congestive Heart Failure (CHF).** We hope this material will help you understand how your doctor, NorthCrest Medical Center, and YOU can best manage your illness.

Because CHF limits the quality of many people's lives, we have developed a special CHF treatment program. One part of this program is a **clinical path.** A clinical path is a general guideline that helps the doctor and hospital plan your care. The "patient version" of the path will help you know what to expect while you are in the hospital. However because your doctor will adapt the clinical path to meet your individual needs, you may not receive everything noted on the pathway. You might also receive treatments or tests that are not part of the path.

Another part of our comprehensive CHF treatment program is **patient education.** Be sure to learn all that you can. Ask questions! Once you leave the hospital, it is important for you to follow your instructions. Diet and other life-style changes will help keep your CHF under control.

A third part of our treatment program is **long-term disease management.** Your doctor and other health care providers will help you monitor and manage your illness. It is important for you to keep all appointments and to call the doctor if you have special problems. Someone from the hospital may call you a few days after discharge to follow-up with you. Never hesitate to call the hospital or the doctor with your questions. Our goal is to keep you as healthy as possible.

Thank you for choosing NorthCrest Medical Center for your care.

NorthCrest Medical Center
100 NorthCrest Dr
Springfield, TN 37172
(615)384-2411
Fax: (615)382-3814

(Courtesy NorthCrest Medical Center, Springfield, Tennessee.)

PATIENT NAME: _____ INITIATED BY: _____ DATE: _____

IN CONJUNCTION WITH: _____ REHAB POTENTIAL: G F P PROJECTED # VISITS: __10__ ACTUAL # VISITS: _____

SIGNATURE _____	INITIALS ____	SIGNATURE _____	INITIALS ____
SIGNATURE _____	INITIALS ____	SIGNATURE _____	INITIALS ____
SIGNATURE _____	INITIALS ____	SIGNATURE _____	INITIALS ____

FOCUS	TARGET DATE	CODE, DATE & INITIALS

DIAGNOSIS: (1) Congestive Heart Failure

OUTCOMES:
1. Demonstrates decrease or absence of edema within 10 visits.
2. Demonstrates no wt. gain >3lbs/day in a 24 hr period throughout plan of care
3. Verbalizes medication regimen within 4 visits
4. Demonstrates compliance with the medication regimen within 10 visits
5. Venipunctures as ordered will have therapeutic levels within 10 visits
6. Verbalizes signs and symptoms of CHF within 4 visits
7. Verbalizes understanding of diet regimen within 4 visits
8. Demonstrates compliance with the diet regimen within 10 visits
9. Demonstrates ability to obtain daily wts. within 10 visits
10. Demonstrates ability to measure edema within 10 visits
11. Verbalizes conditions that exist, requiring physician notification within 10 visits

CODES:	PROBLEMS	OUTCOMES/MEASUREMENT ACTIVITIES
	R-RESOLVED	M-MET	NM-NOT MET
	NR-NOT RESOLVED	MP-MET TO POTENTIAL	R-REVISED
	RP-RESOLVED TO POTENTIAL	ME-MET EXCEPT FOR ONGOING EVALS	DC-DISCONTINUED

(Courtesy NorthCrest Medical Center, Springfield, Tennessee.)

PATIENT NAME: _____ NUMBER: _____

APPROACHES	VISIT	CODES, DATES, & INITIALS
Every visit do these things:		
1. Assess vital signs: B/P, Apical pulse, radial pulse, respirations	1-9	
2. Assess heart tones and breath sounds: Note any advent·ious findings	1-9	
3. Assess skin color	1-9	
4. Weigh patient	1-9	
5. Measure for edema (R/L ankle, R/L calf), Note amount, sites, pitting, non-pitting	1-9	
6. Assess for Jugular Vein distention	1-9	
7. Measure Intake and Output and begin teaching family or patient to perform and record	1-9	
8. Assess for changes in Levels of Consciousness (altered sensorium)	1-9	
9. Assess for response to activity (Instruct on measures to conserve energy)	1-9	
10. Assess effectiveness of medications	1-9	
11. Assess untoward side effects of medications	1-9	
12. Do venipunctures as ordered during the visit schedule	1-9	

CODES:

A. VERBALIZATION	*D. TECHNIQUES*	*F. STATUS*	*H. VARIANCES*
1-PATIENT	1-EXPLANATION	1-COMPLETED	1-IMPAIRED LEARNING
2-CAREGIVER	2-DEMONSTRATION	2-D/C (N/A)	2-DETERIORATION
3-WITH CUES	*E. TEACHING TOOLS*	3-D/C (PATIENT)	3-IMPROVEMENT
4-WITHOUT CUES	1-CAREPLAN	4-D/C (DOCTOR)	4-RX CHANGE
5-%	2-INSTRUCT SHEETS	5-REOPENED	5-MED CHANGE
6-UNABLE	3-VIDEOTAPE	*G. PERFORMANCE*	6-VISIT CHANGE
B. DEMONSTRATION	4-PICTURES	1-ACCOMPLISHED	7-OTHER
1-PATIENT	5-PRINTED DIET		
2-CAREGIVER	6-OTHER		
3-WITH CUES			
4-WITHOUT CUES			
5-%			
6-UNABLE			
C. TOLERANCE			
1-WELL			
2-FAIR			
3-POOR			

(Courtesy NorthCrest Medical Center, Springfield, Tennessee.)

PATIENT NAME:		NUMBER:
APPROACHES	**VISIT**	**CODES, DATES, & INITIALS**
Assigned Visits		
1. Instruct on definition of CHF	1	
2. Instruct on Medication Regimen including dose, frequency, route, side effects, and interactions, to include medication instruction sheet(s)	1-3	
3. Instruct on signs and symptoms of CHF which includes a weight gain of more than 3 lbs. in a 24 hr period, increased SOB/dyspnea, increased edema, presence of or increased orthopnea, development of or increased pulmonary congestion, neck vein distention, decreases UOP, pale, clammy skin, chest pain	1-3	
4. Teach safety and care regarding O_2 therapy when indicated	1-3	
5. Instruct on diet regimen including the effects of sodium in the diet and the need to read food labels for salt content	4	
6. Instruct on supplementing potassium in the diet: Oranges, Bananas, Tomatoes, Dates	4	
7. Instruct on the significance of small, easily digested meals on cardiac function	4	

CODES:

A. VERBALIZATION
1-PATIENT
2-CAREGIVER
3-WITH CUES
4-WITHOUT CUES
5-%
6-UNABLE
B. DEMONSTRATION
1-PATIENT
2-CAREGIVER

3-WITH CUES
4-WITHOUT CUES
5-%
6-UNABLE
C. TOLERANCE
1-WELL
2-FAIR
3-POOR

D. TECHNIQUES
1-EXPLANATION
2-DEMONSTRATION
E. TEACHING TOOLS
1-CAREPLAN
2-INSTRUCT SHEETS
3-VIDEOTAPE
4-PICTURES
5-PRINTED DIET
6-OTHER

F. STATUS
1-COMPLETED
2-D/C (N/A)
3-D/C (PATIENT)
4-D/C (DOCTOR)
5-REOPENED
G. PERFORMANCE
1-ACCOMPLISHED

H. VARIANCES
1-IMPAIRED LEARNING
2-DETERIORATION
3-IMPROVEMENT
4-RX CHANGE
5-MED CHANGE
6-VISIT CHANGE
7-OTHER

(Courtesy NorthCrest Medical Center, Springfield, Tennessee.)

PATIENT NAME: _____   NUMBER: _____

APPROACHES	VISIT	CODES, DATES, & INITIALS
8. Instruct on obtaining daily weights and keeping a log and notifying the health care provider of a 3 lb weight gain or more in a 24 hr period	5	
9. Instruct on measuring edema and keeping a log for comparison	5	
10. Instruct on elevating lower extremities and avoiding pressure under the knees in the presence of edema	5	
11. Instruct on pulse monitoring and safe parameters 60-80 beats/minute	5	
12. Instruct on response to activity levels (e.g. Ability to walk 12-14 steps without dyspnic episodes)	6	
13. Teach alternating rest with activity	6	
14. Teach cessation of activity/unnecessary movement should chest pain occur	6	
15. Instruct on the impact of environmental stress	7	
16. Instruct on the use of assistive devices or assistance with mobility to ensure safety	7	
17. Instruct on other safety factors (slow position changes)	7	
18. Instruct on the need for timely notification of the physician, emergency help, 911, home health agency	8	

CODES:

A. VERBALIZATION
1-PATIENT
2-CAREGIVER
3-WITH CUES
4-WITHOUT CUES
5-%
6-UNABLE
B. DEMONSTRATION
1-PATIENT
2-CAREGIVER

3-WITH CUES
4-WITHOUT CUES
5-%
6-UNABLE
C. TOLERANCE
1-WELL
2-FAIR
3-POOR

D. TECHNIQUES
1-EXPLANATION
2-DEMONSTRATION
E. TEACHING TOOLS
1-CAREPLAN
2-INSTRUCT SHEETS
3-VIDEOTAPE
4-PICTURES
5-PRINTED DIET
6-OTHER

F. STATUS
1-COMPLETED
2-D/C (N/A)
3-D/C (PATIENT)
4-D/C (DOCTOR)
5-REOPENED
G. PERFORMANCE
1-ACCOMPLISHED

H. VARIANCES
1-IMPAIRED LEARNING
2-DETERIORATION
3-IMPROVEMENT
4-RX CHANGE
5-MED CHANGE
6-VISIT CHANGE
7-OTHER

Continued

PATIENT NAME: _____   NUMBER: _____

APPROACHES	VISIT	CODES, DATES, & INITIALS
19. Instruct on the need for medical appointment follow through	8	
20. Provide Discharge Instructions	9	
21. Re-evaluate level of knowledge regarding recall of teaching and reinstruct as indicated	9	

CODES:

A. VERBALIZATION
1-PATIENT
2-CAREGIVER
3-WITH CUES
4-WITHOUT CUES
5-%
6-UNABLE
B. DEMONSTRATION
1-PATIENT
2-CAREGIVER
3-WITH CUES
4-WITHOUT CUES
5-%
6-UNABLE
C. TOLERANCE
1-WELL
2-FAIR
3-POOR

D. TECHNIQUES
1-EXPLANATION
2-DEMONSTRATION
E. TEACHING TOOLS
1-CAREPLAN
2-INSTRUCT SHEETS
3-VIDEOTAPE
4-PICTURES
5-PRINTED DIET
6-OTHER

F. STATUS
1-COMPLETED
2-D/C (N/A)
3-D/C (PATIENT)
4-D/C (DOCTOR)
5-REOPENED
G. PERFORMANCE
1-ACCOMPLISHED

H. VARIANCES
1-IMPAIRED LEARNING
2-DETERIORATION
3-IMPROVEMENT
4-RX CHANGE
5-MED CHANGE
6-VISIT CHANGE
7-OTHER

ICD9 436—Average Number of Visits of 11 per Case
Nursing

	1	2	3	4	5	6	7	8	9	10	11
Consults											
Conduct initial evaluation	X										
Consult MD to finalize orders	X										
Refer to other disciplines	X										
Perform nutritional screen	X										
Diagnostic procedures											
Draw Protime as ordered											
Activity											
Treatment/interventions											
Assess vital signs as ordered	X	X	X	X	X	X	X	X	X	X	X
Assess neuro status	X	X	X	X	X	X	X	X	X	X	X
Equipment											
Assess need for home equipment	X	X									
Assess patient/caregiver's use of equip	X	X	X								
Medications											
Assess knowledge of meds	X	X	X								
Teach med schedule	X	X	X								
Assess compliance of med schedule			X	X	X	X	X	X	X		
Teach side effects, purpose		X	X	X	X	X	X	X			
Adjust Coumadin per MD order											
Diet											
Assess knowledge of diet requirements	X										
Teach specified diet	X	X	X								
Assess compliance			X	X	X	X	X	X	X	X	

Continued

ICD9 436—Average Number of Visits of 11 per Case
Nursing

	1	2	3	4	5	6	7	8	9	10	11
D/C planning											
Develop plan of care with patient/CG	X										
Review CVA carepath with patient/CG	X					X			X		
Assess goal progression		X	X	X	X	X	X	X	X	X	X
Coordinate care among team members	X	X	X	X	X	X	X	X	X	X	X
ID/utilize community resources		X	X	X	X	X	X	X	X	X	X
Teach/Instruct	X										
Instruct s/sx of TIA/CVA	X	X	X								
LFL—bleeding precautions if on Coumadin	X	X	X								
Safety—home environment	X	X									

Outcomes:
No unplanned rehospitalizations
No unplanned ER visits
No deterioration in signs and symptoms
Stabilization of Coumadin therapy
ADL's maintained or improved
Revised 6/27/97

Goals: Pt/CG will verbalize safety measures by 2nd visit
Pt/CG will verbalize s/s of CVA/TIA by 3rd visit
Pt/CG will verbalize s/s of bleeding to report by 3rd visit
Protime will be within limits of _____ by 11th visit
Pt will demonstrate no new neuro deficits by 11th visit
Pt/CG will verbalize knowledge of low Na diet by 6th visit
BP will be within limits acceptable for pt by 11th visit _____
Pt/CG will demonstrate compliance with med regimen and verbalize purpose & side effects of meds by 8th visit

(Courtesy Methodist Alliance Home Care Services, Inc., Memphis, Tennessee.)

ICD9 496—Average Number of Visits of 12 per Case
Nursing

	1	2	3	4	5	6	7	8	9	10	11	12
Consults												
Conduct initial evaluation	X											
Consult MD to finalize orders	X											
Refer to other disciplines	X											
Perform nutritional screen	X											
Diagnostic procedures												
Activity												
Treatment/interventions												
Assess vital signs as ordered	X	X	X	X	X	X	X	X	X	X	X	X
Assess respiratory status	X	X	X	X	X	X	X	X	X	X	X	X
Assess personal needs	X	X	X									
Assess social needs	X	X	X									
Equipment												
Assess need for home equipment	X	X										
Assess patient/caregiver's use of equip	X	X	X									
Medications												
Assess knowledge of meds	X	X	X									
Teach med schedule	X	X	X									
Assess compliance of med schedule		X	X	X	X	X	X	X	X	X	X	X
Teach side effects, purpose		X	X	X	X	X	X	X	X	X		
Diet												
Assess knowledge of diet requirements	X											
Teach specified diet	X	X	X									
Assess compliance			X	X	X	X	X	X	X	X		

Continued

ICD9 496—Average Number of Visits of 12 per Case
Nursing

	1	2	3	4	5	6	7	8	9	10	11	12
D/C planning	X											
Develop plan of care with patient/CG	X											
Give care path to patient	X											
Assess goal progression		X	X	X	X	X	X	X	X	X	X	X
Coordinate care among team members	X	X	X	X	X	X	X	X	X	X	X	X
ID/utilize community resources		X	X	X	X	X	X	X	X	X	X	X
Teach/Instruct	X											
Instruct s/sx of CHF/ COPD complications				X	X	X	X	X				
Safety—home environment, Oxygen	X	X	X									
Instruct in infection control		X	X									

(Courtesy Methodist Alliance Home Care Services, Inc., Memphis, Tennessee.)

ICD9 496—Average Number of Visits of 12 per Case
Physical Therapy

	1	2	3	4	5	6	7	8	9	10	11	12
Consults												
Conduct initial evaluation	X											
Consult MD to finalize orders	X											
Refer to other disciplines PRN	X											
Diagnostic procedures None												
Activity												
Recommend/teach activity levels	X	X	X	X	X	X	X	X	X	X		
Treatment/interventions												
Breathing exercises/pursed lip/diaphragmatic breathing if indicated		X	X	X	X	X	X	X	X	X	X	X
Gait training if indicated		X	X	X	X	X	X	X	X	X	X	X
Endurance exercises if indicated		X	X	X	X	X	X	X	X	X	X	X
Equipment												
Assess need for home equipment	X	X										
Assess patient/caregiver's use of equip	X	X	X									X
Medications—assessed by RN												
Diet—managed by RN												

Continued

ICD9 496—Average Number of Visits of 12 per Case
Physical Therapy

	1	2	3	4	5	6	7	8	9	10	11	12
D/C planning												
Develop plan of care with patient/CG	X											
Give care path to patient	X											
Assess goal progression		X	X	X	X	X	X	X	X	X	X	X
Coordinate care among team members	X	X	X	X	X	X	X	X	X	X	X	X
ID/utilize community resources		X	X	X	X	X	X	X	X	X	X	X
Teach/Instruct												
Teach breathing exercises to pt/CG if indicated		X										X
Teach energy conservation if indicated		X					X					X
Teach home program if indicated											X	X

(Courtesy Methodist Alliance Home Care Services, Inc., Memphis, Tennessee.)

chapter **ten**

Measurement Indicators

Sandra Bassett

Learning Objectives

- Define at least three types of indicators.
- Discuss the dimensions of performance.
- Identify the components of measurement.
- Define indicator reliability and validity.
- Discuss various types of sampling.

The quality management function involves measuring conformance to requirements and reporting any differences accurately. According to Crosby, the cost of quality is divided into two areas—the price of nonconformance and the price of conformance. The price of nonconformance comprises all the expenses involved in doing things wrong or not doing them right the first time. Conversely, the price of conformance relates to expenses of doing things right (Crosby, 1984).

Measurement is the foundation of all improvement activities. How will improvement be recognized without a road map with specific mile markers? According to the Joint Commission on Accreditation of Healthcare Organizations (JCAHO) on improving organizational performance, measuring performance allows people to make informed judgments about the stability of processes, identify opportunities for improvement, and decide if improvements meet preestablished criteria (JCAHO, 1997). Other organizations are publishing standards from which measurement indicators can be derived; state and federal regulations can be used, as well. Some of these are referred to in Chapter 5, "Continuous Quality Improvement (CQI) Principles."

CATEGORIES OR TYPES OF INDICATORS

An indicator is a quantitative measure relating to a process or outcome of care. The five categories of indicators are as follows:

- Structure indicator—A structure indicator relates to the setting or structure in which care takes place. Examples are materials, human resources, and organizational structures.

- Process indicator—A process indicator is used to measure what is actually done in either providing or receiving care, for example, nursing assessment process or medication administration.
- Outcome indicator—An outcome indicator deals with the effects or results of care, for example, customer satisfaction or maternal deaths.
- Rate-based indicator—A rate-based indicator is an indicator that is expected to occur repeatedly over a period of time, for example, percentage of nursing assessments done within 2 hours of admission.
- Sentinel indicator—A sentinel indicator relates to occurrences, usually serious occurrences, that happen infrequently, for example, biopsy needle broken and retained in bone following a bone marrow biopsy.

In health care, process and outcome indicators are used most frequently. The key is determining what, how, and when to measure. The health care professional does not have to be a scientist or statistician to develop indicators. For information relating to research refer to Chapter 11, "Research Design and Implementation."

WHAT TO MEASURE

The leaders identify those areas that are important to organizational improvement. The focus can be on major functions or processes related to patient care or to high-risk, high-volume, or problem-prone areas. Infection control, risk management, and safety are common aspects of measurement. Since the majority of customers relate performance to service, not necessarily clinical, customer satisfaction is at the top of the list of indicators. Dimensions of performance identified by the JCAHO, for example, timeliness, effectiveness, and efficiency, are definite considerations in determining what to measure. (See Box 10-1.) Almost anything, however, can be measured. Authoritative resources should be explored before indicator development; reviewing literature and national, professional, and community standards of care and practice are a few examples.

The real question is how easily the indicator can be measured. If the process or function is being documented in some fashion, the process of measurement is easier to accomplish. If it is not, more time, manpower, and other resources may be required to collect the data. The importance of the indicator to the organization must be considered before implementation.

HOW TO MEASURE

Many ways of collecting data for a particular indicator are available; examples are logs, checksheets, oral or written surveys, observation, and computer software packages. As discussed previously, careful consideration should be given to how the information is to be collected. The mechanism should be simple and straightforward. Is the collection process cost-effective? Is it feasible? Is the indicator understandable to those who will be collecting the data?

Box 10-1

JCAHO's Dimensions of Performance

I. **Doing the Right Thing**

The **efficacy** of the procedure or treatment in relation to the patient's condition

The degree to which the patient's care and services have been shown to accomplish the desired or projected outcome(s)

The **appropriateness** of a specific test, procedure, or service to meet the patient's needs

The degree to which the care and services provided are relevant to the patient's clinical needs, given the current state of knowledge

II. **Doing the Right Thing Well**

The **availability** of needed test, procedure, treatment, or service to the patient who needs it

The degree to which appropriate care and services are available to meet the patient's needs

The **timeliness** with which a needed test, procedure, treatment, or service is provided to the patient

The degree to which the care and service are provided to the patient at the most beneficial or necessary time

The **effectiveness** with which tests, procedures, treatments, and services are provided

The degree to which the care and services are provided in the correct manner, given the current state of knowledge, to achieve the desired or projected outcome for the patient

The **continuity** of the services provided to the patient with respect to other services, practitioners, and providers and over time

The degree to which the patient's care is coordinated among disciplines, among organizations, and over time

The **safety** of the patient and others to whom the services are provided

The degree to which the risk of an intervention and risk in the care environment are reduced for the patient and others, including the health care provider

The **efficiency** with which care and services are provided

The relationship between the outcomes (results of care) and the resources used to deliver patient care and services

The **respect and caring** with which care and services are provided

The degree to which those providing care and services do so with sensitivity and respect for the patient's needs, expectations, and individual differences

The degree to which the patient or a designee is involved in his or her own care and service decisions

From Joint Commission on Accreditation of Healthcare Organizations: *JCAHO's comprehensive accreditation manual for home care,* Oakbrook Terrace, Ill, 1997-98, The Commission.

WHEN TO MEASURE

Before initiating the process, the frequency of data collection is identified. Consideration should be given to the risk involved in the care, the frequency of occurrence of the particular process, and the degree of severity of the problem-prone aspects. For example, the frequency and number of admissions would be considered when deciding whether to assess all of them or a sample. Conversely, an indicator relating to maternal deaths would not occur frequently. Therefore each event would trigger the application of the indicator. The length of data collection would relate to the frequency of the indicator application.

CHARACTERISTICS OF AN INDICATOR

An indicator must be written in an understandable way; it should be concise, specific, and to the point. Those that are too long or have unfamiliar language lead to misunderstanding and confusion. The content should include a measurement component that further enhances the definition of the particular indicator. An example for the home care setting is, "The nursing assessment will be completed and submitted to medical review within 2 working days from the start of care." Another characteristic of indicators is the ability to identify a numerator and denominator for each indicator. The numerator is the number of events as identified by the indicator. The denominator is the number of potential events related to the same indicator. Identifying both the numerator and denominator is extremely important in analyzing the data, identifying opportunities for improvement, and determining improvement. In the nursing assessment example, the numerator would be the number of assessments completed and submitted to medical review within 2 working days. The denominator would be the total number of nursing admissions within the same time period.

INDICATOR RELIABILITY AND VALIDITY

The purpose of indicators is to assist with the improvement process. Therefore indicators are developed to provide a tool that is both valid and reliable. Reliability relates to the consistency of the indicator after repeated usage. Validity means that the indicator measures what is intended to be measured (Leebov and Ersoz, 1991). Indicators that are unreliable and invalid produce confusing, irrelevant, and useless data and information while consuming precious organizational resources (JCAHO, 1990). Reliability and validity are proven through repeated testing. The chances of false negatives and false positives decrease by testing for reliability. False negatives are things that actually happened and failed to be identified by the indicator. Conversely, a false positive occurs when an item that was not an occurrence as it relates to the indicator is identified as an occurrence.

SAMPLING

One decision point for each indicator is to collect the data on the entire population or on a sample of the population. Sampling is reviewing data from a portion of the population. The population comprises all potential occurrences meeting the intent

---

Box 10-2

Types of Probability Samples

- Simple random sampling—In this type of sampling, each item has an equal chance of being selected; this is similar to pulling a name out of a hat.
- Systematic sampling—This kind of sampling is performed by randomly selecting the first case and then assigning a number for further selection. For example, after randomly selecting the first case the researcher would review every fifth case for application of the indicator.
- Stratified random or systematic sampling—This type of sampling is applied to a subset of the population chosen by a criterion such as race, sex, religion, or zip code. Once the subset is identified, the process for random or systematic sampling is applied.

---

of the indicator. Indicators relating to high-volume processes or procedures would lend themselves to sampling. In contrast, sentinel event indicators would not be appropriate for sampling. Sampling allows for making inferences on the entire population based on a smaller number of data. Sampling is less costly and time consuming.

Types of Samples

The two types of sampling techniques are probability and nonprobability samples. The types of probability samples are explained in Box 10-2. Probability sampling necessitates every item having an equal chance to be selected in the sample. Therefore nonprobability sampling does not necessitate equal chance for selection. Bias must be realized and addressed when using nonprobability sampling. The types of nonprobability samples are explained in Box 10-3.

RELATIONSHIP TO STANDARDS

The majority of measurement indicators are developed in response to a broken or cumbersome process. As stated earlier, the professional nurse needs a mechanism to determine when success is achieved. Measuring practice identifies the success or failure of the process. In other instances, professional standards of care or standards of practice can serve as the basis for the particular indicator. A standard is usually written in very broad terms; detailed measurement parameters are ordinarily not a part of the standard. Indicators are developed to address the specificity of measure.

DISPLAYING DATA

Displaying data utilizing tools such as those in Chapter 5 visually conveys important information. It helps to eliminate the sometimes inaccurate perceptions that surround an issue. The tools bring actual practice to the forefront, usually in a way that the majority of staff understand. Displaying data breaks down barriers and decreases defensive behavior; it allows staff to draw accurate conclusions from the

---

Box 10-3

Types of Nonprobability Samples

- Convenience sampling—This type is used for the convenience of the researchers and to gain momentum in the data collection process. The population may or may not totally be in agreement relative to the indicator.
- Purposive or judgment sampling—The population is selected based on certain criteria, which are determined by the researcher's judgment. This process is subjective at best.
- Expert sampling—This method is the same as purposive, but expert sampling involves selecting experts in the field because of their access to the needed information.
- Quota sampling—In quota sampling the researcher makes a decision based on judgment about the best type of sample for investigation. The researcher specifies characteristics of the sample beforehand to increase its representativeness. An example would be 5% or 25 cases, whichever is larger (National Association for Healthcare Quality, 1996).

---

data. By converting the data into pertinent, understandable information, the team can easily move through additional steps of the measurement process. Accurately displaying and understanding data require knowledge and practice.

EDUCATION

Education is required for effective implementation of the measurement indicator. All persons involved in writing, defining, implementing, and assessing the indicator must agree on common language. Much of the confusion is resolved in the testing period. The educational process should include understanding the purpose of the indicator, the definition of all terms, and processes of collecting the data and assessing the information.

Summary

The quality management function involves measuring conformance to requirements and reporting any differences accurately. The price of conformance relates to the expenses of doing things right. Conversely, the price of nonconformance is the expense of doing things wrong or not doing things right the first time. Measurement is the foundation of all improvement activities.

The types of indicators are structure, process, outcome, rate based, and sentinel. In health care, process and outcome are the most common. Attention is given to what, how, and when to measure. Indicators are developed to be both reliable and valid in nature. Various techniques are included in probability and nonprobability sampling.

Education of all involved staff is imperative for successful measurement activities. Core curriculum involves writing, defining, implementing, and assessing indicators. A common knowledge and language among employees is necessary to achieve success.

Discussion Questions

1. What are the various types of indicators? Give at least two examples of each.
2. How does the professional nurse determine what, how, and when to measure?
3. What are the characteristics of an indicator?
4. What is the difference between probability and nonprobability sampling techniques? Discuss examples of each.
5. Why is education relative to measurement indicators important?

Case Study

Customer satisfaction is the key to any organization's success. "The Best Home Medical Equipment Company" wishes to measure its customers' perceptions of service.

Case Study Exercise
1. Discuss the type(s) of sampling technique(s) that could be utilized.
2. Discuss the differences in outcomes when using probability versus nonprobability sampling.

REFERENCES

Crosby PB: *Quality without tears,* New York, 1984, A Plume Book.

Joint Commission on Accreditation of Healthcare Organizations: *Primer on indicator development and application,* Oakbrook Terrace, Ill, 1990, The Commission.

Joint Commission on Accreditation of Healthcare Organizations: *JCAHO's comprehensive accreditation manual for home care,* Oakbrook Terrace, Ill, 1997-98, The Commission.

Leebov W, Ersoz, CJ: *The health care manager's guide to continuous quality improvement,* 1991, American Hospital Publishing.

National Association for Healthcare Quality: *NAHQ guide to quality management,* Glenview, Ill, 1996, The Association.

chapter eleven

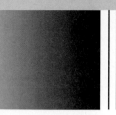

Research Design and Implementation

Susan R. Jacob _____

Learning Objectives

- Explore the impact of research on health care resource management.
- Describe steps in the research process.
- Describe various research methodologies.
- Identify ways that practitioners can participate in the research process.
- Explore issues related to research utilization.
- Consider future implications of research implementation and utilization for nursing and health care professionals.

IMPACT OF RESEARCH ON HEALTH CARE RESOURCE MANAGEMENT

Nursing research is a systematic approach used to examine phenomena important to nursing and nurses. Research can create a strong scientific base for nursing practice and demonstrate accountability for the profession (Talbot, 1995). Research is a process that takes place in a series of steps. The components of the research process are listed in Box 11-1.

The generation and utilization of research in health care agencies and with populations served by these agencies are vital to the delivery of high-quality and cost-effective services. Research can help identify health problems, suggest ways to control them, and measure outcomes. Outcomes from well-designed studies can assist agency personnel in delivering effective care and determining optimal productivity standards. Administrators and managers can use research findings to enhance their decision-making and control strategies. Clients ultimately benefit from research when agency personnel provide effective, efficient care based on research findings from well-designed studies (Cary, 1989). Nursing research findings are translated into health policy (Abdellah and Levine, 1994).

The Agency for Health Care Policy and Research (AHCPR) at an agenda-setting

---

Box 11-1

Components of the Research Process

1. Formulating the research question or problem
2. Defining the purpose of the study
3. Reviewing related literature
4. Formulating hypotheses and defining variables
5. Selecting the research design
6. Selecting the population, sample, and setting
7. Conducting a pilot study
8. Collecting the data
9. Analyzing the data
10. Communicating conclusions

---

conference in March 1992 examined research issues in quality improvement and quality assurance. Participants examined how to better structure research and development to increase the effectiveness of quality improvement (QI) and quality assurance (QA) and their responsiveness to changing health care delivery and public policy (Grady, Bernstein, and Robinson, 1993). Priorities for research focused on four major themes—methods and measures; information technologies; organizational issues; and using QI and QA information.

STUDY DESIGNS

Study designs are plans that tell a researcher how data are to be collected, from whom they are to be collected, and how data will be analyzed to answer a specific research question. The most common designs used in health care research are case study, survey, needs assessment, experimental, quasiexperimental, methodological, meta-analysis, and secondary analysis.

Nonexperimental Designs

Nonexperimental designs include case study; survey; needs assessment; ex post facto design, which includes descriptive correlational design; retrospective design; prospective design; path analysis; and predictive design.

Case study

Case study designs are used to present an in-depth analysis of a single subject, group, institution, or other social unit. The purposes of a case study are to gain insight and provide background information for more controlled, broader studies, to develop explanations of human processes, and to provide rich, descriptive anecdotes (Wilson and Hutchison, 1996). One disadvantage is the expense involved; the cost of studying one case can approach the cost of studying a larger sample. Another disadvantage is the lack of ability to generalize the results. Practitioners or researchers may publish results from a unique case.

Survey

Survey designs are very popular in nursing research studies that are designed to obtain information regarding the prevalence, distribution, and interrelationships of variables within a population. The survey is a good design to use when collecting demographic information, social characteristics, behavioral patterns, and information bases. Surveys might be used by ambulatory clinics to assess demographic information of the population geographically near the clinic to determine what services might be needed by potential clients in the area.

Advantages of surveys include the ability to collect large amounts of information with little expenditure of time and money, the ease of replication, and the standardization of scales and questionnaires. Disadvantages include the low return rate, the possibility that prestructured questions are confusing or irrelevant, and the tendency for data to be superficial because cause-and-effect relationships about study variables are not included (Wilson and Hutchison, 1996).

Needs assessment

Needs assessments are undertaken to determine what would be most beneficial to a specific aggregate group. This design can be used by organizations to determine needs of their employees or by agencies to determine needs of their consumers. For example, employers may conduct a needs assessment to determine the need of employees for on-site child care. An advantage of this type of design is that the needs assessment makes it possible to make changes that reflect the perceived need. Disadvantages include the limitation of people providing input and the potential that it will not be politically correct to institute the change that is desired (Talbot, 1995).

Experimental Designs

Experimental

Experimental designs involve the manipulation of one or more independent variables, random assignment of subjects to either a control or treatment group, and finally, observation of the outcome or effect that is presumably due to the independent variable. Rigor and control of extraneous variables allow researchers to establish cause-and-effect relationships, testing causal relationships (Wilson and Hutchison, 1996). Experimental designs include pretest-posttest control group design, posttest-only design, Solomon four group design, factorial design, randomized block design, and clinical trial. The randomized clinical trial is the premier study design used to evaluate the effectiveness of medical interventions; it is a prospective design in which subjects are randomly assigned to treatment and control groups and effects are measured in terms of statistical significance to the extent that differences in outcomes are the result of interventions (Abdellah and Levine, 1994).

A disadvantage of the experimental design is that it is not always suitable for real world conditions; manipulating some variable is not always ethical or feasible if the standard of care of clients would be compromised, random selection is often not a possibility, and many of the phenomena of concern to nursing are multidimensional and therefore not suitable for a true experimental design (Wilson and Hutchison, 1996).

Quasi-experimental

The **quasi-experimental designs** include one-group posttest-only design, static group comparison, one-group pretest-only design, nonequivalent control group design, and interrupted time series design. The quasi-experimental study design lacks one of the required components of the experimental design; when randomization, the formation of a control group, or the manipulation of one or more variables is not possible, however, this is a useful design. For example, a researcher may design a study to examine the efficacy of different bereavement interventions. Participants could be assigned to one of two or three interventions. A control group might not be appropriate for this study because withholding bereavement intervention from a group of participants would not be ethical. Therefore this study would be quasi-experimental on the basis of lacking a control group.

Methodological

Methodological research focuses on the development of data collection instruments such as surveys or questionnaires; the goal is to improve the reliability and validity of instruments. This work is time consuming and tedious but necessary for the implementation of research studies; when high-quality instruments are developed, they can be used in multiple studies. An example of a methodological study would be the development of a measure of pain, such as a visual analog scale.

Meta-analysis

Meta-analysis is an advanced process whereby research on a specific topic is reviewed and findings of multiple studies are statistically analyzed and expressed quantitatively. Meta-analysis synthesizes quantitative data from different studies, thus enlarging the power of the results and allowing generalizations to be made more confidently than they are in a single study. The larger the sample of studies, the greater the confidence in the results (Abdellah and Levine, 1994). An example of this design could be an examination of the literature and a meta-analysis of findings related to pediatric preparation for hospitalization. The researcher would decide to include published studies exclusively or published and nonpublished studies during specific years of publication. The researcher might also limit the review to studies of specific design such as experimental and quasi-experimental. Other factors would include age of the sample and time frame of the children's experience with hospitalization. By using this research method studies can be compared and conclusions drawn about the topic of study, such as the most effective preparation methods, and findings can be incorporated into practice.

A limitation of meta-analysis is that the findings are only as good as the studies included in the review. In addition, using completed studies as primary data may present a problem because studies that were conducted several years ago may not be relevant to current practice.

Secondary analysis

Secondary data analysis can be valuable for many types of studies. Meta-analysis is a prime example of a research design that utilizes secondary data. Many computerized record systems such as Medicare and Medicaid patient systems contain large data sets that can be used for research studies. Literally hundreds of federal, public, and private databases in the health care field can be accessed for the implementation of outcomes research (Abdellah and Levine, 1994). A researcher might examine the effectiveness of a newly developed statewide managed care program by examining hospital and outpatient records to determine utilization of nursing personnel and services.

Advantages of secondary data analysis include saving time and expense related to data collection (Talbot, 1995). Disadvantages include missing data and the data's not being exactly what the researcher would like.

Although the trend in nursing research has been toward large, complex studies, some situations call for small, simple studies that can be conducted by a single researcher with modest resources. Many issues can be addressed without the involvement of large samples and complex methodology. Esoteric and overly complicated methodology cannot substitute for well-designed and creatively conducted research on important topics (Abdellah and Levine, 1994).

Quantitative and qualitative research are two distinctly different approaches to conducting research. The researcher chooses the method based on the research question and the current level of knowledge about the phenomenon and the problem to be studied (Talbot, 1995).

Qualitative Designs

Qualitative research is a method of research designed for discovery rather than verification; this type of research is used to explore little-known or ambiguous phenomena. The researcher is looking to explain a phenomenon or process rather than verify a cause-and-effect relationship. Qualitative methods are very important to the study of complex human beings. Concepts that are important to health care professionals are often difficult to reduce in a quantitative way. Interviewing is the main technique used in qualitative methods to explore the meaning of certain experiences to individuals. This method is time consuming and costly and utilizes small samples, therefore generalizations cannot be made from findings. However, when exploring issues such as caregiver strain or hardiness, interviewing participants to get their perspective might be more appropriate than sending out a standard questionnaire that might not encompass everything the researcher would discover from personally interviewing the participants. The main types of qualitative research designs include phenomenology, ethnography, and grounded theory.

Phenomenology

Phenomenology is a valuable approach for studying intangible experiences such as grief, hope, and risk taking. Phenomenology is designed to provide understanding of the participants' "lived experience." For example, the researcher might conduct interviews with women who have had breast cancer to attempt to understand their experience of living with breast cancer.

Ethnography

Ethnography is a method used to study phenomena from a cultural perspective. Ethnographers spend time in the cultural setting with the research participants to observe and better understand their experience. For example, a researcher might seek to understand the experience of terminally ill children. To gain insight into their experience with parents, other terminally ill children, and medical staff the researcher might spend time observing them in a pediatric cancer facility. Observation and interview would be the main techniques used for data collection.

Grounded theory

Grounded theory is a method designed to explore a social process that people use to deal with problematic areas of their lives, such as coping with a terminal illness or adjusting to bereavement. Personal interviews conducted in the homes of participants would likely be the main form of data collection.

Although qualitative research studies in health care research are important, qualitative methods are time consuming and costly. One-to-one interviews take time, and the interviews must be recorded, typed, transcribed, and analyzed. Data analysis is conducted by the researcher, who reviews each transcribed interview line by line to group common conceptual meanings; concepts are combined to describe the experience for the group being studied. Since qualitative studies usually have small samples and results are not generalizable, triangulation studies might provide the strength needed to recommend change based on research findings.

Triangulation

Triangulation is the use of various research methods or different data collection techniques in the same study. Triangulation commonly refers to the use of both quantitative and qualitative methods in the same study. This method can be useful when data from multiple sources and methods are needed to provide a relatively complete understanding of the subject matter.

Pilot Studies

Pilot studies are small-scale studies often referred to as feasibility studies. The purpose of the pilot study is to identify the strengths and limitations of a planned larger scale study. Pilot work is preliminary research that can be used to assess a study's design, methodology, and feasibility and typically includes participants similar to those who will be used in the larger research study. By performing each step of the procedures that will be used in a planned larger scale study, the researcher can evaluate the effectiveness of the proposed data collection methods (Hinds and Gattuso, 1991).

Pilot studies can serve to determine the feasibility of utilizing interventions and to discover preliminary trends in outcomes for a particular agency and its personnel and clients (Cary, 1989). Most funding agencies favor research that is based on pilot work. However, a pilot study may not be warranted if the researcher has used the same techniques, instruments, and participants in the same or a similar setting.

RESEARCH UTILIZATION

Currently many are concerned that nurses have failed to realize the potential for using research findings as a basis for making decisions and developing nursing interventions. This concern is based on evidence that nurses are not always aware of research results and do not effectively incorporate these results into their practice (Polit and Hungler, 1993). Major difficulties cited relate to nurses' inability to access and use research findings and having negative attitudes toward research. Opinions that research is not relevant to current practice and views that theory and practice are not related are common (Luker and Kenrick, 1992).

Health professionals should be familiar with two major research utilization projects that were implemented to address the problem of nurses' failing to review and utilize research findings. These formal projects are the Western Interstate Commission for Higher Education (WICHE) regional nursing research development project and the Conduct and Utilization of Research in Nursing (CURN) project. These projects were federally funded for the design and implementation of strategies to promote research use in practice.

WICHE Project

The 6-year WICHE project was funded by the Division of Nursing and directed by Krueger and colleagues (Krueger, 1978; Krueger, Nelson, and Wolanin, 1978). Participants in the project were recruited from various clinical settings and educational institutions to participate in a workshop that focused on improving their skills in critiquing research. Participants selected research-based interventions that they were willing to implement in practice and developed detailed plans for using selected research findings in practice. Participants in the WICHE project also functioned as agents of change in clinical agencies when the research was used in practice. One of the major findings of the WICHE project was that few well-designed clinical studies had clearly identified implications for nursing care (Burns and Grove, 1995).

CURN Project

The CURN project was a 5-year (1975-1980) project funded by the commission's division of nursing and directed by Horsley (Horsley, Crane, and Bingle, 1978). The major goal of the CURN project was to increase the use of research findings in nursing practice by disseminating research findings. Facilitating organizational changes necessary for implementation of findings and encouraging collaborative research (Polit and Hungler, 1997) were also integral to this project. For this project research utilization was looked at as an organizational process rather than a process that should be implemented by an individual nurse. From this perspective clinical agencies have to make a commitment to implement research findings and then develop policies and procedures to guide the implementation process. An outcome of the CURN project was the development of clinical protocols to direct the use of selected research findings in practice. The steps in the research utilization process include synthesizing multiple studies on a selected topic, organizing the research knowledge into a clinical protocol for practice, transforming the protocol into nursing actions, and evaluating the protocol to determine if it produced the desired outcome (Burns and Grove, 1995).

During the CURN project clinical studies were examined for scientific merit, clinical relevance, feasibility for changing practice in an agency, and cost-benefit ratio. Protocols were developed by participants for structured preoperative teaching; reducing diarrhea in tube-fed patients; preoperative sensory preparation to promote recovery; preventing decubitus ulcers; intravenous cannula change; closed urinary drainage systems; distress reduction through sensory preparation; mutual goal setting in patient care; clean intermittent catheterization; and pain. Protocols were implemented in clinical trials and evaluated for effectiveness. Based on the evaluation decisions were made by individual agencies to reject, adopt, or modify the intervention. These protocols are still available for use in practice (CURN Project, 1981-1982).

Clinical Practice Guidelines

In 1992 the federal government again demonstrated support for research utilization activities when the Agency for Health Care Policy and Research, within the Department of Health and Human Services (DHHS), convened panels of experts to summarize research and develop clinical practice guidelines. These panels summarized research findings and developed practice guidelines in the areas of acute pain care management in infants, children, and adolescents; prediction and prevention of pressure ulcers in adults; and identification and treatment of urinary incontinence in adults. These guidelines are free on request from DHHS.

Strategies to Promote Research

Burns and Grove (1995) predict that in the future accrediting agencies will require health care agencies to have protocols that are documented with research. Therefore procedure manuals, standards of care, and nursing care plans will need to reflect current nursing research. Progressive nurse executives are fostering a positive environment for conducting research, as well as implementing findings in practice. To challenge traditional practice an attitude of openness and intellectual curiosity must prevail. Polit and Hungler (1993) suggest that administrators should foster a climate of intellectual curiosity by making staff aware that their experiences and problems are important; offering support by encouraging individual staff, establishing utilization committees, establishing journal clubs, and allowing research studies to be conducted in the agency; offering financial and resource support for utilization; and including research utilization as a criterion in performance evaluation. Administrators with a commitment to research should facilitate the establishment of research committees for the promotion and implementation of research utilization and the review of proposals from employees or others seeking access to subjects for research projects. Administrators also have an obligation to provide staff development and to inform researchers about the agency and its potential research opportunities (Talbot, 1995).

Individual nurses must be empowered to be self-directed and encouraged to initiate innovative care based on research findings from sound, well-designed studies. Evaluation of the overall cost benefit, as well as effectiveness, is imperative before incorporating new techniques.

Polit and Hungler (1997) suggest that practicing nurses promote research by reading widely and critically, attending professional conferences, expecting evidence that a procedure is effective, seeking environments that support research utilization, becoming involved in a journal club, collaborating with nurse researchers, and participating in institutional utilization projects.

Agency personnel are constantly exposed to research findings, whether by allusions to them in the articles in clinical journals or by the actual research studies reported at conferences or in professional journals. A consumer of research has an obligation to critically appraise research reports. Without a critical appraisal practitioners may generalize results and attempt to integrate research findings into their unique practice, often resulting in the failure to produce the same results. Reasons for different outcomes may be related to differences in the method of applying the same research procedures, clients who differ significantly from the original research participants, data collection methods that prevent adequate control of variables, inappropriate statistical methods, or misinterpretation of results (Cary, 1989).

When personnel misinterpret research findings, the resultant opportunity costs to the agency can rob them of the resources of time and money and the clients of time and progress toward optimal functioning or recovery. Administrators must foster a climate in which research is appreciated and the development of personnel as consumers and producers of research studies is promoted. Once personnel have the critical appraisal skills to correctly interpret results, they can make informed decisions concerning aspects of practice or agency operations that can be successfully implemented (Cary, 1989).

Nurse Researcher Roles

Two nursing roles, the **clinical nurse specialist (CNS)** and the **clinical nurse researcher (CNR),** are specifically focused on research.

Clinical nurse specialist

The CNS is a nurse with a master's degree who is an expert clinician with additional responsibility for education and research. The CNS is in an ideal position to link research to practice by assessing the agency's readiness for research utilization, working with staff to identify clinical problems, and helping staff find, implement, and evaluate findings that are relevant to current practice (Pepler in Talbot, 1995). All CNSs are educated in the research process and can conduct their own investigations, as well as collaborate with doctorally prepared nurses.

Clinical nurse researcher

The CNR should be a nurse with a doctorate and clinical and research experience who can focus on either conducting or facilitating of research, using a knowledge of statistics, grantsmanship, evaluation research, and administration. Interpersonal skills such as patience, flexibility, and approachability are imperative (Pepler in Talbot, 1995). The clinical nurse researcher employed by a hospital or home health agency must develop relationships with staff nurses to identify the research questions that staff nurses see as most significant in their particular setting. The CNR should be responsible for designing studies and assisting staff nurses in understanding the implications of the studies. In addition, the CNR should provide guidance to the staff regarding their role in the research process. This role could involve patient recruitment for studies or data collection. The CNR should also be responsible for disseminating findings of the research not only to staff nurses, but also to administrators of the agency so findings can be incorporated into practice. The CNR may also need to communicate results to legislators if the results potentially affect health policy.

An example of findings that could affect health policy is the findings related to the efficacy of hospice bereavement intervention. Currently, legislation mandates that hospice programs provide bereavement services. However, no reimbursement for bereavement is provided by Medicare. When hospice Medicare legislation was enacted in 1986 no well-designed studies documented the effectiveness of bereavement programs. Therefore bereavement programs were not included in the funding to hospice programs provided by Medicare. If bereavement intervention studies are conducted and the intervention is found to have a positive effect on morbidity, mortality, and health care costs, then legislation could be changed to cover bereavement services.

If agencies do not have a CNR, they should be encouraged to develop relationships with researchers in university settings or other agencies. Professors in academic settings are expected to conduct research and are often interested in collaborating with health care agencies that might serve as a site. These agencies often have the patient population that can serve as a study sample. For example, a university professor interested in home health care issues might collaborate with an agency to examine the efficacy of various health care delivery models for patients with congestive heart failure. In a managed care environment it would be essential for the agency to offer care that is the most effective and efficient. Therefore this collaborative relationship would have benefits for both the researcher and the health care agency.

Researchers have an obligation to take steps to ensure utilization of findings. Polit and Hungler (1997) suggest conducting high-quality research; replicating studies; collaborating with practitioners; disseminating findings aggressively; communicating clearly—eliminating jargon; and providing nursing implications as a standard section of research reports and articles.

Many health care practitioners who may routinely read clinical practice journals are unfamiliar with research journals. Busy clinicians who read the occasional research report disseminated through a practice journal may not spend time browsing the library for research. Computerized databases aid the process of locating research relevant to current practice, but often nurses and other health care professionals are not aware of the journals devoted entirely to the publication of research studies. Box 11-2 contains a list of research journals.

One of the significant publications is the *Annual Review of Nursing Research* (ARNR). The purpose of the ARNR is to conduct systematic reviews of nursing literature; provide guidance to graduate students and faculty in specific fields of research; and provide critical evaluations for health policy makers (Abdellah and Levine, 1994). This is an excellent resource for those involved in the development and utilization of research.

Box 11-2

Nursing and Health Related Research Journals

Advances in Nursing Science
Applied Nursing Research
Clinical Nursing Research
Image—the Journal of Nursing
  Scholarship
International Journal of Nursing
  Studies
Journal of Advanced Nursing
Journal of Transcultural Nursing
Nursing Clinics of North America
Nursing Economics
Nursing Policy Forum
Nursing Research
Nursing Science Quarterly

Research in Nursing and Health
Scholarly Inquiry for Nursing
  Practice
American Journal of Public Health
Hastings Center Report
Health Affairs
Health Care Management Review
Health Services Research
Journal of the American Medical
  Association
Journal of Nursing Measurement
Journal of Health Economics
New England Journal of Medicine
Social Science and Medicine

FUNDING OF RESEARCH

Federal funding is available through the National Institutes of Health and the Agency for Health Care Policy and Research. However, since obtaining money for research is becoming increasingly competitive, voluntary foundations and private organizations should be investigated as possible funding sources. Private foundations such as the Robert Wood Johnson Foundation or the W.K. Kellogg Foundation offer program funding for health-related projects (Stanhope and Lancaster, 1996). Investigators should be encouraged to pursue funding for small projects through local sources or private foundations until a track record is established in research design and implementation. After several years of experience in the research arena investigators are more likely to be successful in securing funding through federal sources.

Institutional Review

Although researchers are responsible for examining their own study to ensure the protection of human rights and determine the risk/benefit ratio, eliminating bias is a difficult task. Therefore most health care agencies have established a committee or advisory board to examine research proposals for ethical concerns. This formal committee is often called the human subjects committee or **institutional review board (IRB).** Institutions that receive federal funding or conduct drug or medical device research regulated by the Federal Drug Administration (FDA) are required by federal regulations to establish an IRB. Studies that are funded federally have to meet strict guidelines to ensure the protection of the human rights of subjects, such as self-determination, privacy, anonymity and confidentiality, fair treatment, and protection from discomfort and harm. The IRB is responsible for reviewing the study procedures and process of informed consent to ensure the protection of subjects. The informed consent must include essential study information and statements about potential risks and benefits, protection of anonymity and confidentiality and voluntary participation, compensation, alternative treatment, and the investigator's name and phone number.

Investigators should obtain a copy of the institution's guidelines when writing a study protocol and consent form. These guidelines contain information on how to gain approval, prepare the consent form, and proceed through the review process (Talbot, 1995). Institutional review boards usually do not meet more frequently than once a month or once every 6 weeks. Therefore the investigator needs to determine the meeting times when designing the study so the protocol can be submitted and reviewed by IRB at the earliest opportunity.

The IRB chairperson decides which of the three levels of review—exempt from review, expedited review, or complete review—is indicated for a particular study. Studies that involve no risk at all to subjects are exempt from review. Studies that involve no more than minimal risk (no more than encountered in everyday life) are generally considered in the expedited review process. This process is usually carried out by the chairperson of the IRB or one or two committee members (Burns and Grove, 1995). Studies that involve more than minimal risk to subjects call for a complete IRB review. In these cases the IRB must review the proposal to ensure that risks are minimized, the risk/benefit ratio is reasonable, selection of subjects is equitable, informed consent is sought with each prospective participant and appropriately documented, and adequate provisions are made to protect the safety and confidentiality of subjects.

In institutions where IRB approval is not required for non–federally funded programs the researcher should seek external advice regarding ethical considerations. When IRB is an option, researchers should seek IRB approval because it demonstrates rigor to the audience when the research is disseminated either through presentation or publication. In fact, many research journals will not publish studies that do not have the approval of an institutional review board.

Research Funding Sources
National Institute of Nursing Research
Priority areas for funding by the National Institute of Nursing Research (NINR) include low birth weight infants, HIV infection: prevention and care, long-term care for the elderly, symptom management, information systems, health promotion, technology dependency across the lifespan, interventions for Alzheimer's disease, long-term care and minority aging, nursing and biology interface, dysfunctioning bladder and bowel, home health care and supportive services for older adults, Biobehavioral symptom management, minority youth health behavior research, cognitive impairment, and living with chronic illness. The National Institute of Nursing Research is also interested in facilitating research into the clinical application of intervention strategies to reduce health risks at the community level.

Community-based strategies targeting health problems of rural residents and of underserved minority groups are of particular interest to NINR.

Agency for Health Care Policy and Research

The Agency for Health Care Policy and Research (AHCPR) aims to enhance the quality, appropriateness, and effectiveness of health care services through the establishment of a broad base of research and the promotion of improvements in clinical practice and in the organization, financing, and delivery of health care services (Abdellah and Levine, 1994). AHCPR invites proposals for research **grants** focused on assessment of health care technologies; medical malpractice and liability; delivery of health services in rural areas; availability, accessibility, and quality of care for low-income groups, minorities, and the elderly; alternative delivery systems, providers, and practice patterns with HIV-related illnesses; and the nature, use, and outcomes of different types of in-home health and supportive services.

AHCPR facilitates the development, periodic review, and updating of clinical practice guidelines. In addition, AHCPR supports the design and development of databases for use in outcomes research (Abdellah and Levine, 1994).

Private foundations

Many foundations and corporate direct-giving programs are interested in funding health care projects and research. Computer databases and guides to funding are available in local libraries.

Sigma Theta Tau International

The International Honor Society for Nurses makes research grant awards available to increase scientific knowledge related to nursing practice. Awards are available at the international and local chapter level.

Summary

As costs escalate and funds diminish in our society's rapidly changing health care environment high-quality, cost-efficient care will be the key to survival of health care providers (Koch and Fairly, 1993). Health care research has much to contribute to cost containment and resource management. Well-designed studies must be conducted and significant findings disseminated in a clear way so that practitioners can see relevance to current practice. Research-based practice must occur, and innovative models of patient care must be tested for quality, appropriateness, and effectiveness. Educators must prepare health care professionals to have an appreciation of research and participate in research design implementation and evaluation at the level of their preparation. Health care administrators must facilitate an environment that fosters intellectual curiosity and supports research efforts. Collaborative arrangements between health care agencies and universities must be developed for such activities as student projects, continuing education, development of clinical practice guidelines, and research endeavors. Consumers must be educated about the value of health care research, and policy makers must be informed of pertinent findings so that results can be translated into health policy.

Discussion Questions

1. Identify a research study in the literature that has relevance to your professional practice and evaluate the findings for application to your practice.
2. What factors must you consider in developing a plan to disseminate research findings relative to practice in your particular setting?
3. As a home health nurse you learn that several studies on cultural differences in expression and perception of pain have been done. How would you find this information and use it in your practice?
4. As a head nurse in a critical care unit you would like to change the structured visitation to open visitation. How can research design, implementation, or utilization facilitate this change?
5. As a home health nurse you learn that reports have demonstrated the effectiveness of the use of telephone calls to recently discharged clients to determine if services are needed again. You would like to try the procedure in your home health agency but are uncertain about how effective this approach would be. How would you test the effectiveness of telephone follow-up in your agency? Whom would you involve in the process?

Case Study

Janice, a clinical nurse researcher in a medical center, asks the staff nurses on a pediatric oncology unit to identify patient care problems that should be investigated. The nurses identify pain control as a major problem for the children admitted to the unit. In talking with the nurses on the unit, Janice discovers that the nurses routinely use physiological measures such as heart rate and blood pressure as indicators of pain. The nurses only occasionally rely on parents' reports, but they rarely consult the child.

Janice conducts a review of the literature to determine proven ways to assess pain in children. In the *Western Journal of Nursing Research* Janice discovers a meta-analysis of pediatric pain assessment techniques. Findings from this study indicate that self-report tools are appropriate for most children 4 years and older and that these tools provide the most accurate measure of children's pain. Janice discovers a pediatric pain interview tool in the literature that she thinks would be practical and feasible for use on the unit. She then writes a utilization memo to the nurse manager, citing the problem (inadequate pain control), research findings documented in the literature, and a suggestion for change in practice (use of the self-report pain assessment) on the pediatric oncology unit. Next Janice organizes a meeting with the nurses to discuss conducting a pilot study on the unit to determine the effectiveness of the pediatric pain assessment interview tool and the unit's usual procedures for assessing pain in the pediatric oncology patients. Findings from this study are incorporated into practice by documenting the preferred method of pain assessment in the formal procedures and protocol for the unit.

Case Study Exercise
1. How was the meta-analysis of pediatric pain assessment techniques more useful than multiple articles related to pain assessment?
2. How would the CURN project be useful in this situation?
3. What are the benefits of conducting a pilot study?
4. How would findings from the pilot study affect patient outcomes?

REFERENCES

Abdellah F, Levine E: *Preparing nursing research for the 21st century,* New York, 1994, Springer.

Burns N, Grove S: *Understanding nursing research,* Philadelphia, 1995, WB Saunders.

Cary A: Home health nursing. In Martinson I, Widmer A, editors: *Home health nursing,* Philadelphia, 1989, WB Saunders.

Conduct and Utilization of Research in Nursing (CURN) Project: *Using research to improve nursing practice,* New York, 1981-1982, Grune & Stratton.

Grady M, Bernstein J, Robinson S, editors: Pub No 93-0034, Washington, DC, 1993, U.S. Department of Health and Human Service Agency for Health Care Policy and Research.

Hinds P, Gattuso J: From pilot work to major study in cancer nursing research, *Cancer Nurs* 14(3):132, 1991.

Horsley JA, Crane J, Bingle JD: Research utilization as organizational process, *J Nurs Adm* 8(7):4, 1978.

Koch M, Fairly T: *Integrated quality management: The key to improving nursing care quality,* St. Louis, 1993, Mosby.

Krueger JC: Utilization of nursing research: The planning process, *J Nurs Adm* 8(1):6, 1978.

Krueger JC, Nelson AH, Wolanin MO: *Nursing research: Development, collaboration, and utilization,* Germantown, Md, 1978, Aspen.

Luker K, Kenrick M: An exploratory study of the sources of influence on the clinical decisions of community nurses, *J Adv Nurs* 17(4):457, 1992.

Pepler C: Using research to improve practice. In Talbot L, editor: *Principles and practice of nursing research,* St. Louis, 1995, Mosby.

Polit D, Hungler B: *Essentials of nursing research: Methods, appraisal and utilization,* ed 4, Philadelphia, 1997, JB Lippincott.

Stanhope M, Lancaster J: *Community health nursing: Promoting health of aggregates, families, and individuals,* St. Louis, 1996, Mosby.

Talbot L: *Principles and practice of nursing research,* St. Louis, 1995, Mosby.

Wilson H, Hutchison S: *Consumer's guide to nursing research,* Albany, NY, 1996, Delmar.

chapter twelve

Data Management and Integrated Information Systems

Alice M. Davidson
C. Ben Sanders

Learning Objectives

- State the purpose of a management information system.
- Identify some effects of managed care on information systems.
- Describe the process involved in acquiring new information systems.
- Recognize the factors involved in the cost-benefit equation for information systems.
- Recognize the effects of present influences in changing the adoption and use of information systems in health care.

Information systems have become paramount in the quest for high-quality, cost-effective health care. Data, raw unanalyzed facts, have been collected throughout this country over the past decade in urban and rural health care institutions without ever being subjected to aggregation or analysis. Much of this activity is driven by the standards of external review organizations requiring collection of data or the specific financial needs of the institution, but little beyond that. With the expansion of managed care and increased competition in the marketplace, it has become readily apparent that survival depends on an organization's ability to collect the needed data, analyze the data, and implement changes based on the analysis.

Although organizational performance improvement activities are currently incorporating outcomes management and clinical guidelines development, existing data collection systems within health care delivery organizations are unable to meet current needs, let alone the needs of such integrated systems. Information systems developed for health care organizations have been departmental in nature and therefore create managerial and technical challenges in creating cohesive information systems. To build an integrated delivery system that can offer a full continuum of care, the system must integrate clinical outcomes, information on processes of care, and financial information.

INFORMATION SYSTEMS IN HEALTH CARE

"What is a **management information system?** While there is no universally agreed upon definition, we will define the term as a system used to provide management with needed information on a regular basis." (Small and Lee, 1975) Ensuring reliable and accurate data is only one element in an information system. Order, purpose, and arrangement are important elements in any system. Information systems can be computerized or manual, although in today's world of health care delivery, manual systems are found primarily in small rural facilities, doctors' offices, or inner-city clinics. Cost-related issues force small facilities to keep limits on computer expansion and continue maintenance of manual systems. The important issue is that an effective information system collects data and transforms it into relevant information for use.

Health care automation and management information systems have continually improved over the past few decades. Much of this progress has been the result of technological improvements in computing power and data storage devices. "In 1946 there was one computer in the United States." (Gardner and Kelly, 1981) The first computer that was installed for business application was in 1954. That was the beginning of information management systems. From that beginning until the mid-1960s the processing of data was limited to use in financial departments, collecting and processing data for payroll, accounting, and billing. Management and training responsibilities rested with the financial officer, and expansion of computer systems and personnel training were very limited in focus.

By 1965 managers in other areas, particularly operational activities, began to realize the potential for computers, and with impetus from the middle managers centralized data processing expanded. Centralized data processing, however, was not capable of giving management the current information necessary for organizational decision making.

As we entered the 1980s technology had improved dramatically, and with this improvement came competitive cost. Emerging hardware and software companies began to compete for the market. Personal computers and remote terminals became a cost-effective reality. Information systems became less an accounting tool and more a management and clinical tool. New departments were developed and managed by information systems professionals with the knowledge and skill to move organizations into the information age. This development, however, was not without its problems.

Organizational structure changes invited turf conflicts and divided staff. With the introduction of remote terminals with access to a computer's central processing unit in health care delivery organizations, patient care information became available to a large population of caregivers. Terminals on units and in diagnostic areas provided information quickly and allowed the easy capture of information valuable to both managers and clinical staff.

As the evolution of information management continued, decentralization of data processing became inevitable. Computer logic functions, previously performed by a centrally managed computer system, were being moved to multiple independent and interdependent distributed computer systems. Information control now became the responsibility of the manager. Some managers were enthusiastic about the opportunity to manage and explore their own data, whereas others saw it as an overwhelming situation. Learning to operate a personal computer was a real challenge for many managers, even though they realized it would allow them to make more timely and accurate decisions.

The rapid consolidation of health care delivery into broadly integrated provider groups has dramatically affected provision of care, as well as management of information. Today clinical managers find themselves involved in software acquisition decisions and planning for information support systems. With continuing growth in managed care, expansion of home health and other nonhospital services, and the consolidation of health care provider organizations into integrated delivery systems, information systems must be able to perform in a manner in which they have never performed before.

Mergers and strategic alliances require organizations to rethink health care information system acquisitions. Projections indicate that the industry will have spent more than $13 billion on automated information systems in 1997. An integrated health care organization can spend $25 million to $50 million over a 5-year period to implement a system (Gates, 1996).

The vision for the next decade includes paperless medical records, data repositories, and widespread provider access to on-line medical records including x-rays and other diagnostic information. Although this vision is exciting, it also holds challenges. Security of sensitive medical information must be maintained, and industry-wide standards for these electronic records require continued development. As expected, cost will be an important factor, and (of prime importance for patients and clinicians) these systems must support the provision of high-quality care.

INFORMATION SYSTEM RESOURCE ISSUES

In the health care setting, information systems affect a wide range of clinical and operational management activities.

Clinical Information Systems

Currently, **automated information systems** assist health care personnel and health care organizations in managing a number of processes of care. These areas of clinical process management support include patient demographic information acquisition and maintenance, patient appointment management, and the generation and tracking of requests for laboratory, pharmacy, diagnostic, and supply services.

Clinical data are often supported by information systems in areas such as laboratory test results reporting, medication administration records, and vital signs documentation. Less often one may find automated information systems managing documentation of history and physical examination, progress notes, reports on diagnostic image evaluations, and other types of narrative reports. Also in the clinical arena, information systems are used to maintain data on indicators of quality care (for example, nosocomial infections, adverse care events, readmission rates, and adherence to standards of care).

Clinical information systems are also used to assist caregivers in identifying potential problems in the care of a patient (for example, clinical alerts on laboratory values outside of normal limits) and may assist in making clinical decisions (decision support systems), such as selection of antibiotics appropriate to a patient's specific clinical situation (Burke, Classen, and Pestotnik, 1997). Finally, workload management information systems such as nursing acuity systems and laboratory workload systems are used to help clinical staff plan, manage, and evaluate the impact of clinical demand on personnel requirements. These types of systems bridge the clinical and organizational management arenas.

Management Information Systems

Workload management systems are used by managers to assess and plan staffing and scheduling requirements for their departments. Managers also utilize systems for planning and managing personnel, time and attendance, payroll, supplies, equipment, and other budget-related components. A significant part of the manager's work involves communication. These communication tasks may be supported by information systems in the form of word processing software, E-mail systems, graphics programs, and presentation (that is, slide and transparency) software. Like clinical staff, managers also are involved in the use of quality tracking and management systems.

Costs of Information Systems

Although information systems of various types have been in use in health care for many years and an increased use of such systems is expected, these systems are not without cost. The identification of information system requirements demands the involvement of those with fundamental knowledge of the work processes to be automated. Some of these individuals must be involved in the requirements definition process, and organizations must be willing to invest personnel in this effort.

Once the requirements for information systems are defined, the process of identifying, evaluating, and selecting desired hardware and software must be undertaken. Depending on the size of the organization and the sophistication of the systems to be acquired, this process can require extensive participation from a group of staff members representative of those for whom the systems will be employed. Associated with this selection process are a reduction in productivity for those involved and additional costs for meetings, supplies, travel (for site visits), and possibly consulting fees for special expertise.

Once hardware and software are selected for acquisition, their costs are divided into two sets: the original licensure or purchase costs and the ongoing maintenance costs of the systems. Over a cycle of 5 years, the maintenance costs of systems can equal or exceed the original acquisition cost. The establishment and maintenance of the systems require additional personnel and personnel with specialized skills, so funding will be required for these staff. For the implementation process it is often necessary or expedient to contract for vendor and consultant services to assist in configuration and planning for the system's use (Friel, 1997).

All eventual users of the systems require training to use the systems effectively. That educational process incurs development costs, and the staff in training must be pulled away from their regular work, thus reducing productivity. Additional staff may be required to support normal operations during the training and early implementation periods. A less tangible but very real cost is the burden imposed on the organization by change. Typically, general productivity drops; stress, confusion, and frustration increase. Mitigating the costs and demands of implementing new systems, the benefits are significant and cover a broad range of organizational interests.

Benefits of Information Systems

The benefits of information systems may be found in a number of areas of interest to health care organizations. Most of the benefits may be categorized in relation to their economic, quality of care, or humanistic effects. Humanistic benefits of health care information systems may include the improvement of patient satisfaction. These systems reduce paperwork for patients, such as the repeated provision of personal demographic and insurance information to different care organizations. Integrated information systems also can reduce the duplication of services, such as repeat laboratory work, increase the timeliness of patient services, such as access to appointments, increase access to desired caregivers through more efficient scheduling, and improve the coordination of care among providers by making available information about the patient's care throughout the system.

Another humanistic benefit of **integrated information systems** may be improved professional satisfaction for clinicians. Reductions in paperwork, improvements in communication, and ready access to the right information at the right time and in the right format improve clinicians' ability to serve their clients' needs. These improvements allow more time with clients focused on their perceived needs and provide clinicians with better tools to do their work.

Integrated information systems extend considerable opportunity to improve the clinical quality of care. As mentioned previously, the ready availability of test results reduces duplication caused by missing reports. Through integrated scheduling and reminder systems, transition of patient information and responsibility between care facilities may be improved. Opportunities for increased efficiency may be realized by having multiple caregivers interact with a patient during one visit. The distributed availability of medical record documentation improves communication between providers who collaboratively hold responsibilities for care and helps to reduce errors of duplication. Automated reminder systems assist in reducing errors of omission. Through the integration of guidelines of care in information systems, common standards of care are communicated to all providers, and processes supporting high-quality care are built into a tool used by all (Clayton and Mulligen, 1996).

From the economic perspective, several areas of benefit may be exploited through integrated information systems. Gains in productivity through improved communication and the availability of appropriate information at the point of need can be translated into cost savings and increased revenue (Renner, 1996). For example, electronic medical records require fewer staff to manage record coding, chart building, and chart tracking; lower supply costs for binders, dividers, and paper stock; lower expense for microphotographic storage (microfiche, microfilm); and lower transcription costs. Automated staffing management support systems allow managers to provide appropriate staff and keep costs low.

The increasing use of managed care approaches to holding down health care costs requires the consolidation of disparate data sources to allow the evaluation of care processes in both clinical and economic dimensions. Automated information systems are absolutely essential for supporting those efforts (Davis, Pell, and Pickard, 1997).

HOME HEALTH MOBILE INFORMATION SYSTEMS

Home health service organizations provide care in the home for homebound patients who need assistance managing chronic illness or disability or who require support following hospitalization for acute illness. Under government guidelines, reimbursement is tied to specific items within the clinical documentation and to regular periods of recertification for eligibility. These recertification periods require a review of chart documents for records of visits and procedures, documentation of the plan of care, and the effectiveness of that care. While making visits, many home health professional staff carry selected chart forms, often called "portable charts," for each patient.

These portable chart documents travel with staff while they make rounds of their patients' homes, often many miles from the home office. Home health staff may cover great distances in their work and may not work from the home office. In a paper chart system, gathering patient information and chart documents for future visits, completing and filing chart documents for completed visits, and documenting recertification information usually require the staff member to be at the home office. The agency must pay travel expenses and for the staff member's time for that travel and office work. Much of the documentation is duplicative (for example, patient name, record number, age, gender). It is also common for chart documents to be misplaced, requiring a search for or regeneration of the original.

In addition to difficulties managing chart forms, other types of communication are difficult in home health care. Patients are referred to the home health agency from a variety of providers and provider settings. Communication and coordination of care are made difficult by time and distance and by the variety of persons and organizations involved in that single patient's care. As a result of pressure to reduce health care costs and more tightly manage care, greater levels of service are being provided in the home. Patients are being discharged with significantly more complicated care issues requiring more extensive communication with the referring agency or provider and more sophisticated types of in-home care.

Mobile information systems have been developed to assist home health staff. These systems provide a combination of information capture and management functions including time tracking, charge or procedure capture, clinical documentation, and schedule management support.

In evaluating the acquisition cost of a system of this type, one would consider the following:

- The initial acquisition cost of software
- Cost for the office computer (server) to manage the central data and the mobile data entry/data capture units
- Cost for an interface to the billing software system
- Cost for temporary or permanent staff to install the system
- Cost to train all staff who would use the system
- Ongoing cost of personnel (temporary or permanent) to manage the system
- Annual expense for vendor software support

The offsetting benefits of such a system would include the following:

- Improved patient satisfaction as a result of streamlined coordination of care
- Increased revenues resulting from fewer billing rejections and inquiries
- Improved staff satisfaction resulting from reductions in paperwork and duplication of effort
- Improved quality of care resulting in part from the following:
  —Automation of standards of care and documentation
  —Fewer cases of missing information
  —Improved communication via modem and/or improved availability of contact information
  —Fewer errors in documentation as a result of software edits and required fields
- Savings on expenses for staff time and travel (staff can upload and download information from the field using a built-in modem)
- Improved availability of records
- More efficient care activities allowing greater productivity
- More timely, more efficient, and less costly recertification processes

Creating a model to place dollar values on all of these factors allows one to estimate the relative relationship of cost versus benefit and estimate the time required to achieve sufficient benefits to offset the costs. In home health and most other health care settings, information systems such as these are fast becoming essential tools. In the near future such systems will be ubiquitous.

FUTURE TRENDS FOR HEALTH CARE INFORMATION SYSTEMS

The continued expansion of managed care into health care markets and sharpening competition will continue to press hospitals, physician practices, home health agencies, and other types of care provider organizations to ally with each other, forming integrated delivery systems. Technologies such as interface engines and data repositories will be developed for interfacing and integrating the information systems for these new allies (Golob and Quade, 1993). The goal of these combined information systems will be to develop a longitudinal patient record that accounts for the full continuum of care (prevention to chronic to terminal care) across all sites of care and encompassing the activities of all caregivers (Hughes and Andrew, 1996).

The health care system, in pursuit of lowered cost while maintaining high quality, will make a more complete set of clinical documentation and clinical management capabilities widely available. Purchaser-based organizations such as the National Committee for Quality Assurance (NCQA) and the Foundation for Accountability (FACCT) (Aller, 1996) and accrediting organizations such as the Joint Commission for Accreditation of Healthcare Organizations (JCAHO) (Matthews, Carter, and Smith, 1996) will expand and focus requirements for measuring outcomes. These measures and others chosen by individual organizations will more firmly establish a continuous quality improvement structure in the U.S. health care system. Types of outcomes evaluated will include financial effect, clinical quality, access to service, satisfaction with service, functional status, and quality of life.

In support of capitated contracting for health care services, financial systems will continue to migrate away from orientation to charges and toward orientation to actual costs. Charges will be meaningless in a system that pays for all care on a flat-rate per-case basis or a per-member-per-month basis. The need in a capitated system is to document and manage cost. In a recent survey health care information system leaders indicated that the need to control costs in response to managed care pressures was the most significant driving factor in computerizing their organizations (Elliott, 1996).

Clinical and educational services and information will be brought to the patient or the caregiver in need rather than the latter going to the source of clinical or informational services. The use of Internet technologies will continue to expand in serving patient care, research, and educational ends (Afrin et al., 1997; McCray et al., 1996; Powers, 1996; Zucker et al., 1996). Telemedicine will be exploited as a normal part of health care practice (Nelson, Stewart, and Schlachta, 1996).

Information systems will take on a more central role in the management of daily clinical practice; will be used to provide timely, valid evaluations for outcomes; will provide seamless access to information across allied organizations; will blend information captured by different disciplines, providing that information relevant to each; and will provide clinical and educational information to appropriate individuals wherever they are.

Summary

Historically, information systems in health care were developed to assist with accounting and other financial management functions. Costs for development and deployment have restricted the growth of information systems in the clinical arena.

Current developments driven by market forces for cost control are pressing for information systems to extend into new functions. Information systems in health care organizations are not meeting current demands for cost, process of care, and outcomes information.

Resource demands for information systems may be categorized into (1) one-time outlays for software, hardware, configuration, and training and (2) continuing expenses for vendor support, hardware upgrades, and internal support personnel. Information system benefits may be characterized as economic, clinical, or humanistic. Economic benefits either prevent expense or contribute new revenue. Clinical benefits range from prevention of adverse outcomes to support for best clinical practices. Humanistic benefits include patient satisfaction and professional satisfaction of caregivers.

A home health care information system employing mobile devices illustrates the resource demands and benefits of new technology. Finally, the future of information systems in health care includes continued expansion into clinical practice support, measurement and evaluation of a range of outcomes, and expansion of systems across facilities, disciplines, and distances.

Discussion Questions

1. How might information systems affect a health care manager's job?
2. How has the role of information systems in health care developed?
3. What factors might one consider in evaluating the purchase of an information system?
4. What kinds of technology are being used to bring information to individuals away from the hospital or clinic?

REFERENCES

Afrin LB et al.: Electronic clinical trial protocol distribution via the World-Wide Web: A prototype for reducing costs and errors, improving accrual, and saving trees, *J Am Med Inform Assoc* 4(1):25, 1997.

Aller KC: Information systems for the outcomes movement, *Healthcare Inform Manage* 10(1):37, 1996.

Burke JP, Classen DC, Pestotnik SL: Evaluation of the impact of implementation of a comprehensive computerized antibiotic management program at Intermountain Health Care, *Proc 1997 Annu HIMSS Conference* 1:17, 1997.

Clayton PD, Mulligen E: The economic motivations for clinical information systems, *Proc 19th Annu Symp Computer Application Med Care:* 660, 1996.

Davis A, Pell W, Pickard B: Managing staff resources and costs in changing environments, *Proc 1997 Annu HIMSS Conference* 2:183, 1997.

Elliott J: Managed care spices up the 1996 HIMSS/HP leadership survey, *Healthcare Inform* 13(5):ss2, 1996.

Friel DF: Return on investment (ROI) and its impact on technology planning, *Proc 1997 Annu HIMSS Conference* 1:175, 1997.

Gardner WD, Kelly J: Technology: A price/performance game, *Dun's Rev* 118(2):66, Aug 1981.

Gates M: Information systems for integrated delivery systems, *Health Syst Leader* 3:4, 1996.

Golob RM, Quade BR: Putting it all together: Integration tools, *Healthcare Inform* 10(7):42, 1993.

Hughes S, Andrew WF: Calling all nurses: Report to Jericho, *Healthcare Inform* 13(4):52, 1996.

Matthews P, Carter N, Smith K: Using data to measure outcomes, *Healthcare Inform Manage* 10(1):3, 1996.

McCray AT et al.: The UMLS Knowledge Source Server: A versatile Internet-based research tool, *Proc 19th Annu Symp Computer Application Med Care* (symp suppl):164, 1996.

Nelson R, Stewart PL, Schlachta LM: Outcomes of telemedicine services . . . Patient and medicolegal issues, *Proc 1996 Annu HIMSS Conference* 3:151, 1996.

Powers DE: Internet world wide web bookmarks, *Calif J Health-Syst Pharm* 8(4):9, 1996.

Renner K: Cost-justifying electronic medical records, *Healthcare Financial Manage* 50(10):63, 1996.

Small JT, Lee WB: In search of an MIS, *MSU Business Top* 23(4):47, 1975.

Zucker J et al.: A comprehensive strategy for designing a web-based medical curriculum, *Proc 19th Annu Symp Computer Application Med Care:* 41, 1996.

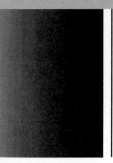

chapter **thirteen**

Maximizing People Potential in Empowered Environments

Lillian M. Simms
Margaret M. Calarco

Learning Objectives

- Describe the nature of empowerment as a personal characteristic.
- Link personal learning to competence and productivity.
- Differentiate between job satisfaction and work excitement.
- Relate work excitement to personal empowerment.
- See patients as partners in an empowered environment.
- Use empowerment principles to create learning environments.

Democracy in the workplace has become the logical extension of political democracy. The right to participate in decision making in one's social, political, and work environments is gradually becoming recognized as a basic human right. In health care settings where doctor-centered care has been the norm for service delivery for centuries, a new wave of thought permeates the environment. Patients, whether known as clients or consumers, are in the driver's seat, and they are unlikely to yield their tight hold on the reins. Through litigation and zealous lawyers, patients are holding health care professionals accountable for their practice. As consumers of health services, patients expect positive outcomes such as recovery, reduction of symptoms, improvement in body function, and even peaceful death without medical interference.

Over time, physicians have maintained a clinician-centered health care delivery model through tight control over entry into and exit from health services. Such a closed system seriously limits the full rendering of health services to people in need of them. Current changes in reimbursement seriously challenge this model, and it is rapidly being replaced by a patient-centered outcome-based model of seamless care. Nurses who are able to function in an outcome-based patient-focused care system must typify a new breed. Increased knowledge and skills alone will not make this new person. There must be a related role change, a change in self-concept whereby nurses see themselves as providers of direct care to clients and families rather than providers of services to institutions. Such a change requires learning new behavior and a personal sense of empowerment that releases a creative energy and sense of excitement about one's work.

The ever-changing health care industry requires workers to be continual learners in their organizations and to focus on serving customers in more clinically innovative and financially efficient ways. The creation of empowered work environments is seen as a way of developing partnerships in health care that enable providers to respond rapidly to customer needs and to the changes in the health care market. This chapter will address the changing concepts of human resource management, productivity, empowerment, and competency development from a customer service perspective and will identify strategies to employ for the creation of an empowered workforce.

DEFINITION OF EMPOWERMENT

Personal and group empowerment reaches its full potential in enabling environments that are designed to nurture continual learning by all workers. The key to empowerment is self-esteem achieved and maintained through learning, self-development, and appreciation of others. Senge (1990) maintains that personal and group empowerment is realized mainly through personal mastery and continual learning. Meade (1995) has defined **empowerment** as "the process of thinking and behaving as if one has power—in the sense of autonomy, authority, control—over significant aspects of one's life and work." To feel empowered in the context of the new employment relationship means to understand the purpose and contribution of our work and to believe that we are ultimately responsible for the work we do, the service we provide, and our own continual development and growth, personally and professionally.

Extrinsic empowerment implies the delegation of official or legal authority by one person to another. It further implies the bureaucratic notion that power lies in the hands of a few (who sit in the right office or wear the right suit) and is granted to others as a reward in selected circumstances. In the view of Smitley and Scott (1994), empowerment is an individual initiative, spelled out in creative thought and courageous action, that is willingly transferred in a flexible organizational environment that nurtures personal and group empowerment.

Group empowerment among nurses was proposed a decade ago. Gorman and Clark (1986) suggested four empowerment strategies: (1) group analyses of reality-based case studies, (2) engagement of unit nurses in planning and implementing needed practice changes, (3) support of nurses by nursing colleagues in application of clinical knowledge and skills (respecting nursing knowledge), and (4) extension of administrative sponsorship. In a training program developed by Gorman and Clark, group learning was encouraged through role-centered case analyses of reality-based unit case studies. The activities of the nurses became highly relevant and visible. Nurses working in heterogeneous groups, representing various parts of each collaborating hospital, acted as teams and selected common problems to address. The training program therefore included both educational and structural solutions for the problems of powerlessness experienced by nurses in the hospital setting. Educationally the program was designed to empower the participating nurses by teaching them the analytical and interpersonal skills they needed to develop and implement plans for change. Structurally it established new lines of communication between staff nurses and nurse managers, linking the nurses to needed resources and giving them more control over their work and working conditions.

PERCEPTIONS OF WORK

The management and business literature is replete with articles and books about empowering others, downsizing, rightsizing, reengineering, coping with job loss, and so on, and yet very little attention has been given to how people feel about their everyday work in life. Essentially empowerment, personal or group, is related to feelings about work. Although work is taken seriously by individuals and society, authors disagree on its meaning. Schurman (1989) believes that the meaning of work is very complex and that work has a different meaning for every individual, allowing for work to be identified as something other than satisfaction. **Work** is viewed as a central human activity in which mind and body unite in actions that not only provide sustenance for the life process but also generate objects, material and ideational, that have meaning and value to both self and others. Attempts to link meaning of work to the organization of work, however, are weak in the literature. Instead, meaning of work is generally associated with job satisfaction, with the former regarded as a reflection of the latter. A distinction between affect about work (that is, meaningfulness of work) and attitudes about work (that is, job satisfaction) has been supported by Sandalands (1988), and he continues to argue for its importance in designing work environments.

Work-enrichment studies often fail to include in their assumptions the meaning of work to the individual. People may view their work as paid employment and not wish to have their jobs enriched. Not all workers choose to find fulfillment in their jobs, and the vast majority of people may choose to find fulfillment outside their jobs (Fein, 1977). Hackman and Lawler (1971) found that workers whose higher-order needs were satisfied performed better and were more positive than those without higher-need satisfaction. Csikszentmihalyi (1990) describes positive work experiences when people are in "flow," linking psychic energy with optimal goal achievement and the work experience. He claims that people make their own optimal experiences happen and that these experiences occur when people stretch their minds to the limit to accomplish something difficult and worthwhile. They become creative and self-motivated when they are in "flow."

The organization of people's work may be a major determinant in shaping their health and well-being outside of work. Karasek and Theorell (1990) attempt to bridge the gap between medical science, psychology, sociology, industrial engineering, and economics to present an approach to the redesign of work organizations to make them more psychologically humane. Citing weaknesses in quality of work life research, Karasek and Theorell propose job redesign strategies that will promote health-related job change. They also support studies of physiological changes among workers as part of any work intervention program. In a study designed to improve competence of patients and personnel, physiological monitoring and educational programs resulted in improvement in patient clinical outcomes and worker health and safety. Toxic work syndrome (work-related illness and absenteeism from work) limits productivity in many organizations.

WORK EXCITEMENT

The concept of work excitement is consistent with current thought from sociotechnological theories that have revived the notion that both social and technological aspects of work are important to the quality of work life in organizations (Simms, Price, and Ervin, 1994; Taylor and Asadorian, 1985). Work excitement was first conceptualized by Simms et al. (1990) in terms of organizational (extrinsic) and individual (intrinsic) factors. A series of early studies in acute, long-term, and home care settings supports five factors as significant predictors of work excitement: receptivity to learning, work arrangements, variety of experiences, working conditions, and change.

Later studies conducted on populations of nurses in military and rural settings confirm the significance of unit culture and opportunities for growth and development (learning). Most recently Erbin-Roesemann (1995), using a large national sample of nurses, advances the validation of the concept through her pioneering doctoral research on the relationship between work locus of control and work excitement. As she postulates, an internal sense of personal control is found to significantly correlate with work excitement. Her study further suggests that low personal control, as well as feelings that powerful others control people's work lives such that they have little influence on their work, significantly correlates with a low level of work excitement. The role of extrinsic and intrinsic forces on personal control of work life is also supported in the empowerment literature and adds further credence to the importance of understanding "work" as well as "job."

The latest validation studies reconfirm the concept of **work excitement** as personal enthusiasm and interest in work evidenced by creativity, receptivity to learning, and ability to see opportunity in everyday situations. Work excitement as postulated then becomes the catalyst for empowerment and learning new behaviors. The conceptual model (Figure 13-1) is permeated with opportunities for learning for caregivers and recipients. For example, self-care and use of high- and low-level assistive technology can be learned and can make a tremendous difference in quality care and successful clinical outcomes. Learning new behaviors should improve clinical competence and the ability to work in flexible groups.

PEOPLE-CENTERED CARE

Mastery of the concept of **patient-centered care** requires an understanding of people-centered work, as well as the work itself. Understanding patient outcomes is

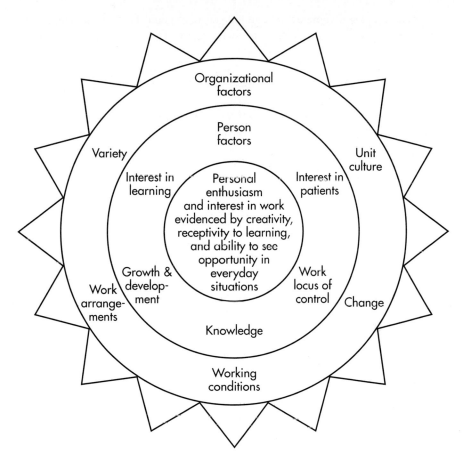

Figure 13-1 The work excitement conceptual model: Organizational and person factors.

an important part of learning how to redesign clinical work and develop clinical outcomes. In a people-centered participatory work environment, a multidisciplinary unit staff can consider the nature of the work to be done and the people and technological resources desirable and available to accomplish the work with the best advantage to patients. Consideration can be given to the following: What pieces of work can or should be done together or by one person? What work can be delegated to other people or equipment? What work should be a patient/family responsibility? What work should be done differently? What work should not be done at all? In other words, what knowledge, skills, and equipment are needed to accomplish quality people-centered care? With the exception of the collaborative practice model presented by Simms, Dalston, and Roberts (1984), which includes patients as care-planning participants, and the Planetree model (Martin, Hunt, and Hughes-Stone, 1990) for training patients as partners in care, patient involvement in care planning is infrequently recognized.

A people-centered approach to care management could facilitate a change from nurse/physician-focused care to patient-focused care. The major goal of the Plane-tree program is to educate patients/families to care for themselves during hospital-ization, after discharge, and in their return to everyday life. Commitments to patient participation in collaborative practice and self-care have been supported in rehabilitation practice for many years. Only recently have health care professionals realized that consumers want more control over their own health. Current concern about rising health care costs has stimulated new interest in patient involvement in decision making regarding their own care.

Not too long ago administrators were not considered part of the patient-care team. Today all participants in care delivery must work in concert with care recipi-ents if we are to maximize human resources in cost-effective ways. Patient-centered care is emerging in new forms of collaborative practice among health disciplines. Some examples of collaborative practice among health disciplines include (1) joint private practices that include nurse practitioners, physicians, social workers, physi-cal therapists, and other caregivers offering patient-required services (rehabilitation engineering has developed as the result of collaboration between engineers and health professionals), (2) hospital-based multidisciplinary clinical units that focus on rehabilitation and seamless care, and (3) multidisciplinary research that links clinical and systems research on reality-based patient problems. Participatory re-search teams that include patients and families are further evidence of interest in linking clinical practice with patient-centered care. The National Ataxia Research Foundation in Wayzata, Minnesota, (*Generations,* 1995) emerged as the result of collaboration among clinicians, researchers, and patients/families.

Successful empowered environments will be built on the collaboration of mul-tiple health-related disciplines. Earlier models focused on nursing and medicine and did not recognize the contribution of other team members or paraprofessionals and support service staff. Collaborative patient-centered practice legitimizes and sharp-ens the roles of each discipline. It also integrates "care" and "cure" philosophies, which are essential in seamless care. Collaborative people-centered care efficiently utilizes personnel in roles they are prepared to assume. Patients/families should be involved in treatment regimens at all points of seamless care from entry into point of service to discharge. Patient involvement has been a part of hospital-based edu-cational programs but only in a passive role. In the future, patient involvement will be increasingly important and should be part of evaluation procedures as well. Clinical outcomes reflecting positive response to therapeutic measures will continue to have a major influence on reimbursement patterns.

THE NEW PRODUCTIVITY

In the 1960s almost one half of all workers in the industrialized countries were in-volved in making things, but by the year 2000, no developed country will have more than one sixth to one eighth of its workforce in the traditional roles of mak-ing and moving things. Currently an estimated two thirds of U.S. workers work in the service sector, and "knowledge" is becoming our most important product

(Drucker, 1993). "The single greatest challenge facing managers in the developed countries of the world is to raise the productivity of knowledge and service workers. This challenge, which will dominate the management agenda for the next several decades, will ultimately determine the competitive performance of companies. Even more important, it will determine the very fabric of society and the quality of life in every industrialized nation." (Drucker, 1991)

Drucker (1991) further suggests that in the knowledge and service sectors, "working smarter" is the only key in increasing productivity. The applications of capital and technology may assist productivity but will never replace knowledge as the critical factor in providing service. Drucker suggests that applying various sets of questions to the work will enable us to understand ways to increase productivity in the service sector.

The first set of questions needs to be, What is the task? What are we trying to accomplish? and Why do it at all? (Drucker, 1991). Defining the task and eliminating nonessential tasks are the first critical steps in addressing service productivity. Once the task is defined, the next step is to concentrate the work on completion of the task. For instance, Drucker (1991) cites the example of the alleged "nursing shortage" in the United States but argues that the issue is that nurses now spend half of their time in completing paperwork and less time in providing direct patient care. This concentration of work on the task is crucial, and asking the questions, What do we pay for? and What value is this job supposed to add? may help in clarifying the task and better aligning the work to the task, thereby increasing productivity.

The third step in improving productivity in the service sector is defining performance. Drucker (1991) delineates three categories of performance in service work that drive the parameters of productivity. The first are service jobs where "performance means quality" (for example, scientists in a research laboratory). The second category includes the majority of knowledge and service workers, including nurses, where quality and quantity together constitute performance. Here, raising productivity in these jobs requires not only asking, What works? but also analyzing the step-by-step process involved in the work to increase efficiency. The third category of service jobs (for example, making beds or filing claims) suggests that performance is measured by quantity and production. Here, work process standards are essential.

The fourth step toward improving the productivity of service work is to create an environment where managers and workers form a partnership to improve performance and become more productive. The goal is to build responsibility for performance and productivity into every job, regardless of skill level. This requires a mutual commitment by managers and workers to continual learning, but more interestingly, Drucker (1991) suggests that knowledge and service workers learn more when they teach, so institutions should become "teaching" entities as well.

This fourth step of improving productivity challenges us to redefine the traditional relationship between management and staff and to commit to a mutually empowering environment. The creation of this new "partnership" will be critical to our future. However, there are no simple or generally accepted criteria for creating partnerships, nor is there a single recognized proper way to go about creating productive work groups. Work can be structured to be performed by individual workers or carried out by a group of workers acting in teams. Effective work redesign can result from interventions with the workers, the work itself, or work group arrangements.

It is therefore important to create **empowered environments** in which work groups can learn as they work on redesigning their own work and work groups. Unit worker learning is essential for innovation and technology transfer. An important aspect of work group culture is readiness to change, and receptivity to innovation may be the critical factor in orchestrating change and learning to use new technology. Excessive stability resulting from low turnover may prevent innovation unless large numbers of people are redistributed or replaced. With a change in organizational culture and a new emphasis on empowered environments, management and staff can become involved in decision making and organization of work at the unit level that improve competent and effective clinical practice.

PARTNERING TO EMPOWER

Acknowledgment, respect, control, and autonomy are key components of an empowered environment. Traditional "human resource management," however, has focused on the creation of organizational systems (for example, compensation systems, selection systems, and performance management systems) to shape employee behavior in support of the organization's goals. Often these traditional structures have created bureaucratic, paternalistic, and dependent relationships between employers and workers that were supported by the implicit agreement between the parties that "if workers were loyal and did the right things for the company, job security would be maintained."

Today, given the continual changes in business and health care, and the subsequent consolidations and "downsizing," the implicit psychological contract of job security has been broken. The task today is to redefine the "employment contract" between workers and employers and create a partnership that centers on customer service. The goal today is to integrate our organizational and personal missions and create a continual learning environment that is self-renewing, empowering, and committed to continual improvement.

In his book, *Healing the Wounds: Overcoming the Trauma of Layoffs and Revitalizing Downsized Organizations,* David Noer (1993) contrasts the implicit assumptions of the "old" and "new" employment contracts. (See Box 13-1.) The **new employment contract** requires us to shift the current paradigm of work from long-term employment in a single career to work that is based on continually developing our skills to serve our customers and to become "employable" in a variety of settings throughout our lifetime. Dependence on our employer for a lifetime career no longer has relevance, and true empowerment will come from recognizing that we are, in many ways, in business for ourselves. With this comes the personal responsibility to understand our own purpose in work and create our own future.

The only way you provide security for yourself is by making sure that your work experience is as up-to-date as possible so that if tomorrow happens, you are able to go out and

Box 13-1

The Paradigm Shift in Employment Contracts

OLD EMPLOYMENT CONTRACT	NEW EMPLOYMENT CONTRACT
Employment relationship is long term	**Employment relationship is situational**
▪ Benefits and services reward tenure	▪ Benefits are portable and flexible
▪ Recognition practices reinforce long-term relationships	▪ Tenure-free recognition systems exist
▪ *Outcome:* Narrow workforce	▪ Blurred distinction between full-time, part-time, and temporary workers
	▪ *Outcome:* Flexible workforce
Reward for performance is promotion	**Reward for performance is based on contribution and relevance**
▪ Linear compensation and status	▪ Job enrichment and participation
▪ Fixed job descriptions	▪ The philosophy of quality
▪ Static performance standards	▪ Self-directed work teams
▪ *Outcome:* Plateaued and demotivated (betrayed) workforce	▪ Nonhierarchical performance and reward systems
	▪ *Outcome:* Motivated and task-invested workforce
Management is paternalistic	**Management is empowering**
▪ Duplicative support systems	▪ Employee autonomy
▪ Long-term career planning systems	▪ No "taking care" of employees
▪ *Outcome:* Dependent workforce	▪ No detailed long-term career planning
	▪ Tough love
	▪ *Outcome:* Empowered workforce
Loyalty means remaining with the organization	**Loyalty means responsible and good work**
▪ Career paths only within the organization	▪ Nontraditional career paths
▪ Voluntary turnover penalized	▪ In/out process
▪ Internal promotion and discouragement of external hiring	▪ Employee choice
▪ *Outcome:* Narrow and nondiverse workforce	▪ Diversity recruiting
	▪ *Outcome:* Responsible, diverse, and more flexible workforce
Lifetime career is offered	**Job contracting is offered**
▪ "Fitting in" counts	▪ Short-term job planning
▪ Relationships are determining factors	▪ Not signing up for life
▪ *Outcome:* Codependent workforce	▪ No assumption of lifetime caretaking
	▪ *Outcome:* Employee and organization are bonded around good work

Modified from Noer DM: *Healing the wounds: Overcoming the trauma of layoffs and revitalizing downsized organizations,* San Francisco, 1993, Jossey-Bass.

get another job because you have the skills people want. That's the only way you have security. You aren't going to get it from the company. It will never be that way again. (Noer, 1993)

Noer (1993) further reminds us that the creation of this new empowered environment will require "culture busting" change. Leadership that positions us for the future will require us to transform the leader role from one of "managing" and sustaining dependence to one of "coaching" and promoting autonomy. The creation of an autonomous workforce that centers on the commitment to customer service is the cornerstone of an empowered environment.

EMPOWERED ENVIRONMENTS

In the current exploration of the organizational literature related to empowerment and in observing the work of self-defined "empowered teams" within organizations, several principles consistently emerge as foundational for the creation of an empowered workforce. These principles include (1) a commitment to customer service; (2) developing a climate of trust and risk taking; (3) continual information sharing; (4) the development of a shared vision, values, and organizational goals; (5) the transition from hierarchies to team development; (6) decision making closest to the level of the work; (7) parameters of clear responsibility and accountability; (8) measurement and feedback; and (9) continual self-assessment and self-directed learning. Figure 13-2 illustrates the bridge to empowered environments.

Customer Service

Commitment to customer service is the hallmark of empowerment in service environments. Although there are a variety of customer groups in health care settings (for example, providers, insurers, payors), it is critically important to identify the primary customer group in health care as the patient and family. Empowerment begins with a clear understanding of the purpose of our work, and in nursing and health care, the purpose of our work is to serve our patient. Many models of patient-centered care are being explored in health care institutions today and represent an attempt to refocus our efforts on providing efficient and quality care to our patients. In addition, as lengths of stay continue to decrease and more and more patients are discharged from inpatient settings in more acute stages of their illness, the family becomes a predominant customer group as well. Assisting the family in caring for their loved one becomes a primary nursing care requirement.

Creating a Climate of Trust and Risk Taking

The second principle underlying empowered environments includes the development of trust within organizations and the encouragement for risk-taking behaviors. Trusting relationships between employers and workers are crucial for the development of empowered environments, but in the era of the new employment contract, we are not calling for a "blind" trust or unconditional loyalty, but what William Morin (1990) calls "nondependent trust."

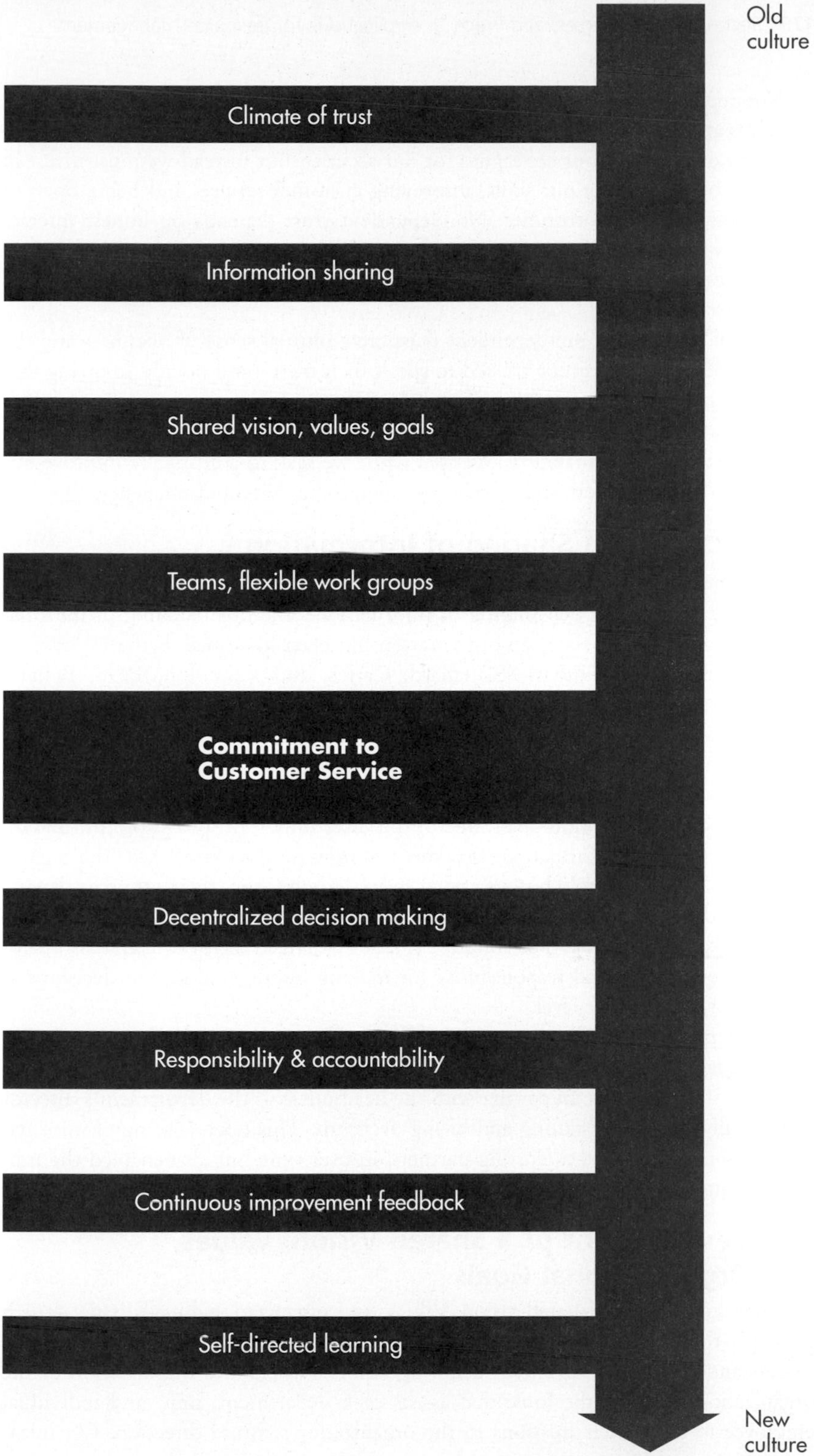

Old culture

Climate of trust

Information sharing

Shared vision, values, goals

Teams, flexible work groups

Commitment to Customer Service

Decentralized decision making

Responsibility & accountability

Continuous improvement feedback

Self-directed learning

New culture

Figure 13-2 The bridge to empowered environments.

Nondependent trust requires that each of us understands that we must care for ourselves and assume responsibility for our future. No longer can we look to our institution, our boss, or our colleagues for our security, but instead we must invest in ourselves by developing our skills, improving customer service, and being open to new employment opportunities. Nondependent trust depends on honest interactions. As workers, we must communicate our needs, our questions, and our expectations openly, and managers must commit to providing honest feedback and information.

Critical elements of nondependent trust are a mutual sense of openness and the belief that individuals can be trusted to speak their own mind openly, knowing that the other party will listen and seek to help. With trust comes the ability to challenge the status quo and to offer innovations in our workplace and in the care we provide. Risk-taking behavior is essential while we seek to continually improve our services to our customers and to increase our productivity and efficiency.

Continual, Open Sharing of Information

Nondependent trust also depends on the third principle of empowered environments: the continual, open sharing of information. The open sharing of information throughout all levels of an organization has been identified as the foundation of empowered environments (Blanchard, Carlos, and Randolph, 1996; Byham, 1994; Noer, 1993).

Workers must have the information they need to perform their work, but they must also have information that helps them understand how their work fits into the broader goals of the organization. In addition to sharing a unified vision of the organization and the business goals, one of the most important pieces of information to share is financial information. Workers not only need to know how the organization is doing as a whole but also need to understand how their unit's or department's budget is determined and how it is maintained. Sharing this information helps workers understand the economic forces that affect health care and also helps engender ownership and responsibility for making resource allocation decisions at the unit or department level.

In a department where all nursing staff were educated about the construction of the budget and were able to review the monthly budget variances on an ongoing basis, the staff were able to partner with the head nurse or the department's director to mutually decide on staffing and hiring decisions. This open sharing of information not only developed a trusting partnership over time but also enabled the unit to make much better staffing decisions and budgetary projections.

The Development of a Shared Vision, Values, and Organizational Goals

The development of a shared vision, values, and organizational goals is the fourth principle that underlies an empowered environment (Baker, 1994; Byham, 1994; Rogers and Ferketish, 1992). An inspiring vision that clarifies the direction of the organization serves as the force that assists each department, unit, and individual employee to align their missions to the organization's future direction. Organizational values describe how the vision is to be achieved and are critical elements for empowered decision making.

Value statements must be clearly defined and reflect action-behaviors that every employee in the organization can understand, commit to, and demonstrate. In addition, it is important to identify the driving value of an organization that must take priority whenever conflicts in values or decisions occur (Byham, 1994; Rogers and Ferketish, 1992). In health care settings "putting patients and families first" may be seen as the driving value of the organization. In the situation in which employees must make a decision while having competing demands placed on them, this driving value should serve as a way of prioritizing decision making. For example, if a housekeeper received concurrent requests to clean a spill in a patient's room, clean a bed after discharge, and clean a physician's office, the driving value of "putting patients first" would assist the housekeeper in prioritizing these requests.

Identification of the organization's business goals is important to communicate so that workers can understand how their specific tasks contribute to the overall goals of the organization. In health care, again, commitment to customer service should be an organizational goal, and all employees can identify how their work contributes directly or indirectly to patient care.

In empowered environments the creation of the vision, values, and goals is often initiated by the organization's leadership but then widely communicated to all workers for discussion and revision. The goal is to develop a mutually shared vision and direction to sustain commitment and focus. This requires active discussion of the vision, values, and goals throughout each level of the organization and requires all employees to determine how they incorporate and demonstrate these values in their daily work.

The Transition From Hierarchies to Team Development

Although several strategies can be employed to assist individual managers and workers in developing skills that enhance communication and problem-solving capabilities, from an organizational perspective the development of participative teams is essential in sustaining empowered environments. Team development crosses the continuum from unifunctional, problem-solving task teams to cross-functional "virtual" teams that are convened to design and implement specified projects. Self-directed teams exemplify the most "empowered" on the continuum.

Team development without the fundamental restructuring of the organization's decision-making process does little to sustain an empowered workforce. The creation of teams that operate in isolation of other units or disciplines only serves to promote existing bureaucracies. Teams that facilitate interaction and interdependence of units and individuals serve to restructure the decision-making system.

Decision Making Closest to the Level of the Work

To sustain an empowered workforce and to truly promote risk taking, creativity, and flexible problem solving throughout the organization, decision-making processes must be streamlined and pushed down to the level closest to the work or issue being resolved. This requires an in-depth examination of existing approval requirements and decision-making structures.

Ashkenas et al. (1995) identify questions that are helpful to ask when determining who should be involved in decision making:

1. Who has the information and skills necessary to make sure this is a high-quality decision?
2. If you had to trust one person in the organization to make this decision, whom would it be?
3. Who will be required to implement and carry out this decision?
4. Have these people been involved?

Ashkenas et al. (1995) have also developed a series of questions to assist managers in examining their decision-making style and assessing the current approval structure. Managers should ask themselves the following:

1. What keeps me from letting my workers make the decision?
2. What keeps me from making this information available to my workers?
3. How often have I reversed or declined to approve a decision of this kind? If the answer is "never" then the question should be as follows:
4. What value am I adding by signing off on every decision of this kind?
5. What keeps me from letting my employee make this decision?

These questions are helpful in understanding the barriers to decision making in organizations and assist us in ensuring the appropriate people are involved in the decision-making process closest to the work. One can see that although this type of decision making may seem "sensible," it often represents a change in the culture of an organization and the need for managers to explore the motivation behind their decision-making styles.

Parameters for Clear Responsibility and Accountability

In the end, empowerment is always an individual choice. The new employment paradigm suggests that the commitment to self-empowerment or self-management is at the heart of empowered environments and productive workplaces for the future. This notion that we are ultimately responsible for our own development, our service to our customers, and our own job security represents a shift in current organizational philosophy that must be addressed.

In organizations self-empowerment occurs within organizational boundaries and structure and is aligned with customer service and the organization's goals. This interplay between individual performance and decision making and organizational boundaries requires clear discussion and decision about parameters for accountability and responsibility.

Blanchard, Carlos, and Randolph (1996) suggest that organizations must identify the "boundary areas for autonomy," which include the organization's purpose, values, image (or vision), goals, roles, and organizational structure. As previously described, the organization's vision, values, and goals clarify the organization's direction and the way work is to be performed. At an individual level, all employees are then responsible for clarifying how their work contributes to the goals.

The essence of **self-empowerment** focuses around one's contribution to work and is assessed by answering the following questions (Vogt and Murrell, 1990):

1. Am I making a difference?
2. Do I have the competencies?
3. Am I making a significant contribution?
4. Am I growing?

Understanding one's personal mission and goals as they relate to the organization is the first step in creating empowered environments.

In addition, there are basic competencies that are required to create and sustain empowered environments. These interpersonal and technical competencies are required for everyone, regardless of role, within the organization. The core competencies that must be addressed by every worker include (1) customer service skills, (2) self-management skills, (3) communication skills, (4) conflict resolution skills, (5) transition management skills, (6) team leader/member and team-building skills, and (7) diversity awareness skills.

Conflict resolution skills are essential for empowered environments because empowerment requires building partnerships between managers and staff, various disciplines, and so on. Conflict is a natural outcome of partnering together and must be resolved constructively. Skill building in this area of performance is essential and builds opportunities for effective self-management and team building.

Continual Improvement Feedback

Personal accountability for performance is critical to sustaining an empowered workforce. It is recommended that workers assess their performance and skill-building needs at regular intervals to create a personal mastery plan. Self-assessment is an ongoing responsibility in empowered environments. Continually improving customer service requires that we continually improve and broaden our skills. The goal in empowered organizations is to be able to match workers to the work that needs to be done across boundaries. This requires clarity of work responsibilities, as well as clarity of required competencies and skill sets.

Once organizational goals have been clarified, all workers must understand how their work contributes to customer and organizational goals. The ability to receive feedback about one's performance in "real time" is critically important in an empowerment process. Organizational systems for measurement and continual performance feedback provide an individual worker with immediate feedback about accomplishments, as well as areas for improvement.

Many organizations have initiated a 360-degree performance feedback system that enables individuals to receive feedback from all constituent groups coming in contact with their work (that is, peers, customers, managers, and so on). For the leadership group, this type of system enables more consistent feedback from staff and lends itself to improved problem solving as a team. From an empowerment perspective, individual employees or teams need to be actively involved in constructing the measurement systems that will be used in the process.

Continual Self-Assessment and Self-Directed Learning

> Learning is the new form of labor. [It's] no longer a separate activity that occurs either before one enters the workplace or in remote classroom settings. . . . Learning is at the heart of productive activity. (Zuboff, 1988)

The key to empowerment is learning and the development of learning organizations. Senge (1990) has espoused five core disciplines essential to building the learning organization: (1) personal mastery, (2) mental models, (3) shared vision, (4) team learning, and (5) systems thinking. These are the glue that integrates the disciplines and fuses theory with practice. Building a shared vision lays the base for widespread grasp of mission and long-term goals. Mental models allow us to create pictures that connect with the real world. Personal mastery fosters the notion of individual responsibility for continual learning. In an empowered organization, people experience metanoia, a shift of mind, as they see their work world differently and their place in the work world as connected. The we/they mindset of management/staff disappears in the people-centered empowered environment. True partnerships can then flourish.

Personal mastery is the phrase Senge (1990) uses for the discipline of personal growth and learning. When personal mastery becomes the spirit of the empowered organization, people become the active force, whether it involves research, product development, or any aspect of the business. So it is in health care delivery settings. If workers themselves do not have excitement about their work and are not personally motivated to participate in the organizational vision, there will be no gain in productivity, no growth, and above all no desire to participate in the "imaginization" (Morgan, 1993) essential to technological innovation.

Senge (1990) further suggests that traditional organizations foster conflicts between work and family and seriously unempower their workers. By failing to recognize the synergy among everyday work, learning organizations, learning individuals, and learning families, traditional organizations limit employee effectiveness and ability to learn. In empowered organizations that have a full commitment to learning and development, the boundaries between what is personal and what is organizational become insignificant.

European society speaks of a **learning society** rather than career education. Europeans propose and view lifelong learning and individual growth as continuing throughout life for leisure and work. Integration of education, work, and leisure is central to their beliefs about how a learning society should be designed. A "learner-controlled" versus a "program-controlled" environment has been found to be a motivating factor in learning (Kinzie and Sullivan, 1989). Drucker (1991) also speaks of continual learning and emphasizes that training is only the beginning of learning. Learning must occur on a daily basis along with teaching. The way work is organized affects the quantity and quality of worker learning.

Changing technology and work environments have created a new potential for worker learning, as well as a need for better approaches to the learning process (Deutsch, 1989). A key point stressed by various researchers is the need for effective organizations to strive consciously toward a participatory work environment to maximize the utilization of resources. Worker learning and the shaping of the work environment are important aspects of acceptance of technological change. The key role of new technology cannot be emphasized enough. The greatest challenge to those involved in worker learning will be to move away from routine inservice education programs to active involvement in learning as an ongoing process (Deutsch, 1989). According to Brown and Duguid (1989), human learning is the bottleneck through which innovation must pass. Learning is not the process of amassing loosely collected data, and productive work is not a series of routine tasks but rather a series of interrelated sense-making, reflective, culture-bound activities carried out for a clearly defined purpose.

Kornbluh, Pipan, and Schurman (1987) define **empowerment learning** as unlimited energy in an organization. Human learning is considered an organizational asset, and in transformed organizations human learning and problem-solving abilities are viewed as vitally important resources in empowering people—a continual source of energy. Participation in transformation is seen as a process, not a goal. A zero-sum conception of power in command and control organizations assumes that power is a finite commodity in which some may gain only if others lose. A radically different approach is suggested by Kornbluh, Pipan, and Schurman (1987): a "non-zero-sum model" of power in which the total amount of power is always expanding. Based on creation of a learning environment, workers are empowered to use their intellectual abilities to individual and organizational advantage.

In this model all organizational participants are workers, and every worker counts. Every worker exerts control over performance and quality of work and life variables. There is no line drawn between professional and nonprofessional work. In empowered metanoic health care organizations, the goal is patient-centered care, and it is everyone's responsibility to participate in building and advancing a shared vision. An empowered organization fosters and nurtures the potential of all its workers and is a combination of intrinsic and extrinsic factors.

Summary

This chapter has defined empowerment and ways to build empowered environments. The ideas expressed are consistent with the thoughts of Adams and Morgan, who pioneered the notions of metanoia and imaginization. Adams (1986) early on presented the idea of metanoic organizations in which both leadership and work are challenged and transformed. Adams and his colleagues challenged the old notions of leadership and management and created the notion of moving beyond single-leader to floating-leadership organizations. Metanoic organizations have experienced a fundamental shift from thinking that people must cope with life and are helpless, powerless, and at the mercy of management to the conviction that people are individually and collectively empowered to create their future and destiny.

Gareth Morgan (1993) spelled out **imaginization** as a new way of thinking and a new way of organizing in which people themselves understand and develop their creative potential. The old ways of management constrain our thinking and prevent imagining new ways of conducting work. The challenge, Morgan says, is to imaginize, a process that will take us beyond bureaucratic boxes and fixed notions of leadership and department. The spider plant, in his view, becomes the perfect structure for seamless pods of responsibility and accountability. The spider plant allows new areas of growth and development to flourish in an environment that benefits the entire organization. In the spider plant organizational environment, empowerment is natural, the term *human resource management* is replaced by *people power,* and personal peak performance for leadership is floating and dependent on the nature of the task and the work groups needed to meet consumer needs.

Managers need to learn the **learning enabler-facilitator** role (Kornbluh and Greene, 1989), a very different role compared with traditional management roles. This new role involves performing the function of enabler of learning and constantly creating the conditions for learning. Learning in groups in organizations has tremendous potential for empowerment. Health care organizations are in a critical state of flux. They must be able to adjust rapidly to change and the acceptance of innovation. Those organizations that are successful will have learned critical skills about creating and expanding their own people resources. Those organizations that can become "learning organizations" will be survivors. The people to facilitate and lead the shift will be those with work excitement (Zavodsky and Simms, 1996).

‖ Discussion Questions

1. What is empowerment, and how do you see its relationship to the development of organizational vision?
2. What is a metanoic organization, and what is necessary to enable workers to develop their own creative sense of empowerment?
3. Describe the predictors of work excitement, and relate the concept to productivity in your work environment.
4. In your work setting, how would you initiate patient-centered care based on principles of empowerment described in this chapter?
5. Why is it important to recognize patients as consumers of health services?
6. Describe and give examples of at least three principles of empowerment that could be applied in your work setting.
7. What happens in an organization in which top management has developed an organizational vision without empowering the staff to participate and suddenly the top team leaves?

REFERENCES

Adams JD, editor: *Transforming leadership: From vision to results,* Alexandria, Va, 1986, Miles River Press.

Ashkenas R et al.: *The boundaryless organization: Breaking the chains of organizational structure,* San Francisco, 1995, Jossey-Bass.

Baker WE: *Networking smart,* New York, 1994, McGraw-Hill.

Blanchard K, Carlos JP, Randolph A: *Empowerment takes more than a minute,* San Francisco, 1996, Berrett-Koehler.

Brown JS, Duguid P: *Learning & improvisation: Local sources of global innovation,* Unpublished manuscript, Ann Arbor, 1989, University of Michigan.

Byham WC: *Implementing a high-involvement (empowerment) strategy,* Pittsburgh, 1994, Development Dimensions International.

Csikszentmihalyi M: *Flow: The psychology of optimal experience,* New York, 1990, Harper & Row.

Deutsch S: Worker learning in the context of changing technology and work environment. In Leymann H, Kornbluh H, editors: *Socialization and learning at work,* Brookfield, Vt, 1989, Gower.

Drucker PF: The new productivity challenge, *Harvard Business Review* 69(6):69, 1991.

Drucker PF: *Post-capitalist society,* New York, 1993, Harper Business.

Erbin-Roesemann MA: *Validation of the work excitement and the work locus of control instruments,* Unpublished doctoral dissertation, Ann Arbor, 1995, University of Michigan.

Fein M: Job enrichment: A reevaluation. In Hackman JR, Lawler EE, Porter L, editors: *Perspectives on behavior in organizations,* New York, 1977, McGraw-Hill.

Generations: The official publication of the National Ataxia Foundation, Wayzata, Minn, 1995, National Ataxia Research Foundation.

Gorman S, Clark N: Power and effective nursing practice, *Nurs Outlook* 34(3):129, 1986.

Hackman JR, Lawler EE: Employee reactions to job characteristics, *J Appl Psychol Monogr* 55:259, 1971.

Karasek R, Theorell T: *Healthy work,* New York, 1990, Basic Books.

Kinzie MB, Sullivan HJ: Continuing motivation, learner control and cai, *Educ Tech Res Dev* 37(2):5, 1989.

Kornbluh H, Greene RT: Learning, empowerment and participative processes. In Leymann H, Kornbluh H, editors: *Socialization and learning at work,* Brookfield, Vt, 1989, Gower.

Kornbluh H, Pipan R, Schurman SJ: Empowerment learning and control in workplaces: A curricular view, *ZSE* J Jahrgang/Heft 7(4):253, 1987.

Martin DP, Hunt JR, Hughes-Stone M: The Planetree model hospital project: An example of the patient as partner, *Hosp Health Serv Adm* 35(4):591, 1990.

Meade RL: *How to empower an organization: Unleash the latent power of your workforce from goals to action,* Minneapolis, 1995, Lakewood.

Morgan G: *Imaginization: The art of creative management,* Newbury Park, Calif, 1993, Sage.

Morin W: *Trust me: How to rebuild trust in the workplace,* New York, 1990, Drake Beam Morin.

Noer DM: *Healing the wounds: Overcoming the trauma of layoffs and revitalizing downsized organizations,* San Francisco, 1993, Jossey-Bass.

Rogers RW, Ferketish BJ: *Creating a high-involvement culture through a value-driven change process,* Pittsburgh, 1992, Development Dimensions International.

Sandalands LE: The concept of work feeling, *J Theor Soc Behav* 18(4):437, 1988.

Schurman SJ: Reuniting labour and learning: A holistic theory of work. In Lehmann H, Kornbluh H, editors: *Socialization and learning at work,* Brookfield, Vt, 1989, Gower.

Senge PM: *The fifth discipline: The art and practice of the learning organization,* New York, 1990, Doubleday.

Simms LM, Dalston JW, Roberts PW: Collaborative practice: Myth or reality, *Hosp Health Serv Adm* 29(6):36, 1984.

Simms LM, Price SA, Ervin NE: *The professional practice of nursing administration,* Albany, NY, 1994, Delmar.

Simms LM et al.: Breaking the burnout barrier: Resurrecting work excitement in nursing, *Nurs Econ* 8(3):177, 1990.

Smitley W, Scott D: Empowerment: Unlocking the potential of the workforce, *Qual Digest* 14:40, 1994.

Taylor JC, Asadorian RA: The implementation of excellence: STS management, *Indust Manage* 27(4):5, 1985.

Vogt JF, Murrell KL: *Empowerment in organizations: How to spark exceptional performance,* Amsterdam, 1990, Pfeiffer.

Zavodsky A, Simms LM: Work excitement among nurse executives and managers, *Nurs Econ* 14(3):151, 1996.

Zuboff S: *In the age of the smart machine: The future of work and power,* New York, 1988, Basic Books.

chapter **fourteen**

Collaboration in Practice

Harriet Van Ess Coeling
Penelope Laing Cukr

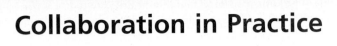

Learning Objectives

- Explain why interdisciplinary collaboration in health care is essential yet difficult.
- List values of interdisciplinary collaboration in terms of cost and quality.
- Identify and give examples of two differences in perspective that can interfere with interdisciplinary collaboration.
- Describe and give examples of five effective communication styles.
- Explain why interdisciplinary collaboration becomes more important as less time becomes available for patient care.
- List and describe five organizational/agency structures that may facilitate collaboration.

THE DILEMMA

Collaboration is a resource maximizing activity in high demand in today's competitive health care economy. It maximizes the resource of human ideas. Humans are an important resource in any organization; they perform work, they make material objects, and they synthesize knowledge to develop new insights and ideas. This last activity is becoming increasingly important as we move forward in the information age. However, it is a very challenging activity because it involves the coordination of efforts among various individuals. Ideas thrive when they are constantly fed and watered by insights from other people. Yet meshing these insights into a new approach is seldom easy. Differing ideas may be rejected or contribute to misunderstanding rather than a solution.

Therein lies one of our modern dilemmas: Increasingly we humans need ideas from others to enhance our own thinking and to function in the most effective and productive manner, yet we are often resistant to receiving these ideas. Tellis-Nayak and Tellis-Nayak (1984) describe a common societal paradox by explaining that though a society segregates its members into stratified groups, society has to bring these distant groups together in a collaborative effort to make the social enterprise possible. The same paradox is found in health care today. We need a variety of disciplines addressing differing concerns. Yet these ideas must come together in a unified plan of care for and with each patient.

Nursing's awareness of this paradox came to the fore in the 1950s and 1960s as nursing leaders emphasized nursing's unique contribution to caring for the patient, a contribution that added to the contribution of physicians who focused on the cure of disease (Weiss and Davis, 1985; Weiss and Remen, 1983). At about this same time a variety of other health care workers were coming on the scene, offering specialized contributions to patient care. This specialization, or differentiation of professional focus, blossomed, and soon hospitals were organizing into a variety of specialized departments, each making a definite contribution to the patient, yet sometimes working in isolation from the other. This explosion of information resulted in complexity of roles and an increased challenge of collaborating among health care providers. Kyle (1995) describes the inevitability that differences of opinion and conflict will arise when strong and talented persons with diverse abilities come together in a complex health care and economic structure.

Hanson and Spross (1996) note that to resolve these conflicts there must be a desire to collaborate and to value and respect others' ideas and actions, as well as a personal belief that complementary knowledge will enhance one's own personal plan for patient care. Nursing's revised Social Policy Statement also emphasizes a need for collaboration that includes respect and recognition of the expertise of others (American Nurses Association, 1995). Ultimately it is a focus on the patient and what is good for the patient that facilitates this respect and brings various disciplines together in a collaborative manner (Lenkman and Gribbins, 1994). Medicine, too, has recognized this need, as evidenced by the following statement made by a former Institute of Medicine president (Iglehart, 1987):

> The issues surrounding nursing are so central to health care that the medical profession can't afford to watch from the sidelines. Physicians must balance their competitive concerns toward nursing with a keener recognition that hospitals cannot operate without nurses. And we must all be sensitive to the fact that what's more important than professional prerogatives is designing a system that best meets the needs of patients.

As early as the 1970s both nursing and medicine saw the benefits and the challenges of the professional specialization that was developing. Values included the development of in-depth knowledge bases and related skills, all of which contributed to the well-being of patients. Challenges included a turning inward toward one's own profession rather than maintaining a focus on the patient. This turning inward toward one's own discipline included a specialized vocabulary and professional goals understood and appreciated primarily by one's own professional membership. This lessened the desire and opportunity for different professionals to dialogue for the benefit of the patient and sometimes led to the fragmentation of patient care. Both medicine and nursing sought to overcome this professional myopia. A desire to improve relationships between medicine and nursing, along with the need to deal with the role overlap between disciplines as advanced practice nurses increased in number, prompted the development of the National Joint Practice Commission (NJPC) to address the traditional problems that affected nurse-physician relationships to establish enhanced role functioning (Lysaught, 1973).

The existence of this commission recognized the paradox of needing both to develop unique bodies of knowledge for different disciplines and to bring specialized ideas together for the good of the patient. Although the work of this particular commission came to a premature closure, attempts to bring together the work of different disciplines continue (Fagin, 1992).

Today the word that most commonly expresses this attempt to merge the contributions of different disciplines is "collaboration." However, there is yet no one commonly accepted definition of this word. Unfortunately, "collaboration" has become an overused word today. It represents an activity that is frequently offered as a solution to a variety of problems without understanding what the inherent interactions really entail.

The purpose of this chapter is to identify behaviors (strategies) and organizational structures that facilitate collaboration so all disciplines can work together for the good of the patient. First, however, the chapter will present findings from recent empirical studies documenting the value of collaboration by showing that it increases the quality of care and decreases costs, thus illustrating that collaboration is indeed worthy of further discussion and development. The chapter will also explain what is generally meant by the word *collaboration*.

VALUE OF COLLABORATION

For years nurses have believed that collaboration between nurses and other professionals improves the quality of patient care. However, only recently have researchers begun to document this relationship. Although most of these studies focus on nurse-physician collaboration, some studies have included other disciplines as well. These studies provide evidence that collaboration improves quality of care, increases patient satisfaction, increases nurse satisfaction, and reduces cost by decreasing length of stay and increasing nurse retention.

Knaus and his research team (1986) studied 13 units and concluded that the degree of coordination significantly influenced the effectiveness of care. Cannon (1988) noted that collaborative practice, facilitated by the agency's professional ethics and practice committee, increased satisfaction of professionals and resulted in improved procedures for the care and treatment of clients. Mitchell et al. (1989) found desirable clinical outcomes such as low turnover, low mortality ratio, no new complications, and high patient satisfaction existed in a unit perceived to have a high level of nurse-physician collaboration, a high level of nursing performance, and a positive organizational climate. Baggs and Ryan (1990) reported an empirical association between collaboration and satisfaction in the specific decision-making situation for nurses. Wandel and Pike (1991) found collaboration between nurses and physicians promoted nurse satisfaction by decreasing moral outrage among nurses faced with moral dilemmas and by developing an alliance between physicians and nurses that enhanced patient care. Knaus's research team later collected data from 42 units and noted that caregiver interaction, as measured by the culture, leadership, coordination, communication, and problem-solving abilities of the unit, was significantly associated with lower risk-adjusted length of stay, lower nurse turnover, higher evaluated technical quality of care, and greater evaluated ability to meet family member needs (Shortell et al., 1992). Alpert et al. (1992) also reported that collaborative efforts contributed to changes in attitudes toward collaboration among caregivers, increased job satisfaction for clinical nurses, and increased patient functional status on discharge.

DEFINITION OF COLLABORATION

Collaboration is often described as the act of working or laboring together. Hansen (1995) gives it a deeper meaning by noting collaboration is not so much an act as a process. Baggs and Schmitt's (1988) comprehensive review of collaboration literature too views collaboration as a process. This review was prompted by their observation that many of the studies of the value of collaboration neither formally defined nor systematically measured this process. The authors corrected this failing in their research by carefully defining collaboration as nurses and physicians cooperatively working together, sharing responsibility for solving problems, and making decisions to formulate and carry out plans for patient care. They also identified three additional behavioral concepts that are important to collaboration: coordination, cooperation, and sharing. Although this definition has guided subsequent work, Brown (1994) notes that the need remains for a commonly accepted and understood definition of collaboration.

Jones (1994) contributes to an overall understanding of collaboration by analyzing collaboration literature in light of nursing's original Social Policy Statement description of collaboration (American Nurses Association, 1980). This statement identifies four behavioral criteria for collaboration: mutual power-control, separate and combined practice spheres, mutual concerns, and common patient goals. However, Jones (1994) goes further by noting that collaboration can be conceptualized not only from this behavioral perspective, that is, what behaviors constitute collaboration, but also from the structural perspective, that is, how health care agencies can be organized to facilitate collaboration.

In summary it is generally agreed that collaboration involves communication. Yet not all communication is collaboration. Collaboration is best seen as a specific type of communication. It goes beyond a mere exchange of information, and it goes beyond a polite listening to the other person (Coeling and Wilcox, 1994). As Siegler and Whitney (1994) note, interdisciplinary collaboration must include *interaction* between members of different disciplines. Specifically, this interaction involves a back-and-forth sharing of ideas in which both parties feel free to either agree with each other or disagree and continue talking with and listening to each other. This latter activity involves speaking up when one has doubts about a decision or a better approach (Devereux, 1981) and continuing the interaction in an attempt to negotiate some sort of settlement regarding what should be done in a given situation (Wandel and Pike, 1991; Weiss and Davis, 1985). Hence the crux of **collaboration** is an exchange of ideas that considers the view of both self and others. It can involve disagreement with an idea, questioning an idea, or acting on the idea by acceptance, compromise, or development of a new plan (Coeling and Cukr, 1997).

What makes collaboration difficult is that each party must engage in these behaviors for an interaction to be truly collaborative. It is important that all parties do so for the ideas of each discipline to be heard. Patients benefit the most when the ideas and insights from a variety of disciplines contribute to their plan of care. Human beings are multifaceted creatures needing many perspectives to enhance their well-being. In addition, it is important to include patients in this collaboration by identifying, verifying, and determining with them which goals are of most importance to their lives. This chapter will now discuss various factors that promote this collaboration in the health care setting. These factors include two specific types of behavior, namely, recognizing different perspectives and achieving effective communication styles, as well as the concepts of time and organizational structure.

FACILITATORS OF COLLABORATION

Scholars are beginning to identify not only the value of collaboration but also the interpersonal behaviors and organizational structures that promote collaboration in the health care setting. The following pages will discuss these factors in turn, explaining them and offering theoretical and research support to motivate the reader to attend to these factors in daily activities. Important as it is to learn these behaviors, it is even more important to develop the desire or motivation to practice them. As Hanson and Spross (1996) and Prescott and Bowen (1985) note, collaboration is an interpersonal process that cannot be accomplished by mandate. Rather, as noted previously, the desire to collaborate must come from inside, and it comes from the desire to do good for the patient.

Recognizing Different Perspectives

Understanding each other would be relatively easy if we all had the same **perspective,** that is, if we all saw the world in the same way. However, common experience tells us that this is not the case. In actuality we see the world and all that happens in it from very different perspectives. These different perspectives arise from our different backgrounds and life experiences, our different personalities and biological makeup, and our different current life situations and future goals. The following section will address two sources of differing perspectives that have important implications in health care communication: professional orientation and gender orientation. Understanding these differences in perspective is a necessary step in collaborating with others.

Professional orientation
Differences in problem solving
Mitroff and Kilmann (1978) have drawn on the work of Jung (1971) to help professionals understand how interprofessional conflict results when different professionals use different approaches to solve the same problem. Jung delineates four

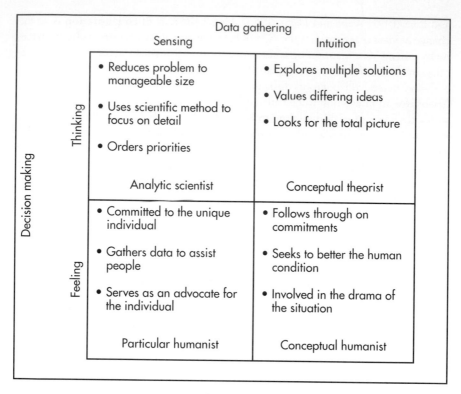

Figure 14-1 Examples of the ways in which different scientists think about and practice science. (Modified from Coeling HV, Wilcox JR: Professional recognition and high-quality patient care through collaboration: Two sides of the same coin, *Focus Crit Care* 18[3]:230, 1991; modified from Mitroff II, Kilmann RH: *Methodological approaches to social science,* Washington, DC, 1978, Jossey-Bass.)

common perspectives used to solve work-related problems. These four perspectives result from differing ways of perceiving the world in both gathering data and making decisions about a given situation. (See Figure 14-1.)

The two ways of taking in data are sensing (attending closely to the details of the situation and reducing problems to manageable units) and intuition (visualizing the entire picture). The two ways of decision making are thinking (explaining things in technical and theoretical terms) and feeling (reaching a decision based on human values and needs). Combining these different ways of taking in data and making decisions yields four modes of practicing science. However, it is important to remember that on a daily, if not hourly, basis every person uses both a dominant mode and a lesser-used mode. No person uses one mode exclusively.

One of these modes is reflected by the **analytic scientist,** who uses the scientific method to focus on detail and ordering of priorities. Another is seen in the **particu-**

lar humanist, who focuses on the unique individual and serves as an advocate for the individual. A third is found in the **conceptual humanist,** who is dedicated to bettering the human condition in general. A fourth is observed in the **conceptual theorist,** who looks for the total picture, exploring multiple solutions and differing ideas. Mitroff and Kilmann (1978) emphasize that all of these modes are scientific and all are important in arriving at the best decision for a complex situation. Although no person consistently acts in one mode or only in one mode, different disciplines favor different modes and educate their new members to practice using the mode favored by the discipline. Hence different health care disciplines will approach the same problem using different modes or perspectives.

Various researchers have documented how different health care disciplines use different modes as they practice their disciplines (Coeling and Wilcox, 1991; McCaulley, 1978; Myers and Davis, 1964). An example of these differing modes may be seen in the cardiac arrest situation. Physicians (documented by the aforementioned sources as being most like conceptual humanists), whose goal is to better the human condition by saving lives, work to restart a stopped heart. In contrast, nurses (described as particular humanists) focus on the individual patient's and family members' expressed preferences in determining the extent of revival efforts. Respiratory therapists (described as analytic scientists) base decisions on technical details such as the amount of oxygen getting to the cells. Finally, professionals such as chaplains and social workers (conceptual theorists) support participants by helping all to see the total picture.

What is important in collaboration is to recognize that each of these modes has value and is in fact necessary to reach the best answer for the patient. Quality care comes from integrating all four modes. Problems arise when professionals do not realize that what is important to them is not always what is important to the person working alongside of them. Insight into each other's mode is essential for working together. Encouraging all team members to verbalize their perspective and then weighing each approach give patients the benefit of many skills and increase the quality of their care.

Differences in organizational perspective

Another professional difference, in addition to the different ways of addressing a problem, is the differing perspective on how the professional fits into the organization. Hodes and Van Crombrugghe (1990) note that some professionals such as nurses are exposed to the "job" environment, including the organizational and managerial aspects of the setting and the need to work with others in the clinical area, early in their academic career. In contrast, physicians learn to be self-sufficient and make critical decisions alone. They are not as encouraged to coordinate their ideas with those of others so that interdisciplinary collaboration can be enhanced. Recognizing disciplinary differences regarding the importance of "fitting in" with the agency or organization can help health care professionals understand each other and appreciate the need to explain to the others where they are coming from.

Differences in use of power

A third difference in perspective relates to one's use of hierarchical power for compliance with one's directives. Again, some professionals such as physicians are inclined to rely on their power in the hierarchy rather than on dialogue with others for implementing their intervention for a given patient. Baggs (1994) refers to the physician's reliance on the hierarchy in comparing Stein's (1967) classic article on the "doctor-nurse game" with the 1990 update of this article by Stein, Watts, and Howell (1990). Baggs (1994) notes that although these authors describe a new relationship of "mutual interdependency" between nurses and physicians, they seem to decry a sense of a collapsing hierarchy, presumably caused by nurse-physician collaboration.

Additional evidence of these different perspectives of power comes from some rather puzzling research findings. Several research groups have found that different disciplines report different perceptions of the amount of collaboration occurring between nurses and physicians in a given situation (Baggs et al., 1992; Giardino, Giardino, and Burns, 1994; Grindel et al., 1996). These studies all note differences in perceptions between physicians and nurses regarding the amounts of collaboration that were occurring at the time of the study. Baggs et al. (1992) suggest that these different perceptions may be a function of one's organizational authority in that even a small amount of collaboration appears to be greater to someone who usually relies on hierarchical authority than to one who relies on "selling" one's ideas to others. Thus one's perception of one's place in the organizational hierarchy affects one's perspective of the amount of collaboration with those having different amounts of power. Again, recognizing this difference in reliance on hierarchical power can help nurses to understand why physicians may need to be reminded to seek input from other professionals. This recognition can also help physicians understand why nurses and other providers find collaboration with them so important and become distraught when they do not believe their ideas are being heard.

Gender orientation

Gender also influences the way we see the world and relate to others. Various scholars have noted that women are more expressive, nurturing, and relationship-oriented than men. In contrast men are more independent and task oriented and see themselves as more precise than women (Katzman and Roberts, 1988; Quinn and Smith, 1987; Tannen, 1990; Tannen, 1995). Tannen has noted that these differences are expressed as different ways of communicating with others. A woman's talk focuses on relationships and connecting herself to others, whereas a man's speech is used to explain things and demonstrate status. Women show they are listening to others by making noises, whereas men make noises to indicate agreement. Women look directly at each other when talking, whereas men tend not to establish frequent eye contact. Tannen reports that these are social behaviors learned at a young age. She goes on to explain that early on girls learn to downplay competition and focus on relationships (involvement, intimacy, and connections). In contrast, boys negotiate their status in the group through demonstrating their knowledge, skills, and scientific understanding.

Tannen (1990) recognizes the dangers of stereotyping gender, noting that these differences are not absolute and when they do exist are usually differences of degree. She warns, however, that pretending these differences do not exist is more dangerous than overemphasizing them because each gender lives in a different (their own) world and judges the other's behavior by their own standards. It is this judging by different standards that mitigates against collaboration.

It is important for health care professionals to recognize these differences because a number of disciplines have traditionally been primarily male or primarily female in nature. Although all health care disciplines today are showing more equal mixes of men and women, many of the professional norms, established when disciplines were dominated by a specific gender, remain. It will take time for these norms to change. Meanwhile it helps to be aware that these norms exist and influence the way we relate to others. It is also important to recognize dangers associated with each perspective.

The danger associated with the female emphasis on relationships is that female health care professionals may have difficulty relating to male colleagues if they do not feel recognized by them. Coeling and Wilcox (1994) note that this may explain why nurses are distressed by lack of feedback when talking with physicians. Nurses expect physicians to show their interest by vocalizing "hmm" and "uh-uh" and to look at them, rather than at the chart, when they are talking to physicians about a patient. Nurses interpret lack of these behaviors as disinterest rather than as a typical male response in which the physician may well be hearing what the nurses are saying. It would be more appropriate for nurses to recognize that physicians are demonstrating a typical male communication pattern when they do this, to accept this pattern as usual, and to learn to continue communicating even when the physician does not seem to be interested in or listening to their comments. Ask physicians sometime to repeat back what you just said when they did not appear to be interested. You may be surprised at how much they really heard. On the other hand, it is important for male providers to accept this female need for recognition and provide it for no other reason than that doing so can help nurses share important information that will improve the quality of the patient's care.

Another danger is nurses' response when they feel physicians are not showing them the affirmation or recognition they expect. As noted previously, men tend to focus on content, whereas women tend to focus on recognition and relationships. Coeling and Cukr (1997) report a study in which some nurses described interactions as noncollaborative because the physician did not communicate in an affirming manner. As one nurse said, "The goal [of the interaction] was accomplished, and the patient was seen, but the doctor demonstrated aggressive behavior." Hence the interaction was judged as noncollaborative. It is important for nurses to recognize that collaboration can occur even in the absence of affirmation. It is equally important, however, for physicians to appreciate nurses' desire for recognition to facilitate nurses' sharing important information.

What physicians desire in communicating with nurses is to have the patient-related information presented rapidly and in an organized manner (Coeling and Wilcox, 1994). The information physicians want the most relates to the medical decisions they need to make. The danger in overemphasizing this type of information is that the physician may miss important psychosocial data relevant to the patient's care. Eventually the nurse gives up trying to share important psychosocial information with the physician, to the detriment of the patient's well-being. The nurse can help the physician listen by providing information in a rapid and organized manner and by sharing information at appropriate times. Organizing data so it can be shared quickly takes mental work and preparation. Yet these activities are part of the nurse's role in sharing relevant information and collaborating with the physician.

In summary, collaboration involves helping the other person to communicate. In health care settings collaboration can be facilitated as the nurse learns to provide information in an organized manner and as the physician learns to show interest in the information the nurse does offer.

Achieving Effective Communication Styles

Another factor that affects collaboration is the **communication style,** or manner of speaking, one uses when speaking to another. Collaboration involves the back-and-forth communication between two or more persons. All parties involved must feel free to speak their mind. Gorden and Infante (1991) describe this as feeling a sense of freedom to voice one's ideas and concerns, especially those relating to efforts to improve a work situation. The style one uses in interacting with other health care professionals affects this sense of freedom to speak up. Styles that have been found to facilitate collaboration include nonaggressive, affirming, listening, confident, and indirect styles. Each will be discussed in turn.

Nonaggressive style

An **aggressive style** of communication is a style that attacks a person's self-concept by attacking the message or the speakers themselves (Infante and Wigley, 1986). Bradford (1989) notes that this aggressive style hinders collaboration by attacking persons to the extent they feel they are not even worthy of sharing their ideas. Research is now beginning to document that nonaggressive behavior facilitates communication (Coeling and Cukr, 1995; Coeling and Wilcox, 1994). Verbal aggression in the workplace is both harmful and counterproductive. Fortunately organizations today are making efforts to actively eliminate all forms of inappropriate aggression, including aggression toward any personnel by other personnel.

Affirming style

In contrast to an aggressive style, an **affirming style** acknowledges, recognizes, and endorses the individual as a human being and demonstrates a desire to hear what the other has to say (Laing, 1969). Norton (1983), who has studied this style extensively, describes it as a style that is relaxed, friendly, and attentive. In this style both parties perceive the other as a willing and receptive listener and refrain from responses that might be taken as negative. One is more likely to share relevant ideas and discuss differences when one feels good about oneself and believes the other person desires to hear what one has to say.

The importance of this affirming style in collaboration is now being documented. Coeling and Wilcox (1994) asked nurses to describe relationship styles that hindered nurse-physician communication. Of the three styles mentioned (aggressive, nonaffirming, and noncollaborating), 73% of the nurses indicated the style that most prevented their communicating with physicians was the nonaffirming style. In another study nurses reported perceived differences in client outcomes when physicians used friendly (p = .01), attentive (p = .0000), and relaxed (p = .0001) styles (Coeling and Cukr, 1995). Nurses also indicated that perceived client outcomes were significantly better (p = .01) when nurses themselves used a friendly style in communicating with physicians.

It is, however, important to recognize that an affirming style may be more important to some participants than to others. Coeling and Wilcox (1994) asked both physicians and nurses what would facilitate communication between the two disciplines. While nurses reported that improved relationships with physicians would best facilitate their communications, physicians stated that the most important factor was providing more factual data in a more organized manner. This difference of opinion may well be related to the different perspectives discussed previously in that men tend to focus on scientific explanations, whereas women emphasize relationships. It is important not only to develop appropriate styles but also to know what is most important to the professional with whom you happen to be speaking at the moment and to be able to adapt your manner of speaking to the needs and preferences of that particular person.

Listening style

Another effective style to promote the needed back-and-forth discussion in collaborating can be described as a **listening style,** that is, a style in which both parties hear what the other is saying. In their discussion of two different schools of communication, Rogers and Roethlisberger (1991) describe the importance of listening to the other person. One school assumes communication between A and B has failed when B does not accept what A has to say as being factual or valid, and the goal of communication is to get B to agree with A's opinions and ideas. In contrast, the other school assumes communication has failed when B does not feel free to express B's feelings to A because B fears they will not be accepted by A. Collaboration is facilitated when A and B are both willing to listen to each other's differences. Prescott and Bowen (1985) reinforce the value of the second school in the health care setting. They observe that physicians and nurses have differing perspectives on many patient care problems. These perspectives are based on the different but complementary orientations of the two disciplines and also on the types of information each possesses. Disagreement between the disciplines often protects patients, bringing various perspectives to light, and should not be discouraged.

Fisher and Ury (1981) and Pruitt (1983) stress the value of listening carefully to the other side as they encourage the collaborator to listen to the other person's interests. Having done this, both participants can work together to create options acceptable to both. This reconciliation comes only after each side hears about the interests underlying each other's proposals. To hear another person out, one must go deep into the other's request rather than rely on initially stated interests. Very often we share only our superficial or socially accepted desires and not our deep desires. Yet achieving our deeper desires promotes more satisfactory goal achievement. Showing a willingness to listen and a desire to hear all of the other's interests before proposing a solution increases the quality of the final agreement.

Professionals may hesitate to listen to others because they do not want to be asked to compromise, feeling they are giving in if they do not get all they want from an interaction. There is a basis in the literature for believing that one must be fully satisfied with the outcome for collaboration to occur. Kilmann and Thomas (1975) warn of the dangers of having neither party fully satisfied if conflict is resolved by compromise. However, negotiation scholars note that it is rare that any one party satisfies 100% of their interests in resolving a disagreement. Feeling you always have to get your way often results in a feeling of failure if you do not get all you wanted. This feeling of failure decreases the self-confidence needed for successful collaboration.

Confident style

Successful collaborators demonstrate a **confident style,** that is, a style that reflects assurance of the value of their own ideas and skills. Professional self-assurance involves a belief in what one knows and can do and the belief that this knowledge can enhance patient care. Weiss and Remen (1983), early researchers on nurse-physician collaboration, report that the behavior of nurses themselves often prevents nursing knowledge and abilities from being maximized. The nurses in this study often (1) lacked identification with the nursing profession in that they had great difficulty articulating the unique skills, knowledge, or philosophy of the professional domain of nursing, (2) invalidated their professional expertise in that they attributed their ideas to personal experience rather than a bona fide body of knowledge, and (3) demonstrated reluctance to assume greater responsibility. Prescott, Dennis, and Jacox (1987) document the influence of self-confidence that comes from experience, noting that the more knowledgeable and experienced nurses demonstrate more collaboration with physicians. Baldwin et al. (1987) also report that self-esteem correlates positively with nurse-physician collaboration. They explain that people who have high self-esteem tend to feel free and accepting of others and are able to state their opinions and hear the ideas of others.

Mariano (1989) notes that a thorough knowledge of one's own discipline is essential in seeing how that discipline contributes to the whole. Evans (1994) adds that assurance of one's competence is essential for development of a sense of internalized independence that is a cornerstone for successful collaboration. This confidence increases professionals' ability to integrate their own ideas and plans with those of other health care workers in a collaborative manner. Team members who feel secure and competent in their particular area can dialogue and communicate their discipline's contributions and limitations.

Thus all health care professionals must develop their clinical knowledge and expertise so they can be confident of their contribution to and participate actively in interdisciplinary dialogue. All health care professionals must believe that what their discipline contributes is necessary for enhancing patient well-being. Nurses must understand what nursing contributes to total patient well-being and take the initiative in explaining to other professionals what nursing is capable of doing. Nursing's Social Policy Statement provides a basis for this understanding (American Nurses Association, 1995).

Indirect style

Although generally a direct style facilitates collaboration, there are times when the indirect style has been found to be effective. This occurs especially in the presence of power differences between professionals. In this **indirect style,** questions or concerns are raised, but direct suggestions are not made. Waldron and Applegate (1994) describe the value of the indirect style by noting that it is a flexible communication style one can use to move the conversation away from the immediate state of disagreement toward the longer-term conversational objective of collaboration.

Several researchers have documented the value of this indirect style. Cunningham and Wilcox (1984) found that the degree of directness used by nurses when they perceived an inappropriate physician order depended on the situation. When there was high risk to the patient in carrying out an order, a certain degree of indirectness served to allow an opening move that then provided opportunity for further discussion. When patient risk was low, nurses used the more direct approach, feeling that if the physician rejected their direct suggestion, the patient would not be seriously harmed. Nurses also reported that they would use the indirect style if they expected a negative reaction from the physician. Coeling and Wilcox (1994) also report that the indirect approach was preferred by nurses as a way of approaching conflict in which they stand a better chance of getting their point across without the physician's getting defensive and leaving the scene before a resolution could be achieved. The value of an indirect style becomes clearer as one learns to view collaboration not as a one-sequence act but rather as a communication process occurring over a period of time.

Some professionals oppose the indirect style, explaining that it reinforces a subservient status. What is important to recognize, however, is (1) there are hierarchical power differences within the health care team and (2) hierarchical differences do not preclude collaboration. Fortunately hierarchical power is not the only source of power. Knowledge and clinical skills are also important sources of power. All competent health care providers possess these sources of power; effective collaboration skills can enhance these sources of power.

Using Time Effectively

A scarce resource to use wisely

Although time is a resource in short supply in most health care agencies, it is a resource that must be available for collaboration to occur. Many professionals are heard to decry the lack of time available to collaborate with their colleagues. Yet few studies have addressed the need for time to collaborate. In one study that did consider the time element, 12% of the nurses and 20% of the physicians reported that spending more time together facilitated communication. In a similar study of nurses only 2 years later, 25% of the nurses believed more time would promote nurse-physician communication, and 45% indicated that lack of time spent communicating hindered interdisciplinary communication (Coeling and Wilcox, 1994). The increasing workload of the past few years seems to allow less time for collaboration. Yet studies cited earlier in this chapter suggest that time spent on interdisciplinary communication has positive payback in terms of increasing quality and decreasing cost. Although one may think one does not have time to collaborate, especially as the pace of work life increases, in reality, one does not have time not to collaborate under these conditions. The less time one has, the more important it becomes to coordinate efforts so as not to waste the time available.

A necessary resource to develop relationships

Another aspect of time involves relationship development. Many professionals indicate that collaboration is easier if the two parties have known each other for some time and have had an opportunity to build a relationship of trust in each other's professional competence. Johnson (1992) notes that collaboration occurs more often when physicians work more closely with the same nurse, as they do in special care units. By being a more frequent observer of what nurses do, the physician is more willing to value the expertise demonstrated and share perceived responsibility. Pike and Alpert (1994) add that collaboration is an evolving relationship that develops over time while trust, mutual respect, and an understanding of the unique and complementary contributions that each professional makes to patient care are established. They also describe the value of facilitating collaboration by having a small number of providers who are able to practice together consistently over time. In their unit they limited the number of physicians who would admit patients to maintain this close relationship between providers.

Restructuring

As Pike and Alpert (1994) note, organizational structures influence the amount of collaboration that occurs. Jones (1994) and Devereux (1981) both review the structural elements recommended by the NJPC (1981) as ways to promote collaboration.

One recommended structural element is that of primary nursing. Primary nursing contributes to collaboration in that one specific nurse is individually responsible for the patient's comprehensive nursing care and can collaborate with the physician who is responsible for the patient's medical care. Having one nurse knowledgeable about all aspects of the patient's nursing care decreases fragmentation of that care and makes it easier for the physician to relate to one, rather than many, nurses relative to a given patient.

Another structural change proposed by the NJPC is that of the integrated patient record. This provides a formal means by which the physician and nurse can document in the same place and increases the likelihood that they will take the time to read each other's notes in doing so.

A third structural change that empowers nurses to enhance their contribution to patient care involves developing policies that facilitate nurses' decision making in their unique spheres of expertise. These policies encourage nurses to use their judgment and increase their self-efficacy in using their judgment. Involving nurses in decision making and collaboration goes hand in hand with joint rounds, which enable nurses and physicians to discuss their mutual concerns in a timely manner.

Also recommended by the NJPC are joint practice committees consisting of nurses and physicians who together monitor the collaborative process and develop standardized procedures for collaboration. Furthermore, the joint record review involves a common appraisal of the level of care, as well as learning to work together while the reviews occur and are processed.

Siegler and Whitney (1994) note that although the previous recommendations are all good suggestions, they have not been adequately tested because of the disintegration of the NJPC and failure of agencies to follow up on these suggestions. They remain worthy ideas that are in use in some agencies today, but they need to be tested further to document their contribution to collaboration. Readers willing to test out the effects of these approaches on collaboration will find Giardino and Jones's (1994) review of instruments for studying collaboration most helpful.

Cost constraints today are forcing providers to look more closely again at these and other structures used to increase collaboration. Allred, Arford, and Michel (1995) identify coordination as a critical element of managed care. They recommend many of the structural elements suggested by the NJPC and add several recent strategies such as critical pathways, discharge protocols, daily face-to-face discussions, and a hospital-community integration position. Hanson and Spross (1996) also identify the need for community-based initiatives at the grassroots level that coordinate hospital and home care efforts. They too state that health care delivery must be collaborative in nature if resources are to be used effectively and health care cost controlled. The need to develop and test out approaches for increasing collaboration has never been greater.

Summary

Evans (1994) notes that the role of the nurse manager is of crucial importance in establishing a structure that facilitates collaboration among all health care professionals. Yet she also addresses the paradox that true collaboration cannot be legislated, dictated, or designed by managers. The structure can be provided, and specific insights and styles can be developed, but the desire and willingness to enter a collaborative relationship with other providers, as well as the patient, have to be valued by each professional. Collaboration ultimately must come from a desire to do what is best for the patient. This may sometimes involve giving up recognition of oneself or one's profession and allowing ideas advanced by another to come to the fore if this is what is best for the patient. Collaboration occurs best when the focus of the collaborative effort is the patient rather than one's own self-interest.

Collaboration, an exchange of ideas that considers the views of both self and others, can maximize human ideas and insights to increase the quality of care and decrease cost. Understanding different perspectives, developing appropriate communication styles, utilizing time wisely, and structuring the environment appropriately all help to facilitate collaboration. These factors contribute the most when the focus of the collaborative effort is on the patient's well-being rather than on professionals themselves.

Discussion Questions

1. Increasingly patients are cared for within a multidisciplinary context, and collaboration may be an answer to efficient and efficacious care. What are the facilitating characteristics of health care providers who support effective collaboration?
2. Identify the variations in definitions of collaboration. What are the positive and negative features of both narrow and broad definitions?
3. Discuss modes of problem solving and identify which of these you believe is your frequently used mode as contrasted to a mode that you use rarely. What mode would you like to further develop, and why?
4. Explain how and to what extent organizational structure contributes to collaboration. Give an example from your nursing experiences. If you could improve this example, how could organizational structure be a modifier?

REFERENCES

Allred CA, Arford PH, Michel Y: Coordination as a critical element of managed care, *JONA* 25(12):21, 1995.

Alpert HB et al.: 7 gryzmish: Toward an understanding of collaboration, *Nurs Clin North Am* 27(1):47, 1992.

American Nurses Association: *Nursing: A social policy statement,* Kansas City, Mo, 1980, The Association.

American Nurses Association: *Nursing's Social Policy Statement,* Washington, DC, 1995, The Association.

Baggs JG: Collaboration between nurses and physicians. In McCloskey J, Grace HK, editors: *Current issues in nursing,* ed 4, St. Louis, 1994, Mosby.

Baggs JG, Ryan SA: ICU nurse-physician collaboration and nursing satisfaction, *Nurs Econ* 8:386, 1990.

Baggs JG, Schmitt MH: Collaboration between nurses and physicians, Image *J Nurs Sch* 20:145, 1988.

Baggs JG et al.: Collaboration in critical care, *Heart Lung* 21:18, 1992.

Baldwin A et al.: Nurse self-esteem and collaboration with physicians, *West J Nurs Res* 9:107, 1987.

Bradford R: Obstacles to collaborative practice, *Nurs Manage* 20(4):72I, 1989.

Brown BJ: From the editor, *Nurs Adm Q* 18(4):vi, 1994.

Cannon P: The professional ethics and practice committee: A step toward the achievement of excellence, *Nurs Adm Q* 12(4):53, 1988.

Coeling HV, Cukr PL: Components of collaboration. Paper presented at the Sixth National Conference of Nursing Administration Research, University of Minnesota, St Paul, Minn, 1995.

Coeling HV, Cukr PL: *Don't underestimate your collaboration skills,* Manuscript submitted for publication, 1997.

Coeling HV, Wilcox JR: Professional recognition and high-quality patient care through collaboration: Two sides of the same coin, *Focus Crit Care* 18(3):230, 1991.

Coeling HV, Wilcox JR: Steps to collaboration, *Nurs Adm Q* 18(4):44, 1994.

Cunningham MA, Wilcox JR: When an M.D. gives an R.N. a harmful order: Modifying a bind. In Bostrom R, editor: *International Communication Association yearbook 8,* Beverly Hills, Calif, 1984, Sage.

Devereux PM: Essential elements of nurse-physician collaboration, *J Nurs Adm* 11(5):19, 1981.

Evans JA: The role of the nurse manager in creating an environment for collaborative practice, *Holistic Nurse Pract* 8(3):22, 1994.

Fagin CM: Collaboration between nurses and physicians, *Nurs Health Care* 13:354, 1992.

Fisher R, Ury W: *Getting to yes: Negotiating agreement without giving in,* New York, 1981, Penguin.

Giardino AP, Giardino ER, Burns KM: Same place, different experience: Nurses and residents on pediatric emergency transport, *Holistic Nurse Pract* 8(3):54, 1994.

Giardino AP, Jones RA: Instruments for studying collaboration. In Siegler EL, Whitney FW, editors: *Nurse-physician collaboration,* New York, 1994, Springer.

Gorden WI, Infante DA: Test of a communication model of organizational commitment, *Communication Q* 39(2):144, 1991.

Grindel CG et al.: The practice environment project, *J Nurs Adm* 26(5):43, 1996.

Hansen HE: A model for collegiality among staff nurses in acute care, *J Nurs Adm* 25(12):11, 1995.

Hanson CM, Spross JA: Collaboration. In Hamric AB, Spross JA, Hanson CM, editors: *Advanced nursing practice: An integrative approach,* Philadelphia, 1996, WB Saunders.

Hodes JR, Van Crombrugghe P: Nurse-physician relationships, *Nurs Manage* 21(7):73, 1990.

Iglehart JK: Health policy report: Problems facing the nursing profession, *N Engl J Med* 317:646, 1987.

Infante DA, Wigley CJ III: Verbal aggressiveness: An interpersonal model and measure, *Communication Monogr* 53:61, 1986.

Johnson ND: Collaboration—An environment for optimal outcome, *Crit Care Nurs Q* 15(3):37, 1992.

Jones RAP: Conceptual development of nurse-physician collaboration, *Holistic Nurse Pract* 8(3):1, 1994.

Jung CG: *Psychological types,* Princeton, NJ, 1971 (originally published 1921), Princeton University Press (Translated by GC Baynes; edited by RFC Hull).

Katzman EM, Roberts JI: Nurse-physician conflicts as barriers to the enactment of nursing roles, *West J Nurs Res* 10:576, 1988.

Kilmann RH, Thomas KW: Interpersonal conflict–handling behavior as reflections of Jungian personality dimensions, *Psychol Rep* 37:971, 1975.

Knaus WA et al.: An evaluation of outcome from intensive care in major medical centers, *Ann Intern Med* 104(3):410, 1986.

Kyle M: Collaboration. In Snyder M, Mirr MP, editors: *Advanced practice nursing: A guide to professional development,* New York, 1995, Springer.

Laing D: *The self and others,* New York, 1969, Pantheon.

Lenkman S, Gribbins R: Multidisciplinary teams in the acute care setting, *Holistic Nurse Pract* 8(3):81, 1994.

Lysaught, JP: *From abstract into action,* New York, 1973, McGraw-Hill.

Mariano C: The case for interdisciplinary collaboration, *Nurs Outlook* 37:285, 1989.

McCaulley MH: *Executive summary: Application of the Myers-Briggs type indicator to medicine and other health professions,* Washington, DC, 1978, U.S. Department of Health, Education and Welfare.

Mitchell PH et al.: American Association of Critical-Care Nurses demonstration project: Profile of excellence in critical care nursing, *Heart Lung* 18:219, 1989.

Mitroff II, Kilmann RH: *Methodological approaches to social science,* Washington, DC, 1978, Jossey-Bass.

Myers IB, Davis JA: Relation of medical students' psychological type to their specialties twelve years later. Paper presented at the 1964 annual meeting of the American Psychological Association, Los Angeles, 1964.

National Joint Practice Commission: *Guidelines for establishing joint or collaborative practice in hospitals,* Chicago, 1981, Neely.

Norton R: *Communicator style,* Beverly Hills, Calif, 1983, Sage.

Pike AW, Alpert HB: On the scene: Pioneering the future—the 7 north model of nurse-physician collaboration, *Nurs Adm Q* 18(4):11, 1994.

Prescott PA, Bowen SA: Physician-nurse relationships, *Ann Intern Med* 103(1):127, 1985.

Prescott PA, Dennis KE, Jacox AK: Clinical decision making of staff nurses, *Image J Nurs Sch* 19:56, 1987.

Pruitt DG: Achieving integrative agreements. In Bazerman MH, Lweicki RJ, editors: *Negotiating in organizations,* Beverly Hills, Calif, 1983, Sage.

Quinn CA, Smith MD: *The professional commitment: Issues and ethics in nursing,* Philadelphia, 1987, WB Saunders.

Rogers CR, Roethlisberger FJ: Barriers and gateways to communication, *Harvard Business Review* 69(6):105, 1991.

Shortell SM et al.: Continuously improving patient care: Practical lessons and an assessment tool from the national ICU study, *Qual Rev Bull* 18(5):150, 1992.

Siegler EL, Whitney FW: Collaboration past and future. In Siegler EL, Whitney FW, editors: *Nurse-physician collaboration,* New York, 1994, Springer.

Stein LI: The doctor-nurse game, *Arch Gen Psychiatry* 16:699, 1967.

Stein LI, Watts DT, Howell T: Sounding board: The doctor-nurse game revisited, *N Engl J Med* 322:546, 1990.

Tannen D: *You just don't understand,* New York, 1990, Ballantine Books.

Tannen D: The power of talk: Who gets heard and why, *Harvard Business Review* 69(6):138, 1995.

Tellis-Nayak M, Tellis-Nayak V: Games that professionals play: The social psychology of physician-nurse interaction, *Soc Sci Med* 18:1063, 1984.

Waldron VR, Applegate JL: Interpersonal construct differentiation and conversational planning, *Communication Res* 21(1):3, 1994.

Wandel JC, Pike AW: Moral outrage and moral discourse in nurse-physician collaboration, *J Prof Nurs* 7:351, 1991.

Weiss S, Remen N: Self-limiting patterns of nursing behavior within a tripartite context involving consumers and physicians, *West J Nurs Res* 5:77, 1983.

Weiss SJ, Davis HP: Validity and reliability of the collaborative practice scales, *Nurs Res* 34:299, 1985.

chapter fifteen

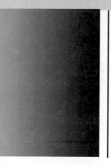

The Impact of Shared Governance on Resource Management

Carol Dobos
Robin Mobley

Learning Objectives

- Identify the characteristics of a shared governance management model.
- Identify nurse manager competencies that foster the success of shared governance.
- Identify nurse manager characteristics that hinder the success of shared governance.
- Explain the resource management advantages of a shared governance management model compared with a traditional bureaucratic hierarchical model.
- Identify one approach to the implementation of shared governance.

NURSING CARE DELIVERY SYSTEM EVOLUTION TO SHARED GOVERNANCE

Nursing care delivery systems and organizational structures have historically changed to respond to both internal and external forces. A series of nursing care delivery changes has led us to the current popularity and prevalence of shared governance. The following history of nursing care delivery systems will illustrate the path to shared governance.

In the early years of this century home care **case management** was the prevalent delivery mode. The nurse contracted directly with the patient or family for private duty nursing care. During and after the two world wars there was an increased demand for inpatient nursing care. **Functional nursing** was the norm based on the industrial model prevalent in the 1950s. During years of subsequent nursing shortages, team nursing was widely implemented.

During the 1970s there was a need to expand the accountability and autonomy of nurses at the bedside. **Primary nursing** was implemented in an effort to improve the job satisfaction and retention of experienced nurses at the bedside, as well as improve the continuity of patient care, which usually meant a greater emphasis on proactive patient teaching and discharge planning. Primary nursing enhanced the professionalism of nurses based on assigning the responsibility to plan, deliver, and coordinate care to a specific nurse rather than a team by function.

Because of the women's movement in the 1980s, women had increasingly more career choices perceived as higher status than the traditional teacher, secretary, or nurse. To attract and retain adequate numbers of registered nurses, equity including collegial status with other health care professionals was sought. Too often, however, nurses viewed themselves as independent practitioners instead of interdependent professionals working in collaboration with other professionals. In addition, many institutions contributed to a shortage of registered nurses and markedly increased the cost of care by erroneously insisting that primary nursing requires an all–registered nurse staff.

More recently the need to contain costs and reconceptualize registered nurses as an expensive commodity led to the redesigning of care delivery systems and roles. The most common structures developed included institutionally trained, multiskilled nonlicensed assistive personnel, or patient-focused technicians developed with the assistance of health care consultants. The present direction moves us toward a registered nurse population-based case manager. The focus is on ensuring predetermined optimal outcomes of care in terms of quality and costs across the continuum with the goal of keeping the patient out of the hospital. **Interdisciplinary care paths** for specific **diagnosis-related groups (DRGs)** within service lines along with accountability for variance monitoring and correction are becoming increasingly prevalent.

To realize essential efficiencies, cost savings, and increased customer satisfaction, the health care delivery team is changing from competition among individuals and professional groups to collaboration. Teamwork and collective decision making are necessary to improve systems and accomplish **continuous quality improvement** to survive in the 1990s. Shared governance was initially implemented within nursing departments to ensure accountability for clinical decision making at the bedside staff nurse level. Currently there is a need to develop a structure that brings out the talent and commitment of the health care team, which includes registered nurses, other professionals, and technical or support staff. Moving beyond only the nursing division, **whole-system shared governance** is being recognized as a mechanism to bring about the collaboration and synergy needed among the interdependent health care team members caring for the patient (Jones, 1994). In the past decade, over 1000 hospitals in the United States have implemented shared governance (Porter-O'Grady, 1992).

SHARED GOVERNANCE AND RESOURCE CONSUMPTION

Shared governance is an organizational management model designed to optimize human resources through an empowering accountability-based structure. Less dependency on bureaucracy and hierarchy for decision making has the potential to unleash the creative forces of staff to reduce costs while also improving patient outcomes.

During this time of diminishing health care resources, creativity and innovation are vital. Within a shared governance framework, leadership emerges from all members of the workforce to create team synergy and increased productivity based on a commitment to shared values and goals. Quality is built in instead of monitored and controlled by managers external to the natural work group.

Savings come from reduced rework, waste, customer dissatisfaction, and other organizational dysfunction. Shared governance encourages, facilitates, and develops staff to be less dependent on others to solve problems, manage relationships, and ensure consistent quality standards and outcomes are met, as well as discover and implement cost-effective strategies. Opportunities for immediate cost savings and value enhancements are lost when staff feel like they have to follow the lead of someone in authority. If they have to wait to be asked for ideas, which then have to be funneled through one or more individuals or layers of management who may not see or have the time to deal with it, the opportunity for savings may be lost or delayed.

Dobos (1994) found that while nurses can identify quality and resource utilization issues, they see the open identification of these issues as putting themselves at personal risk. Risks nurses take are identified as "questioning authority" or "speaking out." Some nurses subversively break rules or bypass the system to meet the needs of their patients instead of openly challenging the system to foster needed change. The fear of falling out of favor with those who have power over the nurse within the workplace prevents some nurses from exerting leadership in solving those problems. Skill development, role modeling, rewarding initiative, and removing barriers are needed. Some nurses fear that if they suggest a solution, they will be seen as stepping out of line or trying to take over the work of the supervisor. Fear of reprisal from peers, as well as management, sometimes exists.

Early in the implementation of shared governance an investment in time and educational resources is required to help staff develop the skills to be successful team leaders and members. The long-term benefits of increased staff accountability for cost containment and improved patient outcomes are well worth this initial investment.

SHARED GOVERNANCE DEFINED

Shared governance is a transitional model that provides a foundation for a more service-driven, horizontal health care organization. As a structure, it facilitates adaptation and accommodation yet provides format and context. Shared governance is a structure utilized in nursing management to build the organization around its service provider and support the relationship between the provider and the customer. All roles that do not directly provide service to the customer are there to support the provider.

Shared governance is a trust-based system empowering the care provider with accountability for predetermined outcomes. Empowerment is a process enabled but not initiated by management; it grows from the grass roots up. The freedom to make decisions, however, depends on the organizational structure and resources that empower the nurse.

The term *shared governance* can be divided to define the concept further. *Shared* is used to recognize the interdependency of people in the organization to meet the goals of the organization. **Governance** links the activities of nurses into the decision-making process of the organization. Shared governance therefore provides the structure for the accomplishment of goals and philosophy through professional decision making that links task with accountability. Shared governance provides staff members who assume both individual and collective responsibility for the adequacy and safety of the nursing care provided. Within the practice group is power, authority, accountability, and decision making related to patient care. The unit work culture is invested in the staff; staff are involved in planning. Decisions should be made closest to where the outcome will be felt. Participants need a sense of ownership for the change.

The staff are ready for shared governance when the culture contains a high degree of trust and there is evidence that staff are capable of managing their practice and work life. Shared governance is a way to see and think about the interactions in our health care system made possible by adding systems thinking to individual competency. **Individual accountability** is a key component. Individual competence and healthy self-esteem are important elements for shared governance to be successful. Staff must feel empowered by overcoming feelings of self-doubt and inequality. A high regard for one's competence, as well as a high degree of **self-efficacy** related to clinical care, is essential. Another essential element is a clear vision for achieving the desired clinical outcomes arrived at jointly and shared among staff.

Shared governance is more than **participative management.** To practice professionally, the individual requires accountability with control, as well as **authority** and **autonomy,** over factors related to the professional work. **Ownership** is key. Participative management by its very definition means allowing others to participate in decisions over which someone else, namely the nurse manager, has control. The staff realize that the decision to participate can be withdrawn at any time. True professionals own their roles demonstrated in their work. This ownership cannot be given or taken away except by their peers only when they have clearly compromised the standards embraced by their role.

ELEMENTS OF SHARED GOVERNANCE

Decisions within shared governance are made within a framework of nonmanagement work groups (usually called councils) that address professional practice issues

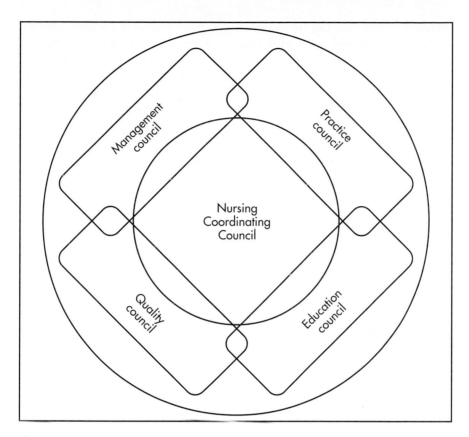

Figure 15-1 Councilor shared governance model. (Redrawn from Westrope RA et al.: Shared governance, from vision to reality, *J Nurs Adm* 25(12):47, 1995.)

and standards, care quality, staff competency, and peer relationships. Research that affects clinical practice is also often a component. A representative from each clinical division is usually found on each council. These councils are usually linked together by an **executive** or **coordinating council** composed of the individual council chairs and the nurse executive, as seen in Figure 15-1.

Councils are different from traditional committees. Committees usually function to advise decision makers and are not decision-making bodies. A council is an authority. The accountability of a shared governance council is clear and well defined, and its membership includes **stakeholders** in the area of specific accountability. Levels of approval are eliminated, resulting in quicker and more effective decisions. Those who must implement the decisions make the decisions. The nurse manager's role changes from being responsible for strategic decision making and controlling quality to strategic coordinator of finances, as well as facilitator for professional practice and teamwork. The aim is to increase quality and reduce costs by empowering all staff members to individually and collectively reach unit, patient care, and institutional and community health goals. Managers are responsible for human, fiscal, material, and system resources, a role vital to driving down the costs of providing care in all health care systems. Staff are accountable for practice and work issues, quality of work, outcomes and results, competence of workers, and decisions of teams. Lateral communication increases within shared governance. When staff take on this role, quality increases, and the manager is freed up to focus on resource issues.

NURSE MANAGER INFLUENCE

With shared governance the manager's role shifts from inspection and punishment to coaching and empowerment. It is the manager who will play the key role in guiding and teaching staff to become proficient in decision making and management of the unit. Managers who perceive themselves to be disempowered are more likely to behave in controlling ways, rigidly adhering to rules and regulations and withholding information in an attempt to preserve control over what little power they think they have. These behaviors interfere with the creation of a climate of trust and respect, which are fundamental to innovative work practices and organizational learning.

Initially, however, sharing power will be time consuming for the manager and difficult to achieve as staff learn to problem solve, communicate results, negotiate, and confront one another when conflict arises. Over time with appropriate support and commitment, staff will collectively develop the skills to effect change within the system; then the manager can redirect focus on maintaining the environment necessary for professional practice. The manager is no longer the ultimate decision maker but coach, teacher, and facilitator. Difficulties arise because it is easier for the staff to have the manager make the decisions. Mentoring staff through the learning curve is very time consuming and frustrating. Under stress power may easily revert back to the manager, and it is important to watch out for this. McConnell (1995) indicates that organizations have to bury at last the notion that the manager is the only person within a work group who is able to think creatively, plan, make decisions, and be accountable for outcomes. She states, "There is, within any given work group, a wealth of capability that will be largely wasted if it is allowed to lie undeveloped." The management model must support the individual and collective capability's being expressed and operationalized.

Porter-O'Grady (1995) indicates that given the opportunity, accountability will tend to escape from its appropriate **locus of control** and will go to the furthest possible point in the organization. The only sure way to ensure that accountability never escapes from the place it belongs is to remove the places or positions to which it can escape. Usually the escape is with the manager. With shared governance, the manager facilitates and enables rather than directs and controls. Learning new behaviors is always more difficult than persisting in existing relationships with known patterns. The successful nurse manager develops staff to leadership roles. A major ongoing **investment** is required in broadening staff's communication, collaboration, conflict management, and problem-solving skills. Significant behavioral changes are required.

The traditional management roles move from leading, organizing, planning, and controlling to the more cohesive roles of integrating, facilitating, and coordinating. Developing staff is also a key management role. The manager becomes a liaison, mentor, and facilitator with a strong sense of self to know when to let go and allow the process to grow in the hands of the staff. **Congruence** among philosophy, strategic plan, and behaviors is essential to build trust.

Drayton-Hargrove (1995) found that changing **organizational structure** to shared governance does not guarantee a changed leadership behavior. She found that although nurse managers desired to be more considerate and open to staff's independence, staff meetings continued to reveal a predominance of directive behaviors—information giving, direction, and criticism. Nurse managers continued to do most of the talking, with staff passively listening. When nurses did initiate conversation, ideas were not clarified or encouraged nor feelings accepted. It is clear that nurse managers need help to change old behavior patterns before shared governance can be truly operational. Manager education to develop supportive and flexible dialogue with staff is needed.

The successful managers of the future need to relinquish control, share decisions, build teams, and communicate well. Self-confidence is key. Those behaviors and roles that are reinforced by successful interactions and feedback of colleagues and managers will be internalized. There also needs to be a commitment to support each other in the spirit of true cooperation, embracing collegiality and interdependency.

Even with skill development and new leadership competencies, staff at the point of care will not remain committed to shared governance unless they see management move out of their way and staff are able to recognize the positive results of their own actions and innovative ideas. Nothing breeds success like success. Staff need to have access to information that allows them to see the outcome of their efforts. This can be done by highlighting staff leadership and involvement in performance improvement initiatives in internal publications, posted storyboards, staff meetings, and more broadly attended communications meetings.

As staff exhibit the desire and skills to accept responsibility for planning, decision making, and problem solving, there is usually less need for management within the organization. Thus a major stumbling block in implementing shared governance is the nurse managers' fear that if shared governance is successful, their role will become obsolete and their position eliminated. There are many opportunities for sabotage in the fragile beginnings of shared governance. In these times of rapid change no institution can promise permanent employment. To realize this is healthy. On the other hand, a manager wrought with fear who clings to the old is more likely to be passed over for new and expanded responsibilities in a redefined manager role more appropriate for today's managed care markets.

IMPLICATIONS AND OUTCOMES OF SHARED GOVERNANCE

Collaboration and Quality

Studies have shown that when shared governance is implemented, many positive benefits occur, affecting the staff, patients, and organization. **Professional collaboration** is a key component of shared governance. Knaus, Draper, and Wagner (1986) found that collaboration among health care team members significantly correlates with decreased mortality rates in hospitalized acutely ill adults. Similarly, Rubenstein, Josephson, and Wesland (1984) report that increased quality of life and decreased mortality in long-term care residents correlates with increased teamwork and planning among care providers. Although not carefully isolated, it is probable that the apparent efficiency and quality associated with professional collaboration may also decrease expenses.

Organizational Commitment

In testing Kanter's (1993) theory of structural power in organizations, Laschinger (1996) found that perceived staff access to opportunity, information, support, and resources found within a shared governance organization are related to factors associated with work effectiveness, such as less burnout and increased **organizational commitment, job autonomy,** and involvement in organizational decision making. By contrast, **hierarchical** and **bureaucratic** work environments have been shown to give only those in higher positions access to work empowerment structures, a situation that demotivates workers. After implementing shared governance, Westrope et al. (1995) demonstrated that staff nurses became more satisfied and more committed to their work environment and role. The staff's participating in important decisions was also linked to greater control over nursing practice and perceived more meaningful work. There was a direct positive effect on staff commitment to their jobs and the organization.

Job Satisfaction

According to Lucas (1991), "An effective practice environment is a critical feature of professional nursing practice designed to provide quality care in a cost-effective manner." **Job satisfaction** is a key variable in an effective practice environment, and increased job satisfaction has been demonstrated to be higher within a shared governance practice model (Vilardo, 1993). Nurses are more likely to be productive when they are satisfied in their position. Nakata and Saylor (1994) show that increased productivity enhances efficiency and improves patient outcomes, with the potential to reduce financial expenditures. Brodeck (1992) reports a significant reduction in hospital expenditures after 1 year with the implementation of shared governance. Morrison, Jones, and Fuller (1997) found that a shared governance organizational structure positively related to job satisfaction. Douglas (1995) found that empowerment positively correlated with outcomes of performance, customer satisfaction, organizational commitment, satisfaction with supervisors, and satisfaction with work. Spreitzer (1995) found that empowerment significantly correlated with innovative behavior and managerial effectiveness, both very necessary for organizations dealing with rapid and dramatic changes. Empowerment is defined as "increased intrinsic task motivation manifested in a set of four cognitions (meaning, competence, self-determination, and impact) reflecting an individual's orientation to his or her work role." (Spreitzer, 1995)

Employee Turnover

Shared governance has been shown to have a great impact on lowering turnover, a major expense for organizations. DeBacia, Jones, and Tornabeni (1993) found that when shared governance was implemented, significant savings resulted from the reduction in costs associated with recruiting, orienting, and training new staff nurses, as well as the use of registry personnel. In addition, increased productivity caused by the implementation of shared governance resulted in a 7.5% decrease in registered nurse hours per patient day as a result of increased **productivity.** Zelauskas and Howes (1992) found that implementing a shared governance model resulted in decreased turnover, decreased sick time used, and decreased cost per patient day. In addition, registered nurses experienced a positive change in perception of promotional opportunities and autonomy. In critical care Volk and Lucas (1991) found that nurses desire a more participative approach to management and when they perceive this increased participation, they are less likely to anticipate leaving their critical care positions. The authors summarize that centralized decision making can no longer be successful in a market-based economy and in critical care units where staff desire to participate. They found that nearly one third of the variance in anticipated turnover can be attributed to management style perceptions in the critical care units, and they recommend ensuring a style consistent with shared governance to keep turnover down.

Jones et al. (1993) evaluated the impact of shared governance on staff nurse perception of management style, group cohesion, job stress, job satisfaction, and anticipated turnover with favorable findings that demonstrate that shared governance improves the nursing practice environment. Within 2 years after the implementation of shared governance, there was a significant improvement in nurses' perception of management style, moving from benevolent-authoritative to a more consultative style. Nursing satisfaction with pay/reward, administration, and task requirements increased significantly, as did staff nurse perception of overall professional job satisfaction. Actual staff nurse turnover declined from 22% to 16%. In another study Ludemann and Brown (1989) conclude that evidence suggests that shared governance provides a system in which nurses perceive themselves working in an environment giving them greater influence, autonomy, and freedom to innovate. They also found job satisfaction increased.

Hastings and Waltz (1995) created a professional practice partnership shared governance model and found that satisfaction with control and responsibility for patient care was one of the strongest predictors of job satisfaction and diminished intent to leave. Variability occurred among units in the degree to which staff members perceived that they had been allowed to participate in decision making, as well as the degree of "letting go" that had been accomplished by the managers.

It is apparent that many outcome studies have reported favorable changes for nurses in autonomy, job satisfaction, collegiality, retention and turnover rates, and cost-effectiveness when shared governance is the organizational model (Hess, 1995). With the implementation of shared governance, organizations can expect increased job satisfaction, increased performance, decreased turnover, and improved patient outcomes, as well as financial savings.

The implementation of shared governance at any institution can be difficult and time consuming, yet the rewards are great. Box 15-1 is an example of how one hospital implemented this concept in its division of nursing.

Box 15-1

Implementing Shared Governance: One Institution's Experience

The Exploration Stage
The Vision

The vision for shared governance in this institution began with the Vice President of Patient Care Services. This nurse executive had been exposed to the concepts of shared governance through the literature, discussion with colleagues, and continuing education. The values embedded in shared governance were consistent with her philosophy of nursing care and nursing practice.

Reaching Consensus

The first stage to implement shared governance was to gain the support of the nursing division leadership. This proved to be a difficult step because of the lack of knowledge about shared governance, as well as the fear frontline managers had of possible elimination of their positions. Empowered staff require less management; this fear led to initial resistance and defensiveness. It was decided to move slowly. In July 1992 the Nursing Leadership Council approved the following goal: "The shared governance version of participative management will be explored." This goal was affirmed again in July 1993 by this body to continue to explore shared governance as a possible organizing framework for the division.

To facilitate this goal attainment, a shared governance task force was created from interested volunteers from all nursing roles, including direct care nurses, unit educators, clinical coordinators, clinical nurse specialists, administrative support staff, education, and management. The charge of the Shared Governance Task Force was to learn about shared governance from the perspective of many authors and institutions; to compare and contrast the philosophy, mission, and core values of the Nursing Division with those found in shared governance organizations; to compare the principles, processes, and structural components of shared governance with those at this institution; to

| **Box 15-1—cont'd**

determine the advantages and disadvantages of moving into a shared governance model; and to make specific recommendations regarding a shared governance model.

A second divisional goal set in July 1992 was to develop a vision statement for the division of nursing. It was determined that this goal was closely tied to shared governance, and thus the Shared Governance Task Force assumed responsibility for this goal.

The Shared Governance Task Force accomplished the following:

1. The creation of a shared vision statement in which all nursing employees took part in the development and validation.
2. The reading of volumes of articles and book chapters, listening to audiotapes, and watching several videotapes about shared governance. All committee members attended a local or national shared governance conference and networked with other nurses who had implemented or planned to implement a shared governance model for their nursing division.
3. The recommendation of and creation of a seminar on resolving conflict while respecting differences, which reinforced acceptance of accountability for problem solving in a direct, respectful, and honest way.
4. Conduction of shared governance focus groups on all shifts in all areas to identify and address staff's concerns regarding shared governance.
5. The sponsoring of a citywide shared governance conference with an internationally known expert on shared governance as the presenter.
6. Initiation of a shared governance communication task force that produced two shared governance communication sheets and published an article on shared governance in the division's employee publication.

The recommendation of the Shared Governance Task Force was very simple and straightforward:

1. To recommend the Shared Governance Task Force initiate a steering committee empowered to design and implement a shared governance structure to begin in fiscal year 1995 and to be fully implemented within 5 years.
2. The Shared Governance Task Force would then disband, with some carryover membership to the steering committee.

At the end of this year the task force determined that the idea of shared governance was something that would enhance not only the satisfaction of the staff but also the efficiency and effectiveness of the patient care they delivered. Once this decision was made, the Nursing Leadership Council decided to vote on the implementation of shared governance. A secret ballot was used to ensure that staff were not subject to peer or management pressure. The committee voted to implement shared governance with an overwhelming majority.

Continued

| Box 15-1—cont'd

The Planning Phase

A steering committee was appointed following the vote to implement shared governance. The charge of the steering committee was to develop a strategy to promote the vision of the nursing division through implementing a shared governance organizational strategy to begin in July 1994 and complete in 1999. To accomplish this charge, a 5-year plan was developed. This plan included the structural model chosen including decision-making bodies. The process was created by the establishment of policies and procedures, which later became bylaws. It was essential to develop communication, education, and feedback mechanisms, as well as develop a plan to work with resistance, misunderstanding, and miscommunication. It was also important to identify and unlearn old non–shared governance thinking and behaviors.

Eleven members made up this steering committee, eight of whom were staff representatives. Each committee member was given the homework assignment of completing their vision of the shared governance model that would work best at this institution. At the next meeting these were reviewed and the councilor model was decided on.

The size of the institution made it reasonable to have representatives from each unit council on each divisional council. Therefore five unit councils became the backbone of the model. Each of these councils sent one representative to the divisional councils, including clinical practice, quality improvement, administrative, research, and education. The chairpersons of each of these divisional councils made up the coordinating council.

Once a model was decided on, the steering committee considered guidelines for choosing membership, meeting times, the scope and responsibility of each council, and their relationship to existing committees, as well as the order in which to implement each council. Members were chosen initially by asking anyone interested in serving on a unit council to complete a form that asked why they would want to serve on a unit council and what they could contribute to a unit council. The responses were posted in each unit, and a vote was taken by members of the staff. Five registered nurses, one nursing care assistant, and one health unit coordinator were elected to the first unit councils. The membership of the divisional councils was made up of a representative from each unit council and others who were interested or involved in a project at the time. The steering committee did recommend that the councils remain small, no more than 8 to 12 members, but that all meetings be open and agendas be posted. It then became the responsibility of each unit council to determine how it would replace members.

One of the most difficult issues with which to deal was meeting times. The goal of the steering committee was to have representation from all shifts. This led to a very frustrating process of finding times that were convenient for all staff members to attend. Initially the steering committee left this decision up

Box 15-1—cont'd

to each unit and divisional council. Once the coordinating council was implemented, it recommended that one day a month be chosen for all shared governance council meetings.

The scope and responsibility of each council was developed by the steering committee and has since become the responsibility of the councils themselves. The relationship of councils to existing committees became important when implementing the councils. Questions were considered regarding the necessity of committees if the councils were picking up these responsibilities. This process went smoothly because most of the people already involved in the committees would also be involved in the council. Therefore several committees were disbanded.

The order in which councils were initiated did not seem to be a difficult issue. However, the steering committee felt very strongly that the unit councils should be initiated before any divisional councils. The steering committee remained intact until all councils were initiated and the coordinating council took over the responsibility for developing and monitoring the bylaws and the process of shared governance at this institution.

The Implementation Phase

Because of divisional redesign and numerous role changes, the implementation of the shared governance model was delayed 1 year until July 1995. The unit councils began in the spring and were functioning well by the time the divisional councils began meeting in July. The coordinating council was implemented in December 1995 and immediately began work on the bylaws.

The first year has been one of tremendous growth and change within the division of nursing. Shared governance has been the guiding force behind meeting the mission of the division, as well as maintaining the vision. Several issues have been difficult. The scope and responsibility of the councils have been the most difficult issue with which to deal. The coordinating council has been able to set up some guidelines that will help each of the councils be successful in the decisions it makes. The guidelines basically move the councils along on a continuum over the 5-year implementation phase. They begin with taking on clinical decisions about patient care, quality, competency, education, how to work together as a team, problem solving, collaboration, and standards of care. By the end of the implementation phase, many issues such as budget allocation and peer evaluation should be within the realm of decision making for council structure.

The process that this institution has used to implement shared governance is only an example of what can be accomplished. The nursing staff have begun to incorporate the idea of shared governance into daily practice. They send appropriate issues to the unit council for discussion.

Summary

It is clear that the old hierarchical, bureaucratic structures long in place for the delivery of care in most hospitals, home health agencies, and nursing homes simply do not work. To increase the survival of health care organizations in today's environment of diminishing health care resources coupled with increased consumer and payor expectations, a shared governance organizational model is an ideal structure to support staff productivity, creativity, and commitment. The organizational management model of shared governance has been shown to increase job satisfaction, employee motivation, staff retention, and productivity. It has the potential to increase staff flexibility, creativity, and commitment. Optimizing human resources and improving patient care are essential for health care systems to thrive in today's marketplace. An investment in time and staff and manager development is key. If managers are unable to change their relationship to staff toward a more collegial coaching style, the structural changes alone may not be sufficient to realize the anticipated gains.

Shared governance is a structure that supports proactive, innovative, and rapid response to the changing market in which health care is being delivered. Organizations must be flexible, fast, and market responsive. As discussed, meeting our internal customer's (staff) needs can enhance our ability to meet our external customer's needs. Shared governance helps us move from a paternalistic position to one with respect for the individual's personal and professional need for autonomy and empowerment.

With an empowered professional staff working as a team to reach clinical outcomes, the manager in a shared governance organization has more time and energy to focus on the external environment, assisting in the marketing of their organization to employers and managed care organizations. These strategies will help ensure the survival of the organization in the health care marketplace. It will continue to be important for management to partner with staff in the redesign of health care organizations and to collaborate in the process of continuous system change structuring (Armstrong and Stetler, 1991).

Discussion Questions

1. Describe the characteristic features of a shared governance management model.
2. What is the role of the nurse manager in a governance model? How does the manager foster or hinder the success of shared governance?
3. Describe and analyze the implications and outcomes of a shared governance model in relation to collaboration and quality, organizational commitment, job satisfaction, and employee turnover.

Case Study

A nursing administrator works in a health care organization that implemented shared governance 3 years ago. All of the units except two have active unit councils, full participation on shared governance councils, and good morale and retention. The nursing administrator has also noted that patient satisfaction, process improvement, and interdisciplinary collaboration have increased in all of the units except two that are managed by the same manager.

Case Study Exercise
1. What approach would the administrator need to take to determine the reason shared governance has not been successful on these two units?
2. If it is determined that the manager is not supportive of shared governance, what are the options to get those two units on track?

REFERENCES

Armstrong DM, Stetler CB: Strategic considerations in developing a delivery model, *Nurs Econ* 9(2):112, 1991.

Brodeck K: Professional practice actualized through an integrated shared governance and quality assurance model, *J Nurs Care Qual* 6(2):20, 1992.

DeBacia V, Jones K, Tornabeni JA: A cost-benefit analysis of shared governance, *J Nurs Adm* 23(7/8):50, 1993.

Dobos C: Personal, situational, and environmental factors influencing personal risk taking in nurses in clinical roles, doctoral dissertation, Memphis, 1994, University of Tennessee.

Douglas CA: Empowering work groups: Development and test of model of the empowerment process, doctoral dissertation, West Lafayette, Ind, 1995, Purdue University.

Drayton-Hargrove S: Changing organization structure alone does not change leadership behavior, *J Nurs Adm* 25(7/8):6, 1995.

Hastings C, Waltz C: Assessing the outcomes of professional practice redesign: Impact on staff nurse perceptions, *J Nurs Adm* 25(3).34, 1995.

Hess RB: Shared governance: Nursing's 20th-century Tower of Babel, *J Nurs Adm* 25(5):14, 1995.

Jones C et al.: Shared governance and the nursing practice environment, *Nurs Econ* 11(4):208, 1993.

Jones PK: Developing a collaborative professional role for the staff nurse in a shared governance model, *Holistic Nurs Pract* 8(3):32, 1994.

Kanter RM: *Men and women of the corporation,* New York, 1993, Basic Books.

Knaus W, Draper E, Wagner D: An evaluation of the outcomes from intensive care in major medical centers, *Ann Intern Med* 104:410, 1986.

Laschinger HKS: A theoretical approach to studying work empowerment in nursing: A review of studies testing Kanter's theory of structural power in organizations, *Nurs Adm Q* 20(2):25, 1996.

Lucas MD: Management style and job nurse satisfaction, *J Prof Nurs* 7(2):119, 1991.

Ludemann R, Brown C: Staff perceptions of shared governance, *Nurs Adm Q,* 13(4):49, 1989.

McConnell CR: Delegation versus empowerment: What, how, and is there a difference? *Health Care Supervisor* 14(1):69, 1995.

Morrison RS, Jones L, Fuller B: The relationship between leadership style and empowerment on job satisfaction of nurses, *J Nurs Adm* 27(5):27, 1997.

Nakata JA, Saylor C: Management style and staff nurse satisfaction in a changing environment, *Nurs Adm Q* 18(3):51, 1994.

Porter-O'Grady T: *Implementing shared governance: Creating a professional organization,* St. Louis, 1992, Mosby.

Porter-O'Grady T: *The leadership revolution in health care: Altering systems changing behaviors,* Gaithersburg, Md, 1995, Aspen.

Rubenstein L, Josephson K, Wesland G: Effectiveness of a geriatric evaluation unit, *N Engl J Med* 311:1664, 1984.

Spreitzer GM: Psychological empowerment in the workplace: Dimensions, measurement, and validation, *Acad Manage J* 38(5):1442, 1995.

Vilardo LE: Linking collaborative governance with job satisfaction, *Nurs Manage* 24(6):75, 1993.

Volk MC, Lucas MD: Relationship of management style and anticipated turnover, *Dim Crit Care Nurs* 10(1):35, 1991.

Westrope RA et al.: Shared governance, from vision to reality, *J Nurs Adm* 25(12):45, 1995.

Zelauskas B, Howes DG: The effect of implementing a professional practice model, *J Nurs Adm* 22(7/8):18, 1992.

chapter **sixteen**

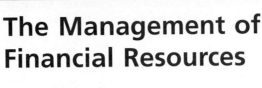

The Management of Financial Resources

Cheryl Slagle King
Ann E. Koliner

Learning Objectives

- Utilize the key nursing financial performance indicators to make effective decisions in the management of nursing financial resources.
- Evaluate strategies to effectively manage financial resources in response to internal and external pressures in the health care environment.
- Describe the budgeting process.
- Recognize the value of external benchmarking in the management of financial resources.

Christine Wilson, RN, the nurse manager of 6 South, left the conference room contemplating what Paula Thompson, the vice president of nursing, had said: "It is the responsibility of every individual employed within the Department of Nursing not only to contribute to the quality of care provided but also to deliver care in a cost-effective manner."

Christine understood the increased pressure on all providers across the health care continuum to reduce costs. Hospitals were once the land of plenty in the days of fee-for-service reimbursement, when every dollar spent was returned to the provider with no questions asked. This system resulted in America's current state of health care affairs, with costs expected to reach 16.2% of the gross national product over the next several years (August, 1995). Today hospitals face capitation under managed care agreements, which pay providers a fixed fee per plan member regardless of the services a patient receives, shorter inpatient hospital lengths of stay, a transition to increased outpatient treatments, and decreasing reimbursements (West, 1996).

Christine reviewed the handout distributed at the meeting by Paula Thompson. It was an outline of a lecture series designed to address the educational needs of the nursing staff on the issue of financial resource management to facilitate high-quality, cost-competitive nursing care. The first section on the outline was "Internal Sources of Information for Resource Management." Christine recently finished working on the budget for 6 South for the upcoming year, so she wasn't surprised to see that the detail under this section included types of budgets, the budgeting cycle, and a systemwide financial overview. Christine also knew that 90% of nursing service budget is allocated to pay the salaries of the nursing staff, demonstrating the need for staff to understand the impact of the utilization of staffing resources on the cost of care. The detail under this section included a series of evaluation measures enabling staff to monitor their units' financial performance.

The next section, "External Information Sources," provided an opportunity to benchmark with health care professionals in other hospitals to share information and, if applicable, exchange performance-enhancing strategies. Christine thought the third and final section, "Strategies to Manage Financial Resources," developed as a case study to encourage interactive learning, would provide an excellent opportunity to address necessary interventions in response to internal and external market pressures.

Paula Thompson had asked the management team to review the draft of the lecture series on financial resource management, make recommendations for revisions, and form a group to focus on applying the concepts at the unit level. Christine was excited about the opportunity to build a foundation of shared knowledge with the staff. She believed if the staff understood why certain decisions and strategies were proposed, generating solutions would become a joint venture between management and staff. Christine returned to 6 South looking forward to finalizing the education plan and initiating staff development.

Two days later Christine entered the conference room to meet with her colleagues to review the staff education plan for the lecture series. Joan Lewis, the nurse educator, prepared an overview for the group. The overview stressed the importance of gathering financially relevant information and data from within the organization and across the continuum of care to make effective decisions about operational performance. The overview also focused on utilizing all sources of information, especially incorporating external benchmarking data sources and environmental data collected from the community.

The group met on a regular basis, completed the content for the lecture series, and prepared a presentation of the material for the entire nursing management team. Christine took one last look at the material.

INTERNAL SOURCES OF INFORMATION FOR RESOURCE MANAGEMENT: LECTURE SERIES—PART I

The first step in the process of efficient management of financial resources is to accurately forecast the organization's operating plan and budgets based on both the short- and long-term operational strategic goals and objectives. Administrators should consider the following factors when forecasting the next fiscal year's operating performance, especially as the health care environment shifts toward managed care and capitation payments (Jones, 1994):

- Historical utilization trends in all settings across the continuum of care
- Costs of delivering a volume of services
- Changes in physician practice patterns
- New or deleted programs, products, or technologies
- Changes in patient acuity and average length of stay
- Managed care contracts and integrated network developments

These factors become the set of assumptions driving the decision-making process and are critical to successful operations. These assumptions reflect management's best judgment, based on present circumstances, of expected future conditions and also serve as the basis for future decisions and actions. Based on these assumptions, goals will be established that will reflect the organization's service volume, revenue, and expense projections for the next fiscal year. Attainment of the goals is expected, although unanticipated events and circumstances may cause the forecast to vary from the actual projection, challenging management to reevaluate and redirect their efforts.

The Profit and Loss Statement

The profit and loss statement is the expression of the hospital's performance for a fiscal year. The profit and loss statement shows the revenue (the money received) the organization generated from (1) operations associated with providing patient care, (2) operations not associated with patient care, and (3) nonoperating sources of income. Allowances for bad debts, or uncollectible bills, charity care, and contractual allowances, the difference between what is billed and what is actually collected, must be included when calculating total revenue (Bertram and Wilson, 1991). Expenses, the costs of being in business and maintaining the organization's operations, are deducted from the adjusted revenue to reflect a profit or loss position. Costs can be broken down into direct and indirect costs. Direct costs such as the nursing salary expense result from providing an actual service. Indirect costs refer to all other costs incurred by the organization that cannot be traced to the provision of patient care, including administrative salaries and utilities (Klann, 1989). See Table 16-1 for an example of a profit and loss statement illustrating declining revenues and increasing expenses.

In preparation for the budget development process, Christine Wilson and the other nurse managers at Yourtown General Hospital (YGH) have gathered their data on the hospital's past and anticipated operating performances. The organization has established the strategic goals of reducing nursing expenses by 5% and reducing total nursing full-time equivalents (FTEs) by 2%. These are aligned with the next year's fiscal performance, based on forecasted projections of the organizational utilization trends. With this information Christine and the other nurse managers are in the position to develop the nursing budget, which will become the template for effective financial and strategic decision making in the next fiscal year.

Table 16-1

YGH Hospital Statement of Profit and Loss for the 12 Months Ending June 30, 1996 (in Thousands)

	FY 1997 Budget	FY 1996 Actual	Increase (Decrease)	Percent Change
Revenue				
Inpatient	$312,448	$311,243	$1,205	0.4%
Outpatient	82,537	82,877	(340)	(0.4)
Physician services	4,340	2,131	2,209	103.7
Other operating	23,547	15,300	8,247	53.9
Nonoperating income	16,343	31,427	(15,084)	(48.0)
Total Revenue	$439,215	$442,978	($3,763)	(0.9)%
Expenses				
Salaries, wages, and fees	154,329	164,283	(9,954)	(6.1)
Fringe benefits	35,947	32,843	3,104	9.5
Patient care supplies	64,812	66,657	(1,845)	(2.8)
Purchased services	94,012	79,451	14,561	18.3
Administrative and general	36,664	33,704	2,960	8.8
Depreciation and amortization	29,637	28,209	1,428	5.1
Interest	14,284	14,907	(623)	(4.2)
Total Expenses	$429,685	$420,054	$9,631	2.3%
Excess of Revenue Over Expenses	$9,530	$22,924	($13,394)	(58.4)%

The Budget

The budget is a written plan for the future developed to allocate resources based on the organization's goals and objectives for the proposed series of programs that will provide patient care services during one fiscal year (Lane-McGraw and Villemarie, 1986). Budgeting should be an action-oriented, continual process of translating a manager's plans into financial terms and an evaluation process using financial and statistical criteria. The budget is a document that represents management's best estimate of the next fiscal year's operating performance, resource requirements, and productivity gains and will provide a standard of comparison, an internal benchmark against which financial performance can be measured. Furthermore, budgeting is a process in which plans are developed, followed by an effort to meet or exceed the plans. Budgets without a system of evaluation to ensure that financial performance objectives are met lose much of their value (Finkler, 1992).

The purpose of the nursing budget is to establish a decision-making mechanism supporting the operations of both the nursing department and the individual units. This is accomplished by the following (Jones, 1994):

- Linking financial resources to human resources
- Determining the department's spending schedule
- Establishing measures of performance
- Analyzing the department's or unit's actual performance
- Evaluating management's performance
- Increasing the manager's and nursing staff's cost awareness

The budgeting process and the "nursing process" share a similar purpose. Both processes are continual systems of assessment, planning, implementing, and evaluating (Bertram and Wilson, 1991).

Budget types

The four most commonly used budgets in health care organizations are as follows (Bertram and Wilson, 1991):

1. The **revenue budget** forecasts the organization's activity for the year. Activity refers to the projected number of patient days, case types, procedures, or visits along the continuum of care.
2. The **capital budget** forecasts the organization's needs for capital equipment for operations and projects such as renovations and improvements or new construction.
3. The **operating budget** projects the organization's day-to-day financial operations for a fiscal year. Revenues from the various payors and other revenue-generating sources, adjustments to revenue, and all the expenses of managing each cost center within the organization are documented in this budget.
4. The **personal budget** is a subset of the operating budget. Health care organizations are extremely labor intensive, requiring careful forecasting of the labor force's requirements and costs.

The operating budget is the primary nursing budget. Nurse managers are most concerned with the expense portion of the operating budget because this is within their realm of control. The revenue portion of the budget, with its associated components of charges, fees, or prices, is not controlled by the nurse manager because reimbursement rates from the various payors are externally driven. However, mid-year changes in these reimbursement rates may result in changes in the expense budget.

Nursing salary costs are a hospital's single largest expenditure and present the opportunity for the most control over the budget (Spitzer-Lehmann, 1994). About 60% of all hospital employees are nursing personnel (Lane-McGraw and Villemarie, 1986). To be fiscally responsible, nurse managers are challenged to efficiently allocate staff during times of fluctuating census. The nursing care delivery model and the skill mix must be clearly defined, and organizational support systems must be in place to facilitate operations to maximize nursing productivity and to minimize expenses.

Box 16-1

Determination of Required FTEs

Method 1—Utilizing Worked Hours per Patient Day
Required FTEs = (ADC × 365 × WHPPD × vacation, holiday, and sickness factor)/2080

Method 2—Utilizing Average Daily Census and Nurse/Patient Ratios
Required FTEs = {[(ADC/ratio days) + (ADC/ratio evenings) + (ADC/ratio nights)] × (8 hours per shift) × (365 days) × (vacation, holiday, and sickness factor}/(2080 work hours in a period)

Budget variance analysis and justification

The nursing budget format establishes a comparison between the revenues and expenses that have been budgeted and those actually experienced for a given period of time, usually using a monthly and a year-to-date time frame. The difference between the budgeted and the actual revenue or expenses represents a variance. Variances present an opportunity to evaluate the effectiveness of operational performance, and they can be expressed as a dollar amount or as a percentage. An unfavorable expense variance reveals that the actual expense was greater than the budgeted expense or that the actual revenue was less than the budgeted revenue; however, the analysis cannot stop with the realization of an unfavorable variance. Additional questions for consideration include, "Why was the expense greater than anticipated?" "Was there offsetting revenue as a result of increased patient activity?" "Did we manage our resources appropriately?", and "How can we do it better?". This process of variance analysis presents a mechanism for the nurse manager to develop accountability and responsibility for the fiscal year's financial goals and objectives (Felteau, 1992).

Full-Time Equivalent Determination

The staffing expense segment of the budget considers the number of FTEs, the number of positions, and the costs of these positions. An FTE is the equivalent of one full-time staff member's normal working schedule, usually 2080 hours per year, or 40 hours per week for 52 weeks (Lane-McGraw and Villemarie, 1986). It is not an actual person or a position. To determine the number of FTEs necessary to staff a unit and their costs, both average daily census (ADC) and worked hours per patient day (WHPPD) must be calculated. In addition to the WHPPD calculation, a replacement factor must be included to account for paid time off for vacation, holidays, sick time, and nonproductive time (Kirk, 1986). This factor represents the amount of time for which an FTE is paid but not the number of hours the FTE actually works. (See Box 16-1.) Organizations usually use a standardized replacement factor value. The replacement factor value ranges from 1.12 to 1.15, depending on the organization's benefit package.

As hospital lengths of stay decrease and as the current trend of increasing numbers of procedures being performed on an outpatient basis intensifies, those patients who are hospitalized will tend to be sicker, requiring a greater number of FTEs per patient. Intensive care units have lower patient-to-nurse ratios than non–intensive care units. In the long-term care environment the minimum number of required FTEs is mandated by the Health Care Financing Administration, the Medicare regulatory agency. In the ambulatory setting the recommended number of FTEs per physician is available from external benchmark data. Usually a specialist practice requires more FTEs per physician than a primary care practice.

Once the number of FTEs has been established, a cost must be assigned. Each FTE has a salary classification and an associated hourly rate. Salary expense for a cost center can be calculated by multiplying the FTEs' assigned hours by their hourly rate. A summation of all salary expenses from all of nursing's cost centers determines the total nursing salary expense.

Key Indicators

The key indicators used for allocating nursing's financial resources are volume, productivity, and cost per unit of service.

Volume

Volume is expressed as a unit of service. The unit of service is a basic measure of an item or service produced by the health care organization (Finkler, 1992). It can be an estimate of the total number of patient days or cases in the inpatient setting or the number of visits in an ambulatory or home care setting in a fiscal year.

The fiscal year can vary among organizations. Some organizations' fiscal year runs from July 1 to June 31, whereas others operate within a calendar year. It is not important how the organization defines its fiscal year for financial resource management; however, a consistent fiscal year ensures a constant basis for comparisons over time.

The total number of patient days in a fiscal year can be divided into numbers of patients in a particular operating period, which can be expressed as a quarter, month, or week. This allows for an internal historical comparison of seasonal variations, which can be indicative of trends. An awareness of trends presents opportunities for nurse managers to allocate their resources in response to these trends. For example, to schedule staff based on volume by day of the week, volume trends on specific days of the week can be reviewed and staffing can be assigned accordingly to maximize the efficient utilization of staffing resources.

Historical health care utilization patterns are changing across the continuum of care, creating a roller-coaster ride for all participants. As illustrated in Figure 16-1, inpatient activity levels, expressed by ADC by quarter, fluctuated significantly because of changes that were attributed to managed care contract negotiations, hospital and physician network development, shorter patient lengths of stay, case management, and transition of patient care services to alternative settings across the continuum.

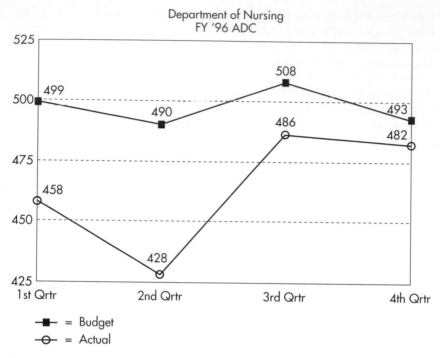

Figure 16-1 Average daily census (ADC) = number of patient days/number of days in a period.

Nursing productivity measures

Productivity is the ratio of output to input. Input such as labor, supplies, and equipment is consumed in the production of an output of goods and services (Kirk, 1986). To increase productivity by creating a greater output of goods and services, the amount and types of input or the processes used to produce the goods or services can be changed (Kirk, 1986). For example, to increase the amount of time that nurses spend providing actual patient care (a desirable output), YGH considered changing its charting practice from a traditional narrative charting format to charting by exception to reduce the amount of time spent on nursing documentation. By changing a process, nursing productivity can significantly be improved. The two most frequently used nursing productivity measures are worked hours per patient day (WHPPD) and the number of FTEs per occupied bed.

The skill mix of the nursing personnel must be aligned with the organization's financial goals. To maximize nursing productivity, organizations may choose to redesign their patient care delivery systems. At a time when health care financial resources are scarce, a greater use of supportive personnel can permit the registered nurse to practice at an advanced level by appropriately delegating clerical and ancillary tasks without affecting the quality of care (Lane-McGraw and Villemarie, 1986).

Box 16-2

Worked Hours per Patient Day (WHPPD) = Total Direct Care Hours Required/Total Patient Days

Steps to calculate the WHPPD for a nursing unit (Kirk, 1986):

1. Direct FTEs = (total FTEs − fixed FTEs*) − (average nonproductive hours paid per FTE)
2. Annual direct care hours = (direct FTEs) × (annual FTE work hours)
3. Budgeted WHPPD = (annual direct care hours)/(projected patient days)

A fixed FTE provides indirect care to the patient, for example, unit secretary or nurse manager.

Worked hours per patient day

WHPPD are the average hours budgeted to provide direct care for one patient for one 24-hour period (Lane-McGraw and Villemarie, 1986). (See Box 16-2.)

The budgeted WHPPD value is usually treated as a unit-specific constant. To determine the appropriate budgeted WHPPD value, data comparisons of the WHPPD national averages from similar institutions, internal historical data analysis, and pilot studies on selected units should be completed (Neely and Strickland, 1995).

WHPPD can vary from unit to unit depending on the patient care requirements. Factors that can influence the WHPPD value include patient acuity, skill mix, standards of care, patient care support systems, and patient average length of stay (Spitzer-Lehmann, 1994). Actual and budgeted worked hours per patient day variances are calculated in the budget. Productivity monitoring or WHPPD variance analysis can assist nursing managers in investigating the implications of a variance on the operations of the units. For example, if the WHPPD value is greater than the budgeted amount, an unfavorable variance, the units may be overstaffed for the actual census level. An increase in case mix index or a change in patient type could also negatively affect the WHPPD statistic. If an earlier discharge from an intensive care unit imposes increased patient care requirements on an acute care unit, WHPPD on the unit will increase. The ultimate goal for a nurse manager is to adjust staffing cost effectively in response to census variations and patient requirements.

Number of FTEs per occupied bed

The number of FTEs per occupied bed is another commonly used productivity statistic. The number of FTEs per occupied bed determines the number of FTEs required to take care of one patient in one bed.

Number FTEs per occupied bed = authorized base of FTEs/ADC

The authorized base can be a nursing statistic, or it may represent the total number of FTEs in the organization. The number of FTEs per occupied bed measure demonstrates the efficiency of the organization or department in providing patient care services. For example, if the ratio of FTE per occupied bed increases when census declines significantly, productivity has declined and an investigation is indicated (Douglas and Mayewski, 1996).

WHPPD and the number of FTEs per occupied bed statistics provide useful information about the amount of nursing time utilized or the number of FTEs employed for a given volume of patients. However, neither statistic addresses the issue of the associated costs. All classifications of FTEs, or direct caregivers, who provide patient care are not paid for their services equally. It is important to remember that a nursing assistant's hourly wage rate is less than that of a registered nurse (RN), and an agency RN or casual pool RN is more expensive than a staff RN. WHPPD and FTE per occupied bed indicators are more effective for making decisions when used in conjunction with financial indicators. Only when indicators based on cost per unit of service are consistently utilized for financial decision making will nursing be able to effectively measure operational performance (Spitzer-Lehmann, 1994).

Nursing Costs Based on a Unit of Service

Nursing salary costs per patient day based on a unit of service

Nursing salary cost per patient day is a key nursing indicator calculated from the nursing budget. The nursing salary cost per patient day is the average cost of providing care to one patient for one day. This indicator is based on volume, which is a unit of service. It incorporates all labor costs, including nursing and noncaregiver salaries, benefits, orientation, and education time for each unit (Walts, 1991). The nursing salary cost per patient day can be calculated for all nursing units so that comparisons can be made between units with similar patient profiles. A significant variance between similar units could alert managers and staff to the possibility that the lower salary cost units may be understaffed or that skill mix may need to be re-evaluated on the higher cost units. The nursing salary cost per patient day and the nursing salary expense can be trended over time and compared with budget for fiscal evaluation. For example, a trended nursing salary cost per patient day can demonstrate the effectiveness of a nursing cost reduction strategy. (See Figure 16-2.) It could identify staffing problems that may interfere with the primary objective of providing patient care (Walts, 1991).

Nursing costs per patient day

Nursing costs per patient day include all of nursing's expenses. This statistic includes labor cost, which is the most significant portion of the nursing budget, plus supplies, support services expenses, and general expenses such as travel, special events, publications and subscriptions, and postage.

Nursing cost per patient day = total nursing costs/total patient days for a time period

This statistic is nursing's global average cost per unit of service. It can be used to look at the entire department's operational performance. If nursing salary expenses

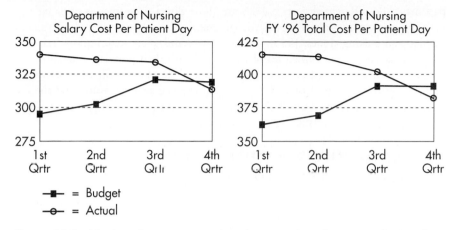

Figure 16-2 Nursing salary costs per patient day = nursing salary expense/patient days for a time period.

per patient day trends are stable and the nursing costs per patient day trends are increasing compared with budget, this provides a signal that the variance can be attributed to other nursing expenses.

Nursing expenses
Trended and point in time comparisons of nursing expenses, both salary and total expenses, can also be valuable tools for decision making, especially when variances between expected and budgeted nursing expenses are analyzed.

Cost per case
As managed care and capitated payment plans make greater inroads in local health care markets, organizations must be able to establish a cost per case, or episode of care, to compete for managed care contracts. The global costs of providing care for a group of patients with a common diagnosis, usually a diagnosis-related group (DRG), across the continuum of care must be determined. For example, a patient may be admitted to an acute care hospital for an orthopedic procedure that will also require long-term care and rehabilitation. The cost per case must include the cost of care provided in each of these settings (Finkler and Kovner, 1993). The goal in product or DRG costing is establishing an equilibrium in which costs are competitive without jeopardizing quality.

Full or total cost per case is the sum of all the costs that are directly related to providing care plus the indirect costs such as utilities and administrative salaries that are not directly traceable to the actual care divided by the number of cases (Walts, 1991). This method of calculation allocates all related hospital expenses, establishing an average cost per case measurement. Direct cost per case, on the other hand, includes only those costs that are directly related to providing the patient care divided by the number of cases. If an organization considers adding a pediatric department, the differential costs, which are those direct costs that vary or change with the implementation of a pediatric program, should be considered relevant in the decision making (Jones, 1995). On the other hand, if an organization desires to accept a managed care contract for obstetrical care for their population of subscribers at a deeply discounted price, total cost per case should be utilized when calculating a contractual price (Jones, 1995). Utilization management teams and the use of critical pathways have been instrumental in managing direct costs and establishing the cost per case statistic.

EXTERNAL INFORMATION SOURCES: LECTURE SERIES—PART II

As organizations are challenged to control costs, managers often look outside of their organization for comparative performance data to direct and support their financial decision making. This is accomplished by benchmarking, which is the process of searching for best practices that lead to exceptional performance (Patrick, 1992). MECON Associates and Voluntary Hospitals of America are examples of organizations that collect and publish data from organizations with demographic similarities from across the country, whereas national, state, and local hospital associations publish data from health care organizations within a region. These data represent a measurement and comparative analysis of operational factors associated with the performance of organizations as a whole, as well as specific functional areas. This analysis identifies better and worse performers in terms of cost and utilization and then determines whether certain organizational and operational factors have a statistically significant relationship with a level of performance (Supplement to Health Care Financial Management, 1995). These benchmarked data are useful to organizations because they can compare their performance, analyze their position relative to a comparative peer group, and set targets for their organizational performance.

Guidelines or benchmarked data are also available for other settings along the continuum of care. Ambulatory care areas that want to determine the appropriate number of FTEs per physician can obtain published data from several sources. Two sources for staffing guidelines are Medical Group Management Association and Medical-Dental Management Consultants; both organizations publish reports showing the average number of FTEs per physician in various specialties (Physician's Marketing and Management, 1994). Long-term care facilities have access to benchmarked data collected by the Health Care Financing Agency for clinical practice patterns, but at this time they do not have access to comparative financial performance data.

Christine planned to contact colleagues who were in high-performing organizations to discuss performance-enhancing strategies that might be implemented at YGH. In addition, Christine reviewed information on benchmarking and anticipated the time when the 6 South staff would be benchmarking internally. Christine moved on to the next section of the lecture series.

STRATEGIES TO MANAGE FINANCIAL RESOURCES: LECTURE SERIES—PART III

The current health care environment changes on a daily basis. It is dynamic and difficult to manage. Capitation, competition, and consumer expectations further complicate the provision of care. Often the solutions to today's problems exacerbate tomorrow's challenges. During the first 6 months of the fiscal year at YGH, the census declined sharply, necessitating the implementation of a set of cost reduction strategies. In the second 6 months of the fiscal year the census rose sharply, creating a new set of challenges with different solutions. Managing financial resources in a volatile and dynamic market is no small or simple task. Staff and management must trust each other and work toward the common goal of high-quality, cost-effective patient care. The following section provides actual examples of strategies to manage both low and high census periods. The strategies listed in Table 16-2 also provide a risk rating and risk detail once a strategy is selected and implemented.

Strategies to Manage High and Low Census Periods

Christine reviewed the census reports for 6 South and also for the total hospital. It was the end of the second quarter of the fiscal year, and Christine studied the numbers. The hospital-wide ADC in the first and second quarters was 8% and 13% under budgeted projections. The ADC in the first and second quarters on 6 South was 12% and 20% under budgeted projections. The RN-per-patient ratio on 6 South was 1:7 on the daylight shift. Typically seven RNs and seven care partners were scheduled from 7 AM to 3 PM to care for the unit's maximum capacity of 44 patients. The actual census on 6 South over the past 12 weeks was 28 patients. Given this lower ADC, Christine had scheduled up to three RNs more than she needed to provide patient care just on the daylight shift. If staffing were not adjusted to reflect the census decrease, total cost per patient day on 6 South would continue to exceed the budgeted cost per patient day, although it would be consistent with the fiscal year's proposed nursing expense budget. If other units in the same situation in the hospital ignored the declining census pattern and did not adjust resource utilization accordingly, the hospital's financial performance could be adversely affected.

Christine opened her file on strategies to use during periods of sustained low census. The strategies were listed in order of low to high risk. A low-risk strategy minimizes the potential for a negative consequence to the unit, staff, physicians, patients, and hospital. A high-risk strategy has the potential to cause a negative ripple effect throughout the organization and must be carefully evaluated to determine whether the negative cost of implementing the strategy is outweighed by the positive benefit.

There were a number of strategic options from which Christine could choose; she could use one or any combination to maximize the overall operational performance, depending on the specific issue. To date, nursing management had implemented the first five strategies and were waiting for the second quarter data before moving ahead with the last three. Christine reviewed the financial performance of 6 South and the Department of Nursing for the first two quarters in light of the de-

Text continued on p. 235.

Table 16-2

Resource Management Strategies for a Decrease in Workload

Strategy	Advantages	Disadvantages	Risk
1. Limit the use of internal per diem staff.	Results in a decrease in paid FTEs and therefore a decrease in overall expenses; also, decreasing per diem hours lessens the impact on regular full- and part-time staff.	If the per diem staff are unable to obtain hours, they may seek positions with other organizations and will not be available if the census increases.	Low
2. Shift staff to busier units in the hospital.	Provides the needed relief to the busier units and allows regular staff to continue to work a full schedule.	This can be a staff dissatisfier if the appropriate orientation is not provided, if this strategy is utilized frequently, or if it is long term.	Low to moderate
3. Place a freeze on hiring and establish a position control system.	Ensures no additional staff are added to any cost center, and therefore additional expenses are not incurred; or positions are added only after intense review by a designated panel following justification by the manager.	This is a staff dissatisfier because their internal transfer opportunities are eliminated. Also, experienced external candidates may be needed in certain specialty areas not serviced by the per diem pool, resulting in stretched ratios or limited admissions; this is also a management dissatisfier because of the lack of flexibility in hiring.	Low to moderate

Table 16-2

Resource Management Strategies for a Decrease in Workload—cont'd

Strategy	Advantages	Disadvantages	Risk
4. Cancel staff on a shift-to-shift basis and allow staff to use benefit time.	Achieves the objective of having the appropriate staffing levels available to provide care, thus meeting the budget targets.	This is a major staff dissatisfier because all of their accrued benefit time could be depleted.	Moderate
5. Cancel staff on a shift-to-shift basis without pay (after benefits are depleted).	Achieves the objective of having the appropriate staffing levels available to provide care, thus meeting budget targets.	This is a significant staff dissatisfier and has a negative impact on morale. The staff begin to question the security of their jobs, and this preoccupation could negatively affect patient care.	Moderate
6. Reassign staff permanently to areas of high census.	Fully maximizes the utilization of internal staffing resources by allocating nurses to the areas of need.	This requires a period of orientation for reassigned staff, and expenses are incurred as a result of lost productivity and training. This is a significant staff dissatisfier because of the disruption in their routine; staff again question job security, and the preoccupation could negatively affect patient care.	Moderate to high

Continued

Table 16-2

Resource Management Strategies for a Decrease in Workload—cont'd

Strategy	Advantages	Disadvantages	Risk
7. Close a nursing unit(s).	Decreases the overhead costs associated with running a nursing unit and maximizes the utilization of existing resources.	This increases the workload for the remaining units, requiring the displacement of staff and a possible reduction in the total nursing workforce (layoff). This requires a period of orientation for reassigned staff, and expenses are incurred as a result of lost productivity and training. This is a significant staff dissatisfier, again raising issues of job security, and the preoccupation could negatively affect patient care.	Moderate to high
8. Reduce workforce (layoff).	Core employees are ensured their total complement of hours worked. Also, labor expenses are maximally managed by matching the required workforce with the actual workload.	This has a long-lasting negative impact, and the remaining employees believe no job is secure.	High

Table 16-3

First and Second Quarter Census and Cost Data

	6 South			Department of Nursing		
Average Daily Census (Volume)						
	Actual	Budget	Variance	Actual	Budget	Variance
1st quarter	30	34	−12%	458	499	−8%
2nd quarter	28	35	−20%	428	490	−13%
Nursing Salary Cost per Patient Day						
1st quarter	$220	$181	−22%	$340	$295	−15%
2nd quarter	$206	$179	−15%	$336	$302	−11%
Total Cost per Patient Day						
1st quarter	$244	$201	−21%	$415	$361	−15%
2nd quarter	$226	$199	−14%	$413	$369	−12%

clining volume. The key indicators Christine tracked comparing budget with actual included the following:

- Average daily census for 6 South
- Average daily census for the department
- Total unit nursing salary cost per patient day
- Total department nursing salary cost per patient day
- Unit cost per patient day
- Department cost per patient day

In spite of nursing management's efforts to reduce expenses by implementing key strategies, 6 South's financial performance at the end of the first two quarters was poor. (See Table 16-3.)

The first-quarter financials on 6 South reflected a nursing salary expense per patient day of 22% above budget, with total cost per patient day 21% above budget. Christine knew that although the number of patients had declined, there was no parallel decline in nurse staffing. The strategies implemented by Christine and the Department of Nursing helped to improve second-quarter performance, although not enough, by decreasing the nursing salary expense per patient day on 6 South to 15% over budget and total cost per patient day to 14% over budget. The second-quarter improvement is also significant from a volume perspective. The second-quarter volume variance was a negative 20% compared with a negative 12% at the end of the first quarter. In spite of a greater decline in ADC in the second quarter, by implementing several key strategies Christine and the 6 South staff were able to improve the unit's financial performance, as reflected in the nursing salary cost per patient day. (See Table 16-3.) At the same time Christine focused on reducing overtime expenses by the following:

1. Implementing an automated staffing and scheduling system to improve scheduling efficiency
2. Developing a scheduling scorecard evaluating the overall efficiency of each unit's schedule
3. Establishing an overtime preapproval process

The Department of Nursing mirrored the trends on 6 South, with second-quarter nursing salary expense per patient day and total cost per patient day improving compared with the first-quarter performance.

Christine was confident 6 South managed financial resources in the most productive and efficient manner possible. However, given the sustained low census, a major reassignment of staff, a reduction in workforce, or a closure of a unit(s) was inevitable.

At the end of the second quarter, nursing management proposed the consolidation of the four surgical units to three. Volume analysis by day of the week and over a 3-month period indicated the opportunity to manage all surgical patients, even on high census days, on three 44-bed units instead of four. Staff were reassigned to the remaining surgical units, and a hospital-wide plan was implemented to downsize the workforce in response to the sustained decrease in patient volume.

Following the reassignment of staff, consolidation of clinical services, closure of one nursing unit, and a reduction in workforce, the census began to climb. Throughout the third and fourth quarters, the gain in census was maintained as a result of the hospital's efforts to increase market share by strengthening physician referral patterns, adding new services, and introducing state-of-the-art technology. Christine and the Department of Nursing were now immersed in managing a significantly higher census compared with the first two quarters, with insufficient base staffing necessitating increased overtime utilization to meet patient care requirements. The strategies Christine considered during a period of sustained high census are shown in Table 16-4.

Christine and the nursing management team utilized the first seven strategies during the third and fourth quarters of the fiscal year. Christine reviewed the last two quarters' financial performance, shown in Table 16-5.

At the end of the third quarter on 6 South, nursing salary cost per patient day dropped to 2% under budget, with total cost per patient day exactly at budget, a remarkable shift from the first and second quarters. In the fourth quarter on 6 South, nursing salary cost per patient day improved further to finish at 4% under budget, and total cost per patient day improved to 2% under budget. The departmental performance was also positive in the fourth quarter, with a 1% under budget nursing salary cost and a 2% under budget total cost performance. Nursing salary costs and total cost per patient day for 6 South and the entire department were under budget again—no surprise given the limited resources and the high volume.

Christine did not experience any satisfaction while she reviewed the financial

Text continued on p. 240.

Table 16-4

Resource Management Strategies for an Increase in Workload

Strategy	Advantages	Disadvantages	Risk
1. Access internal per diem staff.	Provides immediate relief for regular staff by utilizing nurses familiar with the hospital system.	Inability to access the full complement of staff needed to care for the increase in patient volume because of the high demand and limited supply of internal per diem staff; internal per diem staff seek external positions if unable to schedule desired hours internally.	None
2. Increase the hours worked by part-time staff.	Provides immediate relief for regular staff by utilizing nurses familiar with the hospital system.	This is a dissatisfier for part-time staff, who often have other commitments and cannot easily increase the number of shifts they work; staff availability may not meet the demand.	Low

Continued

Table 16-4

Resource Management Strategies for an Increase in Workload—cont'd

Strategy	Advantages	Disadvantages	Risk
3. Preassign internal per diem staff to a specific unit for an extended period of time.	Provides immediate relief for regular staff by utilizing nurses familiar with the hospital system. Decreases the amount of time unit management staff spend on securing adequate staffing numbers.	Limits available staffing resources for other units also in need and decreases the overall flexibility of the per diem staffing pool.	Low to moderate
4. Fill vacant positions.	Eventual relief for the current staff once the new hires are productive and off of orientation.	Increases the unit and departmental position base, necessitating a reduction in workforce if the census drops. This can be a staff dissatisfier related to job security—if we hire today will we have to lay off staff tomorrow?	Low to moderate
5. Stretch existing nurse-per-patient ratios.	Provides the opportunity to immediately care for additional patients.	Staff, patient, and physician dissatisfier if all groups perceive a negative impact on quality of care.	Moderate

Table 16-4

Resource Management Strategies for an Increase in Workload—cont'd

Strategy	Advantages	Disadvantages	Risk
6. Seek approval for unbudgeted additional base positions.	Eventual relief for the current staff once the new hires are off of orientation and productive.	This results in an immediate negative impact to the unit and departmental budgets, although justifiable; this will increase the overall position base, necessitating a reduction in workforce if the census declines.	Moderate
7. Preplan and schedule overtime, including overtime by non-bedside RNs (e.g., educators or managers working as staff).	Provides the opportunity to immediately care for additional patients.	Significant staff dissatisfier; if used long term could negatively affect quality of care and overall relationship with staff; immediate negative impact on the overtime budget, although justifiable.	Moderate to high

Continued

Table 16-4

Resource Management Strategies for an Increase in Workload—cont'd

Strategy	Advantages	Disadvantages	Risk
8. Access external agency nurses.	Provides the opportunity to immediately care for additional patients while relieving internal staff of the overtime burden.	Depending on the internal culture, the utilization of external agency nurses may be viewed negatively from both a cost and quality standpoint; also a process must be put into place to ensure the completion of ongoing evaluation and competency assessments.	Moderate to high
9. Cap and defer admissions to another facility.	Demonstrates to staff a commitment to meeting the established quality care standards by controlling the workload.	This could jeopardize the referral base and damage physician-to-physician relationships and patient referral patterns.	High

performance indicators. Yes, they were positive, but at what cost? Staff burnout from excessive overtime? Questionable quality of care caused by stretched patient ratios? At this point Christine was primarily concerned about getting the right number of nurses on 6 South to meet the patient care needs and was currently evaluating the use of external agency nurses for a short period of time in limited patient care areas.

In addition to addressing staffing issues, Christine worked with a multidisciplinary team to investigate enablers such as stockless inventory, standardization of supplies, lease services, and information support systems that would enable

Table 16-5

Third and Fourth Quarter Census and Cost Data

Average Daily Census

	6 South			Department of Nursing		
	Actual	Budget	Variance	Actual	Budget	Variance
3rd quarter	33	35	−6%	486	508	−4%
4th quarter	34	35	−3%	482	493	−2%

Nursing Salary Cost per Patient Day

3rd quarter	$175	$179	2%	$334	$321	−4%
4th quarter	$167	$174	4%	$315	$319	1%

Total Cost per Patient Day

3rd quarter	$199	$199	0%	$402	$391	−3%
4th quarter	$188	$192	2%	$383	$390	2%

staff and the organization to improve productivity by providing more cost-effective care while maintaining acceptable levels of quality irrespective of volume fluctuations.

Summary

The past fiscal year was the most dynamic and challenging of Christine's 15-year career. After completing her review of the lecture series, Christine reflected on the past and contemplated the future. The world of health care gained complexity with each passing day as a result of growth in technology, heightened consumer expectations, and rapidly diminishing resources. Christine understood that the nursing profession must continue to serve as the ambassador for quality patient care but not at the expense of the financial health of the organization. The development and implementation of creative strategies to maximize resources and maintain quality standards are critical to the ongoing success of any nursing service in any component across the continuum of health care delivery. The nursing vice president was absolutely correct: it is the responsibility of every individual employed within the Department of Nursing not only to contribute to the quality of care provided but also to deliver care in a cost-effective manner.

Health care managers control significant resources that if managed effectively can result in value-driven outcomes for clients and organizations. Developing competence in planning, allocating, and monitoring these resources is essential in today's turbulent health care environment. Understanding key internal and external sources for financial decision making, as well as strategies to manage financial resources in partnerships with staff, will be critical to ongoing success.

Discussion Questions

1. What systems/strategies can be implemented to enhance productivity in any setting where health care services are provided?
2. List key questions to consider when analyzing a variance report. How can a manager use this information to enhance performance? How would these strategies vary at different points within the continuum of care?
3. What additional strategies can nurse managers in settings with rapidly fluctuating client volumes use to ensure the management of the cost-quality link for individuals, populations, and organizations?
4. Questions for discussion related to the profit and loss statement (see Table 16-1):
   - Identify the changes in the hospital's financial performance. (Compare revenue, expenses, and excess revenue over expenses.)
   - Discuss the major contributors to the changes in the financial position.
   - What challenges does the hospital face in implementing the fiscal year 1997 budget?
   - What are the implications for the Department of Nursing given a decrease in

Case Study

YGH is changing its care delivery model from functional to a patient-centered care model, which provides for one RN and one care partner to deliver care to a group of patients on a general medical unit with an ADC of 26.5 and WHPPD of 8.15. The nurse/patient ratios for RNs and the care partners are 1:7 on days, 1:8 on evenings, and 1:9 on nights.

Case Study Exercise
Assume you are Christine and calculate the required number of FTEs using the two methods in Box 16-1. (Answer follows.)

Answer to Case Study
Required RN FTEs (using WHPPD) = $(26.5 \times 365 \times 8.15 \times 1.14)/2080$
$$= 43.22 \text{ FTEs}$$
Required RN FTEs (using ratios) = $\{[(26.5/7) + (26.5/8) + (26.5/9)] \times 8$
$\times 365 \times 1.14\}/2080 = 21.61$ FTEs

In a partnership model the number of partners is equal to the number of RNs; therefore the total number of FTEs required using the ratio method is 43.22 (21.61×2).

budgeted salaries, wages, and fees expenses for fiscal year 1997 compared with fiscal year 1996?

REFERENCES

August JM: Mapping change in health care: Pathways for nursing, *Semin Nurse Managers* 3(2):67, 1995.

Bertram DL, Wilson JL: *Financial management in critical care nursing,* Baltimore, 1991, Williams & Wilkins.

Douglas DA, Mayewski J: Census variation staffing, *Nurs Manage* 27(2):32, 1996.

Felteau A: Budget variance analysis and justification, *Nurs Manage* 23(2):40, 1992.

Finkler SA: *Budgeting concepts for nurses,* ed 2, Philadelphia, 1992, WB Saunders.

Finkler SA, Kovner CT: *Financial management for nurse managers and executives,* Philadelphia, 1993, WB Saunders.

Healthcare Financial Association: From increasing revenues to controlling costs: Bench mark data for strategic planning, *Supplement to Health Care Financial Management,* 1995.

Jones KR: Cost estimation, *Semin Nurse Managers* 2(2):187, 1994.

Jones KR: Cost accounting systems, *Semin Nurse Managers* 3(2):62, 1995.

Kirk R: *Nursing quality and productivity,* Rockville, Md, 1986, Aspen.

Klann S: Mastering the art of budgeting, *Manager* 5(10):10, 1989.

Lane-McGraw C, Villemarie M: Nursing personnel budgets: A step by step guide, *Nurs Manage* 17(11):28, 1986.

Look beyond data for the right number of FTEs per physician, *Physician's Marketing Manage* 85, July 1994.

Neely S, Strickland B: Using a standard staffing index to allocate nursing staff, *JONA* 25(3):13, 1995.

Patrick MS: Benchmarking: Targeting "best practices," *Health Care Forum J* p 71, July/Aug 1992.

Spitzer-Lehmann R: *Nursing management desk reference,* Philadelphia, 1994, WB Saunders.

Walts L: Labor cost-per-patient day: Increasing staff mix flexibility, *Recruitment Retention Rep* 4(4):1, 1991.

West DA et al: Profitable capitation requires accurate costing, *Nurs Econ* 14(3):162, 1996.

part IV

Challenges of Today and Tomorrow

chapter **seventeen**

Achieving the Vision of Professionalism in Practice

Sylvia Anderson Price
Paula R. Jaco

Learning Objectives

- Explore issues that may impede nursing's achieving full professional recognition.
- Assess the influence of leadership in relation to professionalism in practice.
- Describe and analyze the components of a professional nursing practice model.
- Analyze the importance of the nurse manager's role in implementing a professional nursing practice model.

Nursing is in a strategic position to achieve full professional recognition as a viable partner in providing health care services in the twenty-first century. This position has never been more opportune than at the present time. Blumenthal (1994) writes about the challenge to professionalism that the economic issues of the new era of health care will bring. He emphasizes that altruism, a commitment to self-improvement, and peer review are important tenets of professionalism and should continue to be supported and rewarded. If nursing is to achieve full professional recognition as a partner in providing health care during this chaotic time, leaders of nursing must be cognizant of the words of Blumenthal and the key elements of professional practice, including **autonomy, accountability,** and **mastery of a body of knowledge.** As nurses, how we incorporate each of these elements in our nursing practice will determine our survival in today's marketplace and our success in being recognized as professional practitioners.

The dilemma nursing is experiencing centers on several key issues. Nursing has permitted others outside of nursing to gain control in influencing the role of the nurse, perceptions of how care is provided, and the public image of what a nurse is. This has occurred because of our lack of unity as a professional partner in health care. The power and force that nursing could exhibit to the public and other health care providers are disseminated in its own personal agenda. This philosophy does not promote the concept of nursing as a profession. Nursing is under intense scrutiny to justify its worth and value.

Another issue is autonomy in practice, which is sometimes overlooked by nursing. Perhaps this is because with autonomy come accountability and **responsibility.** Some nurses choose not to participate in the autonomous part of their role. They do not want to be held accountable or responsible for their practice. In today's market more nurses are simply "tasking," or performing the routine task. It is much safer, especially when the job market is tight, to maintain a low profile, thus creating as little conflict as possible and not assessing or making critical judgments that may alter the patient's plan of care. An important question is, are the nurses of today not adequately prepared for the evolving health care market, or are they not using their knowledge?

Aiken (1995) suggests that the mix of nurses by educational background is not sufficient to meet the demands of health care today. According to the statistics of the National League for Nursing's *Nursing Data Review 1994,* 68% of the graduates from nursing programs are associate degree prepared. With the increasing level of patient acuity and the critical skills and knowledge required in all health care settings, the quality of education for entry-level nurses must be reevaluated to ensure a level of preparation that will promote accountability and responsibility in nursing practice. As representatives of nursing interacting with other professionals as members of the health care team, we must be recognized for our knowledge and skills as equal partners in the provision of high-quality patient care.

This is best illustrated by Virginia Henderson (1961) when she discusses the nature of nursing:

> The unique function of the nurse is to assist the individual, sick or well, in the performance of those activities contributing to health or his recovery (or to peaceful death) that he would perform unaided if he had the necessary strength, will, or knowledge. And to do this in such a way as to help him gain independence as rapidly as possible. This aspect of her work, this part of her function, she initiates and controls; of this she is master. In addition she helps the patient carry out the therapeutic plan as initiated by the physician. She also, as a member of a medical team, helps other members, as they in turn help her, to plan and carry out the total program whether it be for the improvement of health, or the recovery from illness, or support in death.

Mastery of a body of knowledge is the third issue that must be addressed in our pursuit of full professional status as an equal partner in health care. Are we so naive to believe that we have an insufficient body of scientific knowledge or that we need to continue to prove the need for our existence by defining and redefining this body of knowledge? Nursing's body of knowledge began with the inception of care for the ill and infirmed. Florence Nightingale was the first nurse researcher. This was the beginning of our unique body of knowledge.

Comradeship and collegiality have not been nursing's strengths. There are few mentors who do guide and direct the development of staff nurses. Nurse executives and nurse managers should assist in preparing the practitioners of tomorrow. Sovie

(1987) discusses the nine priorities of exceptional nurse executives and leaders who want to shape the future. Some have greater significance than others, but clearly they reflect on the mentorship role in nursing. These priorities are addressing and solving the nurse shortage, promoting vision and clarifying values, empowering and committing to excellence, enabling participative management, acquiring business savvy, shaping the corporate culture, developing and testing new approaches in nursing practice, educating nurses for the information age, and seeking and forming new coalitions.

The future of health care and nursing is dependent on exceptional nursing leadership not only at the executive level but also in every area in which patient care is administered. For nursing to be recognized as an equal partner in the health care arena, the following components of professional practice are essential: altruism, commitment to self-improvement, peer review, autonomy, accountability, and the mastery of a body of scientific knowledge.

PROFESSIONALISM IN PRACTICE

To achieve the vision of **professionalism in practice,** nursing must continually search for ways to innovate and change, becoming more proactive and responsive in today's competitive marketplace. Leadership is the critical and essential component required to promote the concept of professionalism in the practice environment. Levitt (1988) emphasizes that leaders establish order and discipline and simultaneously foster experimentation and change. To achieve more and better results, more resourcefulness is as important as more resources.

Bennis and Nanus (1985) stress that within the leadership environment three major contexts are (1) **commitment,** (2) **complexity,** and (3) **credibility.** Lack of commitment refers to the tendency to withhold effort from the job, which may be increasing, as evidenced by a gap between the number of hours people are paid for working and the number of hours spent in productive labor. There also is a decline of the work ethic. Complexity refers to rapid and spastic changes or problems, such as the increased complexity of organizations influenced by the business climate: takeovers and bankruptcy. Credibility is at a premium.

Leaders are being scrutinized. Continual attention focuses on welfare, health, education, and the environment through means such as advocacy groups, government regulations, consumer groups, and unions. All are questioning and challenging authority.

Bennis and Nanus found that one of the traits most apparent in leaders is their ability to draw others to them because they have a vision, a dream, a set of intentions, an agenda, a frame of reference. They communicate an extraordinary focus of commitment, which attracts people to them. Leaders manage attention through a compelling vision that brings others to a place where they have not been before.

As leaders, nurse managers must continually pursue opportunities to nurture the growth of the profession to facilitate a learning environment that enhances the delivery of cost-effective, high-quality, client-centered nursing care. Initiating this endeavor is fundamental to leadership.

```
                    ┌─────────────────────────────────┐
                    │         CLINICAL PRACTICE        │
                    │ Quality patient centered care    │
                    │            provision             │
                    │  Primary, long-term and tertiary │
                    │              care                │
                    │ Military, rural, urban and inner │
                    │              city                │
                    │ Hospitals, homes, long-term,     │
                    │           ambulatory             │
                    │         Earth and space          │
                    └─────────────────────────────────┘
```

┌─────────────────────┐   ┌─────────────────────┐
│ **EDUCATION**   │   │ **MANAGEMENT**   │
│ Academic   │   **INTEGRATED**   │ Care coordination   │
│ Lifelong learning   │   **EXECUTIVE BEHAVIORS**   │ Human resources   │
│ Teaching/learning   │   Leadership   │ Economics   │
│ Distance education │   National/international policy   │ Work issues   │
│ Technology diffusion│   Health for all people   │ Informatics   │
│ Writing/publication │   Transformation of people,   │ Assistive technology│
│   │   Work and environments   │ Care systems   │
│   │   Ethical, social, political   │   │
│   │   and economic issues   │   │
└─────────────────────┘   └─────────────────────┘

```
                    ┌─────────────────────────────────┐
                    │            RESEARCH              │
                    │      Scientific initiatives       │
                    │ Theory development, modeling and  │
                    │           simulation              │
                    │  Action/participatory research    │
                    │     Practice-based research       │
                    │ Quantitative and qualitative      │
                    │         investigation             │
                    └─────────────────────────────────┘
```

Figure 17-1 Integrated professional nursing administration. (Modified from Simms L, Price S, Ervin N: *The professional practice of nursing administration,* ed 2, Albany, NY, 1994, Delmar.)

Leadership is an essential component of achieving the vision of professionalism in practice. Professional nursing practice is the application and utilization of knowledge in relation to the biopsychosocial influences optimizing the health of individuals. Professional nursing practice involves accountability, patient advocacy, and autonomy in the provision of comprehensive, holistic nursing care that responds to the needs of patients and their families.

Simms, Price, and Ervin (1994) state that although clinical practice is a major thrust of nursing, other components, including research, education, and management must be considered. The four components of integrated professional nursing administration are (1) clinical practice (application of knowledge), (2) research (development of knowledge), (3) education (learning and transmission of knowledge), and (4) management (care coordination and utilization of knowledge). (See Figure 17-1.) The authors emphasize that these components should be articulated and coordinated toward the attainment of professional nursing practice. The education component affects policy and procedures, which influence research-based clinical practice. Nurse executives, as well as nurse managers, are responsible and accountable for clinical nursing practice, research, and education as they influence professional nursing within an institution.

PROFESSIONAL PRACTICE ENVIRONMENT

An example of a professional practice environment is depicted in the **Magnet Hospital Study** (American Academy of Nursing, 1983), which was designed to identify those hospitals throughout the United States that (1) had reputations for being good places to work and as giving good nursing care and (2) had been particularly successful in attracting and retaining professional nurses. There were 41 magnet hospitals in the final study.

The study focused on attraction and retention of nurses, for example, whether magnet hospitals retain nurses because they are able to give quality patient care and are happier in their jobs and stay or whether they attract nurses for some other reason. The inference and relationship between retention of a qualified nursing staff and quality patient care are evident throughout the report. This study specifically assessed the quality of nursing care of the "goodness" of the hospital; other rankings of hospitals address medical care. The focus was on planned, comprehensive care, continuity of care, and the patients' feelings that they are special because a particular nurse is looking out for them. Competent, personalized, and cost-effective care was one of the major values.

There was a tremendous push for education that was operationalized, and it also related to the drive for a quality product. Because of the staff's ability to solve problems quickly and adopt a proactive stance, a great deal of trust was built between the staff and their leadership team. Treating people with dignity and providing high-performance expectations were emphasized. The expectation was that "if you expect nurses to care about other people, you have to care about them." In magnet hospitals virtually all communication was informal and more or less constant, and much of it was initiated by the staff nurse.

The leaders in the magnet hospitals were highly visible and accessible. They set value standards for nursing departments, not only regionally but nationally. Enthusiasm and excitement were evident in the staff nurses when they talked about their leaders. Top nursing leaders were seen as visionary, enthusiastic leaders in nursing. Magnet hospitals had strong top nursing management teams that shared the values of the chief nurse executive. The team was strong, very cohesive, and together with the management group at the head nurse level, characterized by a genuine liking for one another.

Magnet hospitals have created a mystique and elitism that lead nurses to prefer to work in these hospitals. They are outstanding examples of quality health care environments.

Kramer (1990) reports on a follow-up interview with the chief nurse executives of these magnet hospitals. The data were from telephone interviews with 14 of the 16 chief nurse executives. The hospitals in this sample were acute care, urban, and medium-to-large community or medical center hospitals. The most dramatic changes with regard to staff mix were the debureaucratization of the nursing department through flattening of the structure and increased professionalism through a larger percentage of registered nurses in the work setting. Four out of every five employees in the nursing department were registered nurses in staff positions and were administering direct care to patients.

There was a decrease in the number of nursing administrators. For example, evening and night supervisors were no longer needed to supervise responsible, autonomous staff nurses, who were functioning as assistant hospital nurses. One hospital even eliminated them altogether, and head nurses were on beeper call for consultation on nursing problems that the staff could not handle.

Most of these hospitals had a system of autonomous, self-managed, self-governed operation at the unit level with systematic, participative, representative involvement by unit staff nurses. Their focus was on clinical decision making and nurse-physician collaboration.

The hospitals were redesigning or further developing new nursing care delivery systems, developing programs and activities to enable or empower staff, strengthening collaborative practice, flattening the organizational structure, and strengthening computerization programs, particularly those used for documentation.

Aiken (1995) stresses that when nurses have more autonomy to practice and make the decisions they have been educated to make, when they control the resources that need to be brought together for effective patient care, and when they have trusting relationships with physicians, this will result in better outcomes for patients. In other words, good care outcomes are not primarily a matter of staffing ratios. What nurses do on the units is more important than the number of hands involved in care.

A study by Aiken, Smith, and Lake (1994) that concerned restructuring of hospitals and nursing was an extension of the Magnet Hospital Study. They were interested in determining whether these hospitals achieved better outcomes for patients. The authors wondered if it would be possible to create a similar environment for nurses (increased intra-organizational status, increased autonomy, and more control over the practice environment) with a unit-level reform that could exist in hospitals without unusual top leadership. Magnet hospitals represented hospital-wide top-down reforms. Aiken, Smith, and Lake believe that nurses have not empirically documented sufficiently why nursing care is related to patient outcomes. In their recent study the researchers documented that mortality rates for Medicare patients were lower in 39 of the magnet hospitals than in a sample of 195 nonmagnet hospitals. The magnet hospitals were characterized by decentralized decision making, professional nurse autonomy, and good nurse-physician relationships. The data indicated that lower mortality rates are not simply the result of staffing ratios but that they relate to the organization of nursing that results in greater professional autonomy.

DIFFERENTIATED NURSING PRACTICE

The concept of **differentiated nursing practice** is an important component of professional practice. The National Commission on Nursing Implementation Project

(NCNIP) developed an action plan to differentiate the practice of nursing. Differentiated practice distinguishes professional and technical nursing roles. This enables nurses to perform jobs based on their educational preparation. The professional nurse will require a baccalaureate degree, and the technical nurse will need an associate degree in nursing.

The Midwest Alliance in Nursing (MAIN) sponsored a project to define and differentiate associate degree in nursing (ADN) and baccalaureate degree in nursing (BSN) competencies. Dr. Peggy Primm was the project director. Practitioners in nursing education and service designed the competency standards. Standard competencies were generated for ADN and BSN graduates in three components: (1) provision of care, (2) communication, and (3) management of care. The distinctions between the two roles focus on complexity of decision making, timeline of care, and structure of situation and/or setting. For example, the BS nurse provides direct care for patients (and their families) with complex interactions of nursing diagnoses from pre-admission to post-discharge in structured and unstructured settings and situations, whereas the AD nurse provides direct care for patients (and their families) with common, well-defined nursing diagnoses for a specified work period in structured settings and situations (Primm, 1986).

The boards of the American Organization of Nurse Executives (AONE) and the American Association of Colleges of Nursing (AACN) concurred that differentiation of the scope of nursing practice had not yet been completed. Significant progress over the past 8 years through the work of NCNIP, the American Academy of Nursing, and other groups pointed to the complexity and long-term nature of activities needed to achieve differentiation in practice. Variations in geographical location of nurses, different educational preparation, and long-standing utilization patterns in the field continue to complicate these issues. However, because health care networks are becoming the predominant patient care delivery infrastructure, there is even a greater need to differentiate nursing practice. The AONE and AACN stress that work to differentiate nursing practice calls for both educational and practice intervention (American Association of Nurse Executives, 1994).

PROFESSIONAL PRACTICE MODELS

Implementing Differentiated Practice

A professional nursing practice model at Sioux Valley Hospital (SVH), a 475-bed tertiary care hospital, implemented a patient care delivery system based on differentiated practice on five demonstration units. The project was designed to position nurses as true business partners with other major individuals in the health care industry (Koerner, Bunkers, and Nelson, 1991; Koerner et al., 1989). The professional practice component of the model was addressed by differentiating the roles of nursing, which was based on the American Nurses Association (1965) and Midwest Alliance in Nursing statements (Primm, 1986). In an effort to recognize and use the abilities of the nurse, SVH selected factoring as the mechanism for placing nurses in their respective roles. Registered nurses on each model unit were factored into either the ADN (case associate) or BSN (case manager) job description in collaboration with their head nurse. Individuals were "frozen" into their selected job description for a minimum of 3 months. Then positions were reopened, allowing for transfer to the alternate role if a staff nurse or manager felt uncomfortable with the job description originally selected.

Staff were requested to be more autonomous and accountable, and management to change their behavior from directing and controlling to one of facilitating staff to manage their own practice. Koerner et al. (1989) imply that a critical factor in the success of implementing differentiated practice lies in adequate and repeated staff development programs. This differentiated nursing practice model has shown that factoring allows currently licensed nurses to use the competencies they have developed through professional activities and experiences since graduation.

Redesigning Nursing Practice

The nursing leadership at the Robert Wood Johnson University Hospital developed the **Professional Advanced Care Team (ProACT),** an alternative nursing practice and care delivery model. ProACT is an expanded role, not a differentiated practice model (Tonges, 1989). The role of the nurse is expanded by increasing the extent to which nurses can fully practice their profession. The three roles for nurses in this model are as follows:

1. Clinical care manager (CCM), a registered professional nurse with at least a baccalaureate degree who manages the entire hospital stay of a case of patients through coordination of care with physicians, nursing staff, and other health professionals; the objective is to achieve patient outcomes within the established time frame and resource consumption guidelines
2. Primary nurse, a registered professional nurse who manages patients' nursing care on a 24-hour basis, consults with the CCM regarding patients' condition, delegates to licensed practical nurses and aides, and prepares patients and families for discharge
3. Licensed practical nurse, who functions in the associate role, practicing under the supervision of a registered nurse, and provides input to the primary nurse for the nursing care plan

Provision of related professional and ancillary services (for example, pharmacy, housekeeping, and dietary) was restructured at the unit level to provide maximum support for the delivery of patient care and to improve the quality of service. One of the essential requirements for successful implementation of this model was the willingness and desire of other departments to reach out to assist and support staff in the delivery of patient care. This model combines traditional support service work with a number of tasks previously assumed by nursing personnel.

Blouin and Tonges (1996) state that this model combines two different roles for registered nurses, one of which is a unit-based manager, with expanded clinical and nonclinical support services decentralized from other departments within the hospital to the unit level. ProACT represents an integration of elements from different registered nurse roles, care management, and assistive personnel. According to Blouin and Tonges (1996), "A key feature of this model is the inclusion of multiple departments in a redesigned care delivery system that frees nurses to focus on the complexities of clinical nursing practice and the management of patient care."

THE ROLE OF THE NURSE MANAGER IN CREATING AN ENVIRONMENT FOR THE PRACTICE OF PROFESSIONAL NURSING

The nurse executive and nurse manager are in a strategic position to facilitate an environment that promotes professional nursing practice. This environment will enable staff nurses to use their knowledge, become integral in the decision-making process, and be accountable for decisions affecting their practice. Autonomy, accountability, and authority are essential components of a professional practice model.

Nurse managers must have an internalized idea of themselves to function effectively in their role. One of the major obstacles is reconciling the role of clinician with that of manager. These managers are often selected because of their clinical excellence. However, they may lack the education, experience, or personality for the supervisory role. Overall goals formulated at the administrative level are funneled to the nurse manager, who then must translate them into specific plans of action. It requires managerial acumen to interpret these concepts and apply them to specific situations. These managers must integrate clinical and managerial knowledge while determining measurable outcome criteria. Another important element is their relationship with staff: communicating, coaching, managing of information, and delegating tasks that are critical to goal attainment (Sanders, Davidson, and Price, 1996).

With decentralization, shared governance models, more important decisions focusing on the organization's vision, mission, philosophy, and goals are being implemented at the unit level. Lack of support from staff, economic issues, inadequate preparation of staff, and unclear role definitions converge to form an untenable situation. It is imperative that nursing clarify the nurse manager's role and the competencies required in that role, not only as it currently exists but also as it is projected to evolve.

The evolving trend in health care is interdisciplinary in nature. Barriers between departments can no longer exist. All of the individuals involved in the provision of client care must have a stake as a member of the team. Because nursing is the focal point in interdisciplinary care, nurses must demonstrate a leadership role in this care. It is nursing that has accepted the responsibility to ensure that each patient has been comprehensively assessed and plans of care formulated, implemented, and evaluated. This framework, which has been the core of nursing, is now being adapted by other colleagues who are involved in patient care. This is an exciting adventure and an opportunity for nurses to assume leadership roles in the planning and provision of care in the health care enterprises of the twenty-first century.

Nurse leaders are in a pivotal position of making a difference in the delivery of patient care. It is imperative that these nursing practitioners and faculty members respond by preparing practitioners who will meet the challenges by achieving equal partnership with other health care disciplines in the twenty-first century.

Summary

In many health care institutions nurse executives, as well as nurse managers, have added responsibility for patient care–related services in addition to nursing that reflects both cost and quality issues. Do nurse managers envision themselves as increasing their extent of responsibilities by minimizing their nursing frame of reference or identification? In the health care arena is nursing responding to threats rather than reacting to changing the health care system to reflect both cost and quality from a nursing perspective?

Health care executives often view nurses as caregivers rather than partners. Health care administrators, nurses, physicians, and other practitioners must work together as a team. They need to listen and communicate effectively, recognize the unique contributions of each professional area, provide feedback, explore strategies, discuss and debate issues, and formulate and implement recommendations.

Discussion Questions

1. What are the major barriers to nursing's achieving full professional recognition? In view of today's health care market, what is the potential for nursing to achieve this professional recognition?
2. Why is leadership an important element of professionalism in nursing?
3. What are the essential components of a professional nursing practice model?
4. Why is it important that nurse managers be facilitators in implementing a professional nursing practice model?

Case Study

Change and innovation within an organizational enterprise are resourceful ideas or approaches to existing challenges. They are usually proposed to improve some aspect of the operative units of the organization. You are to propose an innovation that should be responsive to promoting a professional nursing practice model that will provide cost-effective, high-quality nursing care in your health care agency.

Case Study Exercise
Describe the present situation and identify the rationale for the change. Include the design of your plan, the process for implementation, projected timetable for each phase, proposed budget (estimate of costs for human and physical resources), and the evaluation process.

REFERENCES

Aiken L: Transformation of the nursing workforce, *Nurs Outlook* 43(5):201, 1995.

Aiken L, Smith HL, Lake ET: Lower Medicare mortality among a set of hospitals known for good nursing care, *Med Care* 32(8):771, 1994.

American Academy of Nursing: *Magnet hospitals: Attraction and retention of professional nurses,* Kansas City, Mo, 1983, The Association.

American Association of Nurse Executives: Differentiated competencies for nursing practice, *Nurs Manage* 25(9):34, 1994.

American Nurses Association: Educational preparation for nurse practitioners and assistant nurses; a position statement, Kansas City, Mo, 1965, The Association.

Bennis W, Nanus B: *Leaders: The strategies for taking charge,* New York, 1985, Harper & Row.

Blouin A, Tonges M: The content/context imperative: Integration of emerging designs for the practice and management of nursing, *J Nurs Adm* 26(3):38, 1996.

Blumenthal D: The vital role of professionalism in health care reform, *Health Aff* 13(1):252, 1994.

Henderson V: *Basic principles of nursing care,* London, 1961, International Council of Nurses.

Koerner J, Bunkers L, Nelson B: Change: A professional challenge, *Nurs Adm Q* 16(1):15, 1991.

Koerner J et al.: Implementing differentiated practice: The Sioux Valley Hospital experience, *J Nurs Adm* 19(2):13, 1989.

Kramer M: The magnet hospitals: Excellence revisited, *J Nurs Adm* 20(9):35, 1990.

Levitt T: The innovating organization, *Harvard Business Review* 66(1):7, 1988.

National League for Nursing, Division of Research: *Nursing data review 1994,* New York, 1994, National League for Nursing.

Primm P: Entry into practice: Competency statements for BSNs and ADNs, *Nurs Outlook* 34(3):135, 1986.

Sanders B, Davidson A, Price S: The unit nurse executive: A changing perspective, *Nurs Manage* 27(1):42, 1996.

Simms L, Price S, Ervin N: *The professional practice of nursing administration,* ed 2, Albany, NY, 1994, Delmar.

Sovie M: Exceptional executive leadership shapes nursing's future, *Nurs Econ* 5(1):13, 1987.

Tonges M: Redesigning hospital nursing practice: The Professional Advanced Care Team (ProACT) model Part 1, *J Nurs Adm* 19(7):31, 1989.

chapter **eighteen**

Financial Challenges and Economic Implications

Peter I. Buerhaus

Learning Objectives

- Identify forces that are responsible for the transformation of the health care industry.
- Identify recent developments in the measurement of the quality of health care.
- Identify and discuss the economic roles that professional nurses play in the production of patient care.

Health care delivery organizations are in the business of producing mostly medical treatments and personal health care services to satisfy society's demand for health care. They purchase nonhuman and human resources (capital and labor) and combine them to produce a given quantity and quality of treatments and services. Not only does it cost organizations a certain portion of their financial assets to acquire resources, but they also incur other costs whenever resources are used in the production process. That is, there are alternative ways to combine and use resources, and some are more costly than others. From the economic point of view of the organization, professional nurses are inputs in its health production process and therefore are a resource cost. From the economic perspective of nurses, at a certain wage they sell a portion of their time to organizations and use that time to supply nursing services required to produce the desired amount and quality of patient care (Buerhaus, 1997).

Professional nurses play another important economic role when they make decisions concerning how nonnursing resources purchased by the organization are combined with nursing services to produce patient care. These other resources, both human and nonhuman, can be configured and used in alternative ways to achieve the same or similar clinical outputs. Once again, some configurations are more costly than others and have a different impact on quality and clinical outcomes. Thus nurses are a vital input in the production process and at the same time make important decisions on how other resources are combined and used in the clinical

259

production process. These two roles place professional nurses at the center of the organization's production process.

As discussed throughout this book, the health care industry has undergone a remarkable transformation during the 1990s. A variety of financial and economic forces have converged to create a strengthening wave of economic discipline in the delivery and financing of health care (Buerhaus, 1997). Never before have health care organizations felt more pressure to lower their costs and improve the quality of services. Since the early 1990s nurses in all sectors of the health care industry have felt these pressures in both their input and clinical resource management roles. On into the next century, professional nurses and their physician colleagues can anticipate that these forces will continue strengthening and bearing down ever harder on their capability to produce health care more efficiently and of higher quality, however quality is defined.

This chapter briefly reviews the **financial and economic forces** that are responsible for the transformation of the health care industry and suggests how they will pressure organizations and professionals during the foreseeable future. The implications for professional nurses' input and clinical resource management roles will then be considered in terms of the economic and clinical imperatives to lower costs and improve quality.

FINANCIAL AND ECONOMIC FORCES AFFECTING HEALTH CARE ORGANIZATIONS

For the health care industry, history will likely record the last decade of the twentieth century as the time when economic discipline slowly, if not painfully, gripped health care delivery organizations and the professionals who make their living providing health care (Iglehart, 1995). Others might declare that this was the time when the "new economics" in health care emerged (Shortell, Gillies, and Anderson, 1994). No one single event or force is responsible for this continuing transformation; rather it emanates from forces arising in both the public and private sectors of our nation, within the health industry itself, and through the intellect and activities of clinicians and health services researchers. These forces have become increasingly aligned and thus more powerful in changing the way organizations and health care professionals think about and produce personal health care services. Although described in greater detail elsewhere (Buerhaus, 1996a; Buerhaus, 1996b), six transforming forces are briefly discussed in this section.

Intensifying Public Sector Cost Containment

There can be no doubt that federal and state governments are becoming more aggressive and adept in limiting their expenditures on health care. Motivating their resolve is the massive federal budget deficit (over $5 trillion), which has accumulated over the past two decades and now requires nearly one-fifth (over $200 billion) of each year's entire federal budget simply to pay annual interest charges (Congressional Budget Office, 1995). Unfortunately, each year's new deficit spending adds billions more to the public's debt. Congress and the administration have seemingly moved closer toward enacting a balanced budget amendment, as well as adopting other measures to reduce the budget deficit (namely, shrinking the size of the federal government by eliminating certain programs and departments). However, because interest payments must be paid every year to avoid default, other social programs, including health care, will not receive the financing that they would otherwise obtain. States, which have experienced their own budget problems, though not as severely as the federal government, expect to be given the responsibility but not the full funding to sustain many social programs previously controlled by Washington.

To deal with the budget deficit, the federal government has little choice but to target the largest and fastest-growing areas of the budget: the **Medicare and Medicaid programs.** Together they compose nearly 20% of each year's federal budget, and each is growing at an annual rate that more than doubles the rate of inflation (Prospective Payment Assessment Commission, 1996). Both programs have targeted providers, namely hospitals and physicians, as the recipients of efforts to constrain the growth of their budgets. Thus for the foreseeable future providers can expect stingy payment amounts, elimination of regulatory loopholes, and the expansion of prospective payments for care provided to beneficiaries in non-inpatient settings.

As these public sector financing constraints grip organizations and health professionals in the years ahead, nurses can anticipate that payments to home health care providers will become tighter as well. Since 1990, home health care has been the fastest-growing sector of the health care industry (Levit et al., 1994) and, since 1992, the fastest-growing sector for registered nurse (RN) employment (Buerhaus and Staiger, 1996). As patient care revenues become increasingly constrained, the value of each dollar received by health care organizations will increase, causing employers to more carefully weigh their decisions concerning the number and mix of nursing personnel to employ and the kind of work they will perform.

Growth of Managed Care

Because the development and effects of managed care are discussed in greater detail in Chapter 7, only a few points are offered here. First, nurses should realize that in addition to constraining payments to providers, the Medicare and Medicaid programs are taking actions to rapidly increase enrollment of beneficiaries in health maintenance organizations (HMOs) and other managed care organizations (MCOs) (Vladick, 1996). Some observers (Taylor, 1996) expect that essentially all Medicaid recipients and a large proportion of Medicare beneficiaries will be enrolled in MCOs in the near future. In 1995 33% of 35 million Medicaid recipients and 10% of 37 million Medicare beneficiaries were enrolled in some form of managed care plan (Rowlan and Kristina, 1996; Welch, 1996). Expanding HMO enrollment will further constrain patient care revenues and place even greater pressure to reduce hospital utilization and patient length of stay. Second, enrollment of commercial populations in MCOs will continue expanding, with most of the growth occurring in network and group HMOs, which place more restrictions on choice of providers but have lower out-of-pocket costs and greater assurance of quality compared with indemnity plans (Taylor, 1996). Third, the managed care industry has rapidly evolved in terms of organizational structures, utilization control techniques, and incentives to guide clinician and subscriber behavior. New organizational forms will continue to be developed, particularly as integrated health care delivery systems grow. And fourth, research (Buerhaus and Staiger, 1996) on the influence of managed care on the nurse labor market shows that since 1990, RNs and licensed practical nurses (LPNs) (but not aides) experienced slower employment growth in states with high HMO enrollment compared with states with lower HMO enrollment. Also, the decline in the fraction of RNs working in hospitals was larger and occurred earlier in states with high HMO enrollment, as did the increase in the fraction of RNs working in home health care.

Increasing Economic Competition Among Producers

Unlike the 1980s when HMOs competed on everything but the price of a subscriber's premium, **real price competition** has begun to develop in many areas of the country during the 1990s. This trend was developing before the Clinton administration, but with the demise of its national health care reform strategy in 1994, the level of economic competition has accelerated (Blendon, Bodie, and Benson, 1995).

As discussed elsewhere (Feldstein, 1994), in an effort to reduce employee health care costs, large employers began to self-insure in the 1980s. By the end of the decade employers were using their purchasing power to obtain price discounts from HMOs and preferred provider organizations. These providers responded by stepping up actions aimed at identifying and correcting the behaviors of high-cost clinicians, as well as focusing on the processes creating inefficiencies in organizational components of the health plan. Beyond taking steps to reduce costs within their own organization, MCOs directed considerable effort at reducing subscribers' use of hospital care, the most costly component of covered services.

Above and beyond ever-tightening federal and state cost containment measures discussed earlier, the actions of MCOs forced hospitals to focus on high-cost medical treatments and procedures, the practice patterns of physicians, and inefficient care delivery processes, including nursing services. Hospitals realized they had to lower their costs so that they could offer MCOs a lower price in exchange for access to the HMO's subscribers. At the same time, hospitals had to rapidly find new ways to reduce length of stay and eliminate inappropriate consumption of resources so that they could obtain some earnings not only from their managed care contracts but also from the care provided to Medicaid and Medicare populations. As a result, the era of restructuring and reengineering swept the hospital industry (Buerhaus, 1992).

From an economic perspective, hospitals' restructuring efforts represent attempts to minimize the costs and increase the benefits associated with producing the kind of patient care demanded by MCOs and public sector payors. As both inputs in the production of patient care and as decision makers in the production process, it is inevitable that nurses would be intimately involved and affected. As employers intensify their pressure on MCOs, who in turn pass some of the pressure and risk on to hospitals, nurses can expect that they will be even more closely involved in future restructuring initiatives.

Increased Demand for Improved Quality

At the same time that public and private sector cost containment pressures have increased, so have pressures to improve the quality of health care. In part, pressures arose during the decline of federal, state, and local health planning initiatives in the 1980s. Many proponents of health planning and regulatory intervention believe that the quality of health care can only be ensured by forcing organizations and individual practitioners to comply with regulations (Cohodes, 1994; Feldstein, 1983). Others have argued that the production of high-quality health care is inconsistent with the incentives that drive managed care and price competition, believing that providers' motivations to protect the interests of patients will be subverted by a concern for increasing their own income (Relman, 1993). Further, because some hospitals and physicians experienced substantial shortfalls in Medicare and Medicaid payments in the late 1980s, concern was raised over issues of access to care and the possibility that the quantity of services could be reduced.

Despite the vast majority of studies* on Medicaid and Medicare beneficiaries, as well as commercial populations enrolled in managed care systems, which found that outcomes (variously measured) do not differ from those in fee-for-service systems but that costs are lower, there is widespread skepticism that managed care and the development of economic competition in health care will improve the quality of care (Angell and Kassirer, 1996). Ironically, early in the 1980s Feldstein (1983) predicted that to overcome such skepticism, health care organizations would be especially motivated to improve quality, and therefore the development of competition in health care would lead to a real enhancement in the quality of care. Thus it is not surprising that when real economic competition began developing in the late 1980s and early 1990s, a variety of public and private sector developments aimed at improving the quality of health care began to unfold.

Chief among public sector initiatives, the federal government created the **Agency for Health Care Policy and Research (AHCPR)** in 1988. Since then, much of the AHCPR agenda has focused on investigating issues related to the cost-effectiveness, appropriateness, and quality of common medical interventions and disseminating the results of studies. A current AHCPR initiative is examining consumers' assessments of their health plans. More important to the development of serious actions to measure and improve quality, however, has been the actions of employers and business coalitions.

After seeing pressures on MCOs pay off in terms of slowing down the price of health insurance premiums, employers have begun focusing attention on the outcomes of care and on how satisfied employees are with their health plan. Consequently, employers are collecting data on quality and using their purchasing power

---

*Angell and Kassirer (1996); Carey, Weis, and Homer (1990); Carey, Weis, and Homer (1991); Carlisle et al. (1992); Chassin (1996); Clement et al. (1994); Freund et al. (1989); Greenfield et al. (1995); Hillman, Pauly, and Kerstein (1989); Hohlen et al. (1990); Lurie et al. (1992a); Lurie et al. (1992b); Miller and Luft (1995); Murray et al. (1992); Retchin and Brown (1990a); Retchin and Brown (1990b); Retchin and Brown (1991); and Retchin et al. (1992).

to pressure MCOs to compete not only on price but also on the basis of measurable and comparable indicators of quality (Buerhaus, 1996b).

Other important private sector efforts have developed during the 1990s. The membership of the **Association of Health Services Researchers** has grown rapidly, and its research agenda has increasingly focused on studying outcomes and quality-related issues. The Joint Commission on Accreditation of Healthcare Organizations (formerly the **Joint Commission on Hospital Accreditation**) transformed itself, not just in name but in mission and scope, to become a more authentic overseer of quality. The tools of total quality management developed and used effectively in non–health care industries have been applied in health care organizations with gusto and determination. The **National Committee for Quality Assurance** began to accredit managed care plans and launched its initial version of the **Health Plan Employer Data and Information Set (HEDIS)** to collect and compare data on plan performance in the early 1990s (Iglehart, 1996). Numerous philanthropic organizations changed their funding priorities to emphasize quality-related studies, particularly with respect to managed care, and thousands of research and quality improvement organizations, institutes, and private firms have sprung up to assist health care delivery organizations in developing the capacity to measure the quality of care (Blumenthal and Epstein, 1996). These and many other private sector actions have inundated the health care industry, each playing a role in strengthening and shaping the demand to measure, monitor, compare, and improve the quality of health care. Never before in the history of the health care industry has there been more effort—and the majority originating in the private sector—aimed at improving the quality of health care.

The Emerging Science of Quality Measurement

Closely related to the increasing demand for quality improvement has been the development of new analytical tools and methods to measure the technical characteristics of quality patient care and interactions between providers and patients. For example, the application of clinical epidemiology methods has identified (though not explained) wide variation in the processes and outcomes of care among patients receiving routine treatments for the same health care problem and clarified the implications of differing patterns of clinical practice (Blumenthal, 1996b). Advances in sociology and psychometrics have spurred the growth of outcomes research, particularly the assessment of patients' functioning, values, and preferences for different functional states and quality of life (Blumenthal, 1996b). The adoption of quality management techniques practiced in non–health care industries, combined with advancements in information systems and computer technology, has made it cheaper, easier, and faster for researchers and other concerned parties to gather and analyze data from multiple sources—medical records, administrative and claims databases, surveys, and so on (Brook, McGlynn, and Cleary, 1996).

Quality assessment methods are evaluating quality on the basis of structure, process, and outcomes of care in the Donnebedian sense and are being used to focus on quality at the individual, organization, and health plan levels (Blumenthal, 1996a). Advances in risk adjustment accounting for severity of illness, cost-effectiveness, provider profiling, critical paths, and the study of errors in systems have also contributed significantly to the emerging science of quality measurement. Taken together, these advances are enabling quality to be measured on the basis of objectivity and scientific methods. Gone are the days when "expert" opinion was accepted in assessing quality; today credible evidence is required by providers, payors, and consumers.

Capitation and Integration of Health Care Delivery

Providers are finding that to produce the entire range of services—inpatient through home care—in a cost-effective manner, there must be greater **coordination and communication** among health care organizations. Close coordination can eliminate time-consuming and expensive redundancies, reduce costly duplication of services and facilities, ensure that appropriate care is provided at the right time during the progression of a subscriber's course of treatment, and offer opportunities to obtain economies of scale (for example, access to loans at lower interest rates and to lower malpractice insurance rates) (Feldstein, 1994). To achieve the benefits of increased coordination and communication, organizations need to be closely linked together, both administratively and clinically. In many parts of the country MCOs, hospitals, and various non–acute care organizations have begun to align themselves through various forms of affiliation into what is being referred to as **integrated health care delivery systems (IDS)** (Shortell, Gillies, and Anderson, 1994).

The organizations and practitioners composing an IDS must avoid working against each other (as has frequently been their tendency) if they are going to prevent fragmentation of care, which is not only costly but also negatively affects quality. This can be achieved if each provider faces the same financial incentives. Under **capitated arrangements,** the IDS knows what its revenue will be at the time a contract is negotiated: the total amount of revenue equals the fixed price per subscriber multiplied by the number of subscribers. This means that whenever health care services or treatments are provided, costs are generated that in turn reduce the amount of the system's total revenue (Buerhaus, 1996b). Consequently all facilities (not just hospitals) used to provide care become cost centers; there are no profit- or revenue-generating centers under **capitation.** As Shortell, Gillies, and Anderson (1994) point out, "Cost centers do not generate revenue as in the old world of indemnity-based fee-for-service medicine. Then, more volume meant more profit; now, more volume means less profit." Capitating the system aligns the financial incentives facing all components and providers in the system, thereby stimulating coordinated behavior and information flow.

Capitated arrangements also provide the economic incentives that make it financially worthwhile to keep people well. Preventing illness through case finding, early diagnosis, education, and health promotion is valuable under capitation because it helps reduce subscribers' use of higher-cost components of the system, namely hospital care. Furthermore, to reduce the length of stay for patients who require hospital-based care, the IDS must have in place the full range of non–acute care organizations and personnel who are capable of guiding the transition of patients through the system. By facing the same financial incentives, all providers are motivated to minimize the costs of care by using the most appropriate resources and emphasizing programs that keep patients healthy.

Because the development of quality measures is rapidly evolving and quality assessment will be used to compare individual providers, organizations, and health plans, IDSs will face strong incentives to avoid any lapse in the quality of care provided by components of the system. In fact the ability to develop cost, quality, and outcomes monitoring systems is presumably made easier under an IDS (Feldstein, 1994).

In sum, the **transformation in health care** is being driven by a transition away from a system dominated by health planning, reliance on regulations, runaway costs, rapidly accelerating spending, and acceptance of "expert" opinion to assess the quality of health care. In the 1990s the health care system has given way to vigorous public sector cost containment initiatives, expanding enrollment in managed care, adoption of market-oriented incentives and economic competition, and the emergence of integrated delivery systems. These forces are creating economic discipline in the production of health care as practitioners, organizations, insurers, and even consumers are beginning to be held financially accountable for their decisions. Not surprisingly, the rate of increase in total national expenditures on health care has declined since 1992. In fact, in 1994, the latest year for which comprehensive data are available, growth in health expenditures dropped to its lowest rate in more than 30 years (Levit, Lazenby, and Sivarijan, 1996; Levit et al., 1994).

At the same time that the new economics in health care has emerged, so too has the new science of quality measurement. Efforts to compare quality across individuals, organizations, and health plans, as well as to adopt the methods of quality improvement, dominate the landscape. Together, these developments are creating powerful incentives for organizations to continue to lower their costs, improve quality, become more innovative, and do a better job satisfying consumers. These changes are moving the health care system in a direction that promises to offer society greater value for its substantial expenditures on health care.

IMPLICATIONS FOR NURSES

As discussed at the outset of this chapter, nurses are a vital input and at the same time important decision makers in determining how other human and nonhuman resources are combined and used in the clinical production process. The six forces transforming the health care system have important implications for nurses in both of these roles.

Nurses as Inputs in the Production Process

As **economic competition** takes hold, organizations that are not price competitive (obtained by lowering their costs) or are perceived as lacking in quality (as determined by objective measures and compared with other organizations) will go out of business. Lowering costs and improving quality are the realities of health care for the foreseeable future. This suggests two important implications for professional nurses in relation to their roles as inputs in the production of patient care.

First, nurses can anticipate that employers will face strong economic incentives to purchase only those resources that are the most valuable in terms of how effectively they help the organization lower its production costs and improve the quality of care. As they consider the amount and kind of nursing personnel to purchase, organizations will carefully compare the cost and contribution toward quality of advanced practice nurses, RNs, LPNs, and nursing aides. Obviously, professional nurses cost more, and organizations will therefore have a certain level of resistance to employ them over nonprofessional nursing personnel, especially if they believe that the latter's productivity can be increased inexpensively by cross-training and providing additional education. On the other hand, organizations must also consider which category of nurse labor is most productive in improving the quality of patient care. In addition, organizations must weigh the preferences of physicians and the perceptions of purchasers—large businesses, MCOs, and individual consumers—who typically associate professional nurses with high quality, rather than nurse aides and LPNs. Thus organizations must strike a balance between employing lower-cost nursing personnel and those who are more productive in improving higher-quality care.

Second, given the **economic pressures** facing organizations and their effect on decisions concerning the purchase of all categories of resources, professional nurses should realize that for their own good they need to increase their value to the organization. Organizations will rationally pursue actions to lower the costs of providing nursing care and at the same time try to enhance their quality improvement capabilities. Moreover, nurses need to recognize that in the near future new measures of quality are likely to establish more precise linkages between different kinds of professional and nonprofessional nursing personnel and the technical and personal interactive components of quality, as well as clinical outcomes. Perceptions of nurses' contributions to quality will soon be replaced by empirically determined evidence. Thus professional nurses must comprehend that it is in their own interest to be included in the way organizations measure quality. After all, this will become the way that organizations form an understanding of what quality is, how it is produced, and the way nurses contribute to the production of high quality.

To increase their value to an organization, professional nurses need to see themselves as **resources** in the production of clinical care. In the eyes of their employers, nurses' value will increase the greatest when they are seen as finding new ways to lower the costs of producing nursing care and at the same time improving quality. Hence nurses must examine and reexamine all structures and processes under their control and those with which they interact to discover where costs can and must be removed without harming quality. Organizations will reward those who take leadership for eliminating waste and redundancies, abandon inappropriate activities, and enhance the quality of care. Using their creativity and unique knowledge of patient needs, nurses can excel in these activities without compromising professional ethics.

Nurses must also find out what quality means in the eyes of their employers and understand how it is being measured. This will provide nurses with needed information about institutional priorities and motivations and enable a better understanding of the organization's knowledge about the relationship between nursing activities and the production of varying levels of quality. Nurses also need to learn about the tools the organization is using to measure quality and discern if and how nursing interventions are being adequately captured and properly analyzed. These activities can be readily accomplished without much time or effort and will greatly help nurses develop their agenda and set priorities with respect to the actions needed to improve the quality of nursing care, address possible misconceptions of nursing held by those in charge of quality measurement, and become more visible and positively associated with the organization's quality improvement initiatives.

Nurses' Clinical Management Roles

Every day nurses make important decisions on the kinds and amounts of organizational resources that are used and the way that they are combined to produce patient care. Moreover, as inputs into the production process, nurses decide how they themselves interact most effectively with other resources to achieve desired outcomes. As new technology is acquired by the organization, the price and productivity of other resources change, and new measures and standards of what constitutes quality care for different patient conditions are developed, nurses will need to become better at managing and creatively combining resources to meet these standards in the least costly way. Indeed, data will be collected to show how well they perform their management role and whether they are using the organization's resources wisely. Thus not only does the changing environment in health care require professional nurses to improve their value as resources used in the production process, but it also compels them to improve their management of the production process.

To improve their management capabilities, professional nurses have to master the new tools and techniques of quality measurement that were briefly identified earlier and are discussed extensively in Part III and Chapter 21. Nurses are not alone in needing to gain competence in these areas; physicians face even more pressing demands, and many must work through skepticism about what may seem like yet another organizational directive to improve quality. Nevertheless, the discussion of the forces transforming health care discussed in this chapter strongly suggests that the measurement and reporting of quality indicators will be what Blumenthal and Epstein (1996) call "an enduring feature of our new health care system." But by mastering these techniques, nurses can more effectively work with physicians and management, enrich their knowledge of quality measurement, and in the process create opportunities to take greater control over their practice.

Finally, improving nursing's input and clinical management roles is a long-term activity that requires commitment by the profession's educators, researchers, and policy makers. The value of nurses will be enhanced only if members of the profession possess the right knowledge and can apply it competently. Therefore the curriculum of nursing education programs should integrate the emerging science of quality measurement within clinical and management courses. Graduates must also be knowledgeable about health care economics, understand the incentives and objectives of managed care and capitation, and appreciate how integrated delivery systems are emerging and the opportunities they present for professional nurses. At a minimum, future graduates must be able to conduct a basic-level cost-effectiveness analysis. In addition, nurse researchers and policy makers should pursue a quality improvement and cost reduction agenda in their efforts to advance the knowledge base guiding the practice of nurses and create a more supportive environment for practitioners.

Summary

The forces transforming the health care system are profoundly affecting the way organizations produce patient care. The forces are causing nurses and organizations to recognize more clearly nursing's economic roles at the center of the production process and hence their impact on costs and quality. As both resources and decision makers guiding the use of other organizational resources, professional nurses can neither escape these forces nor succumb to the pressures and challenges they present. Rather, nurses have the opportunity, if not the responsibility, to participate in making sure these forces lead to positive outcomes.

This chapter has argued that positive outcomes can only be accomplished if nurses take decisive actions to discover new ways to lower their costs while pursuing strategies that demonstrate how they contribute to and improve the quality of care. In this way, nurses increase their value as resources and managers of resources, thereby enabling organizations and the broader society to obtain a greater return on their investments in the nursing profession.

Discussion Questions

1. What is the relationship between cost containment in health care and annual federal budget deficits? What are the implications of accumulating public debt for health care organizations and professionals?
2. What is the origin of hospital restructuring? In economic terms, what is the objective of these initiatives?
3. Explain in clinical terms how nurses contribute in the production of patient care. Now explain in economic terms how nurses function as economic resources.
4. How are economic forces transmitted from employers to MCOs and from MCOs to health care delivery organizations? How are nursing personnel in MCOs, hospitals, and other organizations affected?
5. From an economic perspective, why should the development of economic competition in health care result in improvements in the quality of health care services?
6. Explain the meaning of the following statement: "Nurses should raise their economic value in the eyes of organizations that purchase nursing services to pro-

duce patient care." What can nurses do to increase their value? Beyond the strategies presented in this chapter, what other ways can nurses raise their value?

7. What is an integrated delivery system? Explain how financial incentives are aligned under capitated arrangements. What opportunities do integrated delivery systems offer the nursing profession?

REFERENCES

Angell M, Kassirer JP: Quality and the medical marketplace—Following elephants, *N Engl J Med* 335:883, 1996.

Blendon RJ, Bodie M, Benson J: What happened to American's support of the Clinton plan? *Health Aff* 14(2):7, 1995.

Blumenthal D: Quality of health care. Part 1: Quality of care—What is it? *N Engl J Med* 335:891, 1996a.

Blumenthal D: Quality of health care. Part 4: Origins of the quality-of-care debate, O—What is it? *N Engl J Med* 335:891, 1996b.

Blumenthal D, Epstein AM: Quality of health care. Part 6: The role of physicians in the future of quality management, *N Engl J Med* 335:1328, 1996.

Brook RH, McGlynn DA, Cleary PD: Quality of health care. Part 2: Measuring quality of care, *N Engl J Med* 335:966, 1996.

Buerhaus P: Nursing, competition, and quality, *Nurs Econ* 10(1):21, 1992.

Buerhaus P: Understanding the economic environment of health care. In Disch J, editor: *The managed care challenge for nurse executives,* AONE Leadership Series, American Organization of Nurse Executives, Chicago, 1996a, American Hospital Association Publishing.

Buerhaus P: The value of nursing care: Creating a new place in a competitive market, *Nurs Policy Forum* 2(2):13, 1996b.

Buerhaus P: What is the harm in imposing nurse staffing regulations in hospitals? *Nurs Econ* 15(2):66, 1997.

Buerhaus PI, Staiger DO: Managed care and the nurse workforce, *JAMA* 276:1487, 1996.

Carey T, Weis K, Homer C: Prepaid versus traditional Medicaid plans: Effects on preventative health care, *J Clin Epidemiol* 43:1213, 1990.

Carey TS, Weis K, Homer C: Prepaid versus traditional Medicaid plans: Lack of effect on pregnancy outcomes and prenatal care, *Health Serv Res* 26:165, 1991.

Carlisle DM et al.: HMO vs fee-for-service care of older persons with acute myocardial infarction, *Am J Public Health* 82:1626, 1992.

Chassin MR: Quality of health care. Part 3: Improving the quality of care, *N Engl J Med* 335:1060, 1996.

Clement DG et al.: Access and outcomes of elderly patients enrolled in managed care, *JAMA* 271:1487, 1994.

Cohodes DR: The slippery slope of health care reform, *Inquiry* 31(1):4, 1994.

Congressional Budget Office, Public handout, U.S. Congress, February 1995.

Feldstein PJ: *Health care economics,* ed 2, New York, 1983, John Wiley & Sons.

Feldstein PJ: *Health policy issues: An economic perspective on health reform,* Ann Arbor, Mich, 1994, AUPHA Press/Health Administration Press.

Freund DA et al.: Evaluation of the Medicaid competition demonstrations, *Health Care Finance Rev* 11:81, 1989.

Greenfield S et al.: Outcomes of patients with hypertension and non–insulin-dependent diabetes mellitus treated by different systems and specialties: Results from the Medical Outcomes Study, *JAMA* 247:1436, 1995.

Hillman AL, Pauly MV, Kerstein JJ: How do financial incentives affect physicians' clinical decisions and the financial performance of health maintenance organizations? *N Engl J Med* 321:86, 1989.

Hohlen MM et al.: Access to office-based physicians under capitation reimbursement and Medicaid case management findings from the Children's Medicaid Program, *Med Care* 28:56, 1990.

Iglehart JK: A conversation with Leonard D. Schaeffer, *Health Aff* 14(4):131, 1995.

Iglehart JK: The national committee for quality assurance, *N Engl J Med* 335:995, 1996.

Levit KR, Lazenby HC, Sivarijan L: Health care spending in 1994: Slowest in decades, *Health Aff* 15(2):130, 1996.

Levit KR et al.: National health spending trends, 1960-1993, *Health Aff* 13(5):14, 1994.

Lurie N et al.: Does capitation affect the health of the chronically mentally ill? Results from a randomized trial, *JAMA* 267:3300, 1992a.

Lurie N et al.: The effects of capitation on health and functional status of the Medicaid elderly: A randomized trial, *Ann Intern Med* 120:506, 1992b.

Miller RH, Luft HS: Managed care plan performance since 1980: A literature analysis, *JAMA* 271:1512, 1995.

Murray JP et al.: Ambulatory testing for capitation and fee-for-service patients in the same practice setting: Relationship to outcomes, *Med Care* 30:252, 1992.

Prospective Payment Assessment Commission: Medicare and the American health care system, report to Congress, Washington, DC, June 1996.

Relman AS: Controlling costs by "managed competition"—Would it work? *N Engl J Med* 3228:133, 1993.

Retchin SM, Brown B: Management of colorectal cancer in Medicare health maintenance organizations, *J Gen Intern Med* 5:110, 1990a.

Retchin SM, Brown B: The quality of ambulatory care in Medicare health maintenance organizations, *Am J Public Health* 80:411, 1990b.

Retchin SM, Brown RS: Elderly patients with congestive heart failure under prepaid care, *Am J Med* 90:236, 1991.

Retchin SM et al.: How the elderly fare in HMOs: Outcomes from the Medicare Competition Demonstrations, *Health Serv Res* 27:651, 1992.

Rowlan D, Kristina H: Medicaid: Moving to managed care, *Health Aff* 15(3):150, 1996.

Shortell SM, Gillies RR, Anderson DA: New world of managed care: Creating organized delivery systems, *Health Aff* 13(5):46, 1994.

Taylor R: The future of managed care. Presentation given at the Harvard Nursing Research Institute's Conference on Executive Nursing Leadership in Academic Health Centers and Major Teaching Hospitals, Cambridge, Mass, June 20, 1996.

Vladick B: The future of Medicare. Presentation given at The Harvard School of Public Health, Boston, Jan 24, 1996.

Welch PW: Growth in HMO share of the Medicare market, 1989-1994, *Health Aff* 15(3):201, 1996.

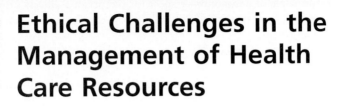

chapter **nineteen**

Ethical Challenges in the Management of Health Care Resources

Maureen Goode

Learning Objectives

- Identify the major moral principles that are linked to the management of health care resources.
- Identify some of the major dilemmas regarding the allocation of scarce resources so that nurse managers may engage in critical dialogue.
- Discuss some of the major medical expenditures that have led our health care system into a state of crisis.
- Identify some immediate nursing interventions that nursing managers must implement to allow patients to begin to limit their use of medical resources.

MAJOR MORAL PRINCIPLES

On almost any given day there is at least one story in the press or on television resulting from the advancement of medical practice, ethics, or litigation. Margaret Brazier (1992) notes the ironic dichotomy of being in the limelight: " . . . one day the doctor is hailed as a savior . . . the next he is condemned as authoritarian and uncaring."

The field of **medical ethics** is far from new. Beginning with the formulation of the Hippocratic oath in Ancient Greece to the present day, health care providers have debated among themselves the codes of conduct that should govern the science of medicine and the art of healing. These ethical codes of conduct for professional practitioners were derived from the more basic universal moral principles that serve as guidance when making ethical decisions:

1. The principle of nonmaleficence—"Above all, do no harm."
2. The principle of beneficence—we should act in ways that promote the welfare of other people.

3. The principle of utility—we should act in ways that bring about the greatest good for the greater number of people.
4. The principle of autonomy—respect for the personal liberty of others.
5. The principle of veracity—truth telling between the health care professional and the patient.
6. The principle of justice—the concepts of justice and equality.

The professional nurse manager of the 1990s must deal with an array of health care ethical dilemmas. The issues of informed consent for patients, staffing decisions that must balance cost and quality, and confidentiality and reporting concerns must all be addressed by today's nurse manager. Successful nurse managers will use the ethical principles of beneficence, nonmaleficence, veracity, and respect for autonomy as they apply to both the patients they serve and the professional nursing staff they employ.

The principles of utility and justice, however, may provide the largest challenges to professional nurse managers, who are charged with the management of health care resources. Any commodity or service that is in short supply relative to the demand raises issues of fairness and distributive justice. Munson (1996) notes that " . . . the basic question, of course, is who shall get it and who shall go without?" Nurse managers must take an active role in ensuring that citizens have access to our health care, coupled with the management of our resources that emphasizes cost-effective delivery while maintaining quality nursing care in a system that is morally just.

The following example illustrates the difficulty in determining the distribution of scarce resources.

You are the head nurse of a busy dialysis unit that can accommodate 12 patients. At the present moment there are two openings for a dialysis machine and four patients who are waiting to be treated. You cannot select on the basis of "first come, first served" because all four referrals showed up in your unit at the same time.

Mr. Jones is a 24-year-old husband and father of two children. It appears that he will require dialysis for only a short period following injuries he sustained in an auto accident. His job is the primary source of income for his family, and he has medical insurance.

Ms. Quinn is a 30-year-old single mother of three who is unemployed and on welfare. She is requiring dialysis following rare complications of a new research drug for the treatment of AIDS.

Mr. Smith is a 75-year-old retired physician from your hospital. Just recently he made the local news, having been arrested for drunk driving on the evening that he and his wife had hosted a benefactors' party for the hospital. He is covered by an extensive insurance plan. Mr. Smith was just recently diagnosed with malignant nephrosclerosis.

Miss Ross is a 6-year-old girl who is awaiting her third kidney transplant, the first two having failed. Both her parents are unemployed, and her medical expenses have been covered by a combination of Medicaid and the state's crippled children assistance plan.

What criteria would you use to select your two patients? Would you use age alone as a criterion? How about those with dependents? What about ability to pay? Did you place any value on their contribution to society? What about those whose disease might be linked to social behavior? Perhaps none of the aforementioned criteria should be used, and in its place the "best recipient" in terms of predicted successful medical outcome should be the only criterion you would want to use.

THE ALLOCATION OF SCARCE RESOURCES

It wasn't until the 1960s and the introduction of the artificial kidney that attention was first paid to the issue of scarce medical resources. From the moment of its inception, there were many more candidates for dialysis than there were available units. In response to this, centers such as the Artificial Kidney Center in Seattle, Washington, set up a committee to select patients who would receive this service (Munson, 1996). The committee was put into place to decide, just as you were asked in the previous case example, who would receive this service when there are limited spaces available.

The crisis drew national attention as other dialysis centers faced similar dilemmas, and this eventually led to the passage of Section 299-1 of Public Law 92-603 by Congress in 1972. This law guaranteed that those with end-stage renal disease who require hemodialysis or kidney transplants would be covered under Medicare. Munson (1996) notes that currently more than 195,000 patients receive dialysis under the Medicare system at a cost of $8 billion per year. By the end of the century it is predicted that some 350,000 patients will be enrolled in the program at a cost of more than $10 billion.

Concerns throughout the 1960s regarding the allocation of dialysis are similarly reflected in the 1980-1990s issue regarding organ transplants. Although the use of the drug cyclosporine dramatically improved the success rate of organ transplants, the scarcity of organs available for transplantation remains critical. Numerous options for improving the pool of available organs range from the open-market approach (this would, however, require a repeal of the 1984 National Organ Transplantation Act, which made the sale of organs for transplant illegal in the United States) to a policy of presumed consent, which has been adopted by several European countries.

It was recently reported that the organization that makes rules regarding the allocation of livers for transplants has decided to introduce rationing. In the past, the United Network for Organ Sharing had always used "the sickest patient" as the criterion for top priority on the transplant list. This group of top priority patients, however, would include both patients whose livers had suddenly failed from a viral infection or toxin and those whose livers have been deteriorating for decades, like people with alcoholic cirrhosis or viral hepatitis, the latter having only half as likely a chance to survive as the former (New York Times, 1996).

According to the *New York Times,* (p. 2, 1996), the new rule for the distribution of livers for transplant will be according to this relative likelihood of success criteria. William Payne, a member of the board of directors of the United Network for Organ Sharing and the director of the liver transplant program at the University of Minnesota, was quoted as saying that this new rule is difficult because it means doctors can no longer ask, "What's best for my patient?" but instead, "Who's the best recipient for this liver?" (New York Times, 1996) This shifts the focus of the historical physician-patient relationship based on the ethical principle of beneficence to one of medical pragmatism.

The problems with transplant and dialysis programs involve the difficult issue of the allocation of scarce medical resources at the micro allocation level. There are, however, less ominous micro allocation decisions made every day: Who will get the bed in the intensive care unit? Which surgery will be canceled to make room for the emergency admission? Which patient who calls an outpatient setting demanding to see the physician will get in that day? All of these micro allocation dilemmas will be challenging to the nurse manager, who must learn to balance the ethical conflict between the patient's interests and the organization's interests.

Along with this are the broader social issues that are connected with the access to and utilization of our medical resources: What kind of health care will be available? How will the costs be distributed? Who will regulate the delivery of these services? Who will get it and on what basis? Although macro allocation decisions are more the domain of Congress, state legislators, insurance companies, private foundations, and health care organizations, today's successful nurse manager must be congnizant of the larger ethical issues affecting the ever-increasing demands for health care resources.

THE HEALTH CARE CRISIS

It has long been recognized in the United States that our system of health care delivery is in a state of crisis. "Despite the widespread expectation in 1994 that either the 'Clinton plan' or some other legislative proposal would deal with the crisis and drastically alter the way American health care is funded and utilized, this did not happen. The crisis remains unresolved." (Munson, 1996)

It is estimated that

. . . In 1950 the United States spent about the same amount on health care as on national defense. Around half that amount was spent on education. Now education and defense spending are about equal, while the costs of health care take more of the gross domestic product than the other two added together. (Munson, 1996)

Edge and Groves (1994) point out that

. . . Health care spending per family each year is approximately $6,535, of which two-thirds ($4,296) is paid out by the families, and one-third ($2,239) is paid by businesses. The cost of health care in 1992 jumped by 11 percent to $817 billion—or 14 percent of the gross national product (GNP). It is estimated that, if current spending trends continue, by the year 2020 health care spending could consume as much as 36 percent of the GNP, or one dollar out of every three.

Even though the health care expenditures in the United States far exceed those in any other industrialized country, we have not, so to speak, received "much bang for our buck"! We rank seventeenth in the world in infant mortality, and teenage pregnancy continues to be on the rise. Japan (which spends only 6.8% of its GNP on health care) and Greece (4.8% of its GNP) have life expectancies that exceed ours. It is also estimated that single-payor plans such as Canada's spend approximately 12% on administration costs, whereas the United States, with our multiple-payor system, spends approximately 25% to 30% of our health care dollars on administrative costs.

Along with the enormous expenditures are the impediments to access. In 1993 the Bureau of Census reported that public and private health insurance protected 220 million Americans; however, 40 million people remained without health insurance coverage. Of these noninsured individuals, 55.5% were employed but by firms that do not offer coverage. Millions of others were poor but did not qualify for Medicaid (*Source Book of Health Insurance Data 1995,* 1996).

Even those who believe themselves to be well insured often discover that their insurance does not cover major items. One in particular is home nursing care. Moreover, this lack of coverage is coupled with the recent drastic reduction in hospital length of stay, pushing increasingly sicker patients back into the community with neither the resources nor support from their insurers.

While attempts at health care reform have been criticized as really being "wealth care reform," the crisis is not to be shouldered completely by insurance companies. "The tyranny of a prince in an oligarchy is not so dangerous to the public welfare as the apathy of a citizen in a democracy." This statement by Montesquieu was reflected in a poll conducted by the Public Agenda Foundation, which found that although 90% of American citizens believe that everyone should have the best possible health care, few were willing to "put their money where their mouth is." Only 10% of those polled said that they would accept a $125 tax increase to support a national insurance program that would cover catastrophic illness (Edge and Groves, 1994).

We must also consider whether this reluctance to pay out for the health care that we desire is problematically compounded by the mind-set of "the American dream" when it comes to health care. Most Americans expect to access and use "the latest and greatest" that medicine has to offer based on our wants rather than our needs.

SETTING LIMITS AND PRIORITIZING

"The widespread belief that we can all get all we need if only we deliver health care efficiently is hopelessly wrong, a deep and fundamental illusion." (Callahan, 1990) This accurate statement by Daniel Callahan begs the question, How do we go about rationing or setting limits to health care?

> As a society we need to address the issue of limits in health care as well as the issue of priority setting with respect to meeting health needs. And the framework within which this must occur is the framework of justice and equal respect for the rights of all. (Fleck et al., 1994)

Nursing must take an active role in ensuring that proper limits are set and the prioritizing of health care needs is accomplished within this framework.

There are several theoretical positions surrounding the moral principle of justice that apply to our debate over the allocation of health care resources.

Egalitarian Theories

Edge and Groves (1994) point out that " . . . these theories emphasize equal access to goods and services. In some of its more radical forms, egalitarianism holds that any deviations from absolute equality in distribution are unjust." This principle is rather ideal and does not correspond well to the way that most health care is distributed in our capitalistic society.

Libertarian Theory

Libertarians emphasize personal rights to social and economic liberty. They are not as concerned with, nor do they outline the requirements of, how the material goods and services are to be distributed, only that the choice of allocation system be freely chosen. In the United States, outside of our charity, social welfare, and military medical services, we have chosen for the most part to allocate health care goods and services using the free-market approach. (Edge and Groves, 1994)

This free-market approach is played out in our current environment, in which health care systems compete for contracts and clients.

Edge and Groves (1994) further assert that even if in the future we were able to develop some sort of national health care plan that would provide all citizens with a "decent minimum," it is likely that it will coexist with our free-market libertarian ideals.

Health care might be considered a social good that is similar to the social goods of education, transportation, housing, and so on. And if we provide the "decent minimum" to citizens via a national health care plan, those with the purchasing power to obtain more health care should be allowed to do so. Such is the nature of our capitalistic society.

Cindy Rushton (1990) describes such a scenario in her article entitled, "Balancing the Benefits and Burdens of ECMO: The Nurse's Role." In this article she asks us to imagine a scenario in which two imperiled newborns require extracorporeal membrane oxygenation (ECMO); one family has the ability to pay for this costly high-tech treatment, and the other does not. If we were to prioritize those treatments that we as citizens would wish to include in the "decent minimum" we want to provide for all citizens, the intervention of ECMO may well be one that we could not afford to offer. Rushton notes that although the family who cannot purchase the expensive procedure may feel that this is "unfair," it does not necessarily follow that this is "unjust" in our capitalistic society. If we believe that this is unjust (as we might want to consider health a different sort of social good that carries a more significant moral claim to it than education, housing, and so on), then we must be willing as a society to pay for the highest level of care for all. This appears quite unlikely, however, because we have been unwilling so far to pay for even a lower level of care for all.

Utilitarian Theory

The principle of utility is sometimes called the "greatest happiness principle." Another way to define utilitarianism is that actions will be judged as right that produce the greatest happiness for the greatest number of people.

There are many examples of the utilitarian principle within our laws and social policy. We restrict individual liberty and autonomy by the traffic laws that we impose to promote safety and our policy of "no smoking" in public buildings. Even something as simple as a "do not walk on the grass" sign is designed on the utilitarian principle that not doing so will result in the greater good for the greater number of people.

Daniel Callahan has proposed a utilitarian rationing system for health care known as the natural life span argument (Edge and Groves, 1994). "He feels that such a rationing scheme is necessary to stave off the ever-widening gap between resources and our expanding health needs caused by the flaws in our current system, as well as the increased needs generated by an aging population." (Edge and Groves, 1994)

Fleck et al. (1994) note that "Currently the elderly have 3.5 times the health needs of the nonelderly. They make up 12% of the U.S. population now but account for 34% of all health spending per year, about $230 billion in 1990. And by the year 2030 the elderly will represent 20% of the U.S. population."

That we presently concentrate the largest portion of our health care dollars in the last years of people's lives begs the question, How much health care are we morally obliged to provide the elderly? Callahan's proposal is that once the following criteria have been met (usually between the ages of 78 and 82 years) we would not be morally obliged to offer life-extending technologies. The four criteria are as follows (Edge and Groves, 1994):

1. One's life work is completed.
2. One's moral obligations to those for whom one has responsibility have been discharged.
3. One's death does not seem to others an offense to sense or sensibility or tempt others to despair and rage at human existence.
4. When the process of dying is not marked by unbearable and degrading pain.

Keep in mind that Callahan does not suggest that we need not provide medical care and treatment to the elderly, but merely proposes that we need not provide expensive, invasive life-extending technologies. While there may be some elderly patients who still desire such treatments, we should, at the very least, allow those who are ready to limit their use of resources to do so.

A research study published in the *Journal of the American Medical Association* (SUPPORT Principle Investigators, 1995) revealed some disappointing results despite the passing of the Patient Self-Determination Act of 1990.

The researchers at five teaching hospitals looked at some 4000 patients to determine a baseline of care for the terminally ill. The patients suffered from one of nine terminal illnesses, and 50% survived less than 6 months. The researchers found that only half of the patients who didn't want to be resuscitated had a "DNR" (do not resuscitate) order entered in their chart, and in 47% of these cases the doctors were aware of their preferences. Among the patients who died with a DNR order, 46% were written within 2 days of their death, indicating that they likely had already received treatment that could have been withheld. Approximately 38% of those who died had spent at least 10 days in an intensive care unit.

The second phase of the study involved another 4000 patients who met the same initial criteria. Half of the patients were given the usual medical care, and the other half were assigned to the intervention program. This intervention program consisted of an intensive care unit nurse, educated in the issues and principles of medical ethics, who could provide information and support to patients and families and could serve as a liaison between patients/families and physicians.

The results of this intervention program revealed that there was no improvement in the use of DNR orders, no reduction in days spent in the intensive care unit, and no reduction in the use and cost of life-sustaining services (SUPPORT Principle Investigators, 1995).

Although the results of this study are indeed a disappointment, they emphasized the enormous amount of further work and intervention that are needed to begin to limit the use of our scarce resources. The continued use of a nursing intervention program such as the one described in the study is of vital importance, and nurse managers and leaders must continue to emphasize the significant consequences if we fail to intervene. Moreover, although an intervention program such as this is designed to address the issue of scarce resources "one patient at a time," a more systematic fix is needed to change the practice of our health care delivery to the elderly and the dying.

The last issue regarding utilitarian principles that will be addressed is, much like the last example, also tied to the principle of autonomy. Throughout the 1970s and 1980s the majority of cases brought before ethics committees and the courts were regarding issues of termination of treatment. The Karen Quinlin case (regarding the removal of artificial respiration) and Nancy Cruzan case (regarding the removal of artificial nutrition and hydration) are just two of the thousands of cases in which patients or family members sought approval to limit the intrusion of modern medicine.

What is interesting, and somewhat disturbing in light of our limited resources, is the 1990s trend of those patients' and family members' demanding care. The case of Baby K is just one example among many.

Baby K was born anencephalic at Fairfax Hospital in Virginia in October 1992. Her mother, believing that "all life should be protected," wanted her child to receive mechanical ventilation when she developed respiratory distress. The hospital physicians disagreed because the national standard of care for anencephalic newborns is to allow such infants to die from respiratory failure and provide "comfort care only" treatments such as nutrition, hydration, and warmth.

Following the discharge of Baby K to a nursing facility (after successful extubation), the hospital sought a declaration from the court that would allow them not to reintubate Baby K should she develop respiratory distress in the future, concluding that such treatment was "medically and ethically inappropriate." Although the physicians may be correct in that further treatment is "medically" inappropriate, the question of whether it is "morally" inappropriate is arguable.

The court, based on its interpretation of the Emergency Medical Treatment and Active Labor Act (EMTALA), otherwise known as the federal antidumping law, found in favor of Baby K's mother, who wished for further treatment of Baby K when needed.

What was extremely disappointing about this case, among other things, was that the U.S. Court of Appeals allowed the case to turn on this broad interpretation of the EMTALA law with little discussion with respect to the religious aspect of this infamous case.

The case regarding Baby K begs a difficult question that we as Americans must address regarding the allocation of our medical resources. Baby K's mother invoked the "absolute sanctity of life" principle as her reason for asking that all be done for Baby K medically. The First Amendment of our Constitution guarantees the freedom to practice one's religion. What we need to ask ourselves is this: Does the freedom to practice your religion in the United States guarantee you the right to use any and all of our scarce medical resources?

In an article that deals with this religious perspective, Stephen Post (1995) cleverly proposes an option. Post suggests that those in the United States who hold the position that all of life should be saved regardless of the quality of life, the medical futility of the intervention, or the cost, should form their own high-risk sanctity of life insurance pools! This would "surely test the degree of moral conviction." (Post, 1995)

Summary

Although the U.S. health care system is one of the best in terms of quantity, that has not necessarily led to the quality outcomes one might expect. The increasing demands placed on this system by citizens who have come to expect it as a "right" without carefully considering the "duty" obligations to pay for, limit, and prioritize our health care threaten to overwhelm the system entirely.

Are we prepared as a society to offer the best to everyone? Or should we instead attempt to offer a "decent minimum" to all that is accomplished within the moral framework of justice? We must be willing to acknowledge that this "just" health care system would not necessarily be one of "equality" for all our citizens.

Nurse managers and leaders must recognize the need for nurses to play a vital role in the education of consumers and health care professionals regarding setting limits and prioritizing our health care needs. Nurse managers must set a precedence for the recognition of patient advance directives and must implement innovative nurse interventions that can lead to successful respect for and adherence to this "limit-setting" tool.

The moral principles of utility and justice must serve to guide us in achieving our future health care policies. It is time for the professional nurse manager to undertake a much more active leadership role in the development of position papers and public discourse on the management of our scarce health care resources.

Discussion Questions

1. What two major moral principles relate to managing scarce health care resources?
2. Which of the major medical expenditures are responsible for our current health care system crisis?
3. Why is it important that consumers prioritize and set limits for the utilization of health care resources?
4. What vital nursing interventions should nurse managers implement within their clinical area that might allow patients to set limits on their utilization of health care resources?

REFERENCES

Brazier M: *Medicine, patients and the law,* ed 2, London, 1992, Penguin Group.

Callahan D: *What kind of life: The limits of medical progress,* New York, 1990, Simon & Schuster.

Edge R, Groves J: *The ethics of health care—A guide for clinical practice,* Albany, NY, 1994, Delmar.

Fleck L et al.: *Just caring: Conflicting rights, uncertain responsibilities,* Lansing, Mich, 1994, Citizen Forums for Health Care Reform, Michigan State University.

Kolata G: New rules on liver transplants, *New York Times,* section 4, p 2, Nov 17, 1996.

Munson R: *Intervention and reflection—Basic issues in medical ethics,* ed 5, Belmont, Calif, 1996, Wadsworth.

Post S: Baby K: Medical futility and the free exercise of religion, *J Law Med Ethics* 23:20, 1995.

Rushton C: Balancing the benefits and burdens of ECMO: The nurse's role, *Crit Care Nurs Clin North Am* 2(3):481, 1990.

Source Book of Health Insurance Data 1995, Washington, DC, 1996, Health Insurance Association of America.

SUPPORT Principle Investigators: A controlled trial to improve care for seriously ill hospitalized patients: The study to understand prognoses and preferences for outcomes and treatments (SUPPORT), *JAMA* 274(20):1591, 1995.

chapter **twenty**

Diversity in the Workforce

Marylane Wade Koch

Learning Objectives

- Identify emerging trends in the workforce demographics.
- Discuss implications for nursing practice.
- Describe implications for resource management.

Health care professionals need to recognize trends affecting society today and develop strategies to address these changes as they relate to health care practice. The U.S. population is growing more diverse in age, gender, sexual orientation, race, physical and mental abilities, and ethnicity. Future issues in expanding human **diversity** include such aspects as financial status, education, marital and family status, religious beliefs, military experience, geographical location, and hobbies. These and other issues of continuing diversity will affect how and by whom health care is delivered, how health care dollars are procured and allocated, and how health care services are valued. Globalization and emerging cultural values will change the way health care professionals are educated and provide health care services in this country.

EMERGING TRENDS

External forces influence businesses and organizations in many ways. Factors such as public opinion and legislation can directly affect societal norms and thus affect organizational practices. A technique for predicting emerging issues is "environmental scanning." (Keen, 1994) This practice includes systematic scanning of various resources such as journals, newspapers, public speeches, current, as well as unenacted, legislation, opinion surveys, and agendas of powerful interest groups to assess changes in the environment. These are usually categorized as demographics, economics, social mores, political norms, and technologies, to name a few (Keen, 1994). Decision makers look to these emerging trends to understand the future implications. Usually these issues come to light in the media, courts, and regulatory agencies and as a result of government and consumer requirements.

WORKFORCE DEMOGRAPHICS
The Age Shift

There is a shift occurring in the U.S. demographics of today's environment. The workforce is aging. The largest workforce group is between 35 and 44 years of age. The next group, ages 45 to 55, will become the second largest group by the year 2000. These baby boomers will account for 49% of the U.S. workforce by the turn of the century. This will affect " . . . everything from health care costs and training to compensation and discrimination claims." (Keen, 1994) For example, the use of health care resources increases greatly after age 40. Likewise, after age 40 discrimination claims are more likely because of the Age Discrimination in Employment Act (ADEA). This group generally is making higher wages and is more productive as a result of age and experience. Formal education has often been past for some time, so supplementary training is needed. Child care as a focus gives way to elder care concerns. These workers want better pension and retirement options. Stability in the job rather than opportunity is more important. Contention may occur while these changes happen. The workers aged 35 to 54 years will increase by 17 million by 2000, one in seven workers will be over 55 years of age by 2005, and workers under 35 years of age will drop from 46% to 38% by the year 2000 (Cejka, 1993).

The Cultural Shift

Another major change is in ethnic diversity. For instance, the workforce pool of the past was about 87% non-Hispanic white, compared with today's 75%. The workforce of the future, those currently 15 years old or younger, will decline to about 68% non-Hispanic white by the year 2000 (Keen, 1994). In fact, it is estimated that by the year 2000, 92% of the growth in the American workforce will be women, minorities, and those of foreign origin. Along with this, 34% of American workers will speak English as a second language (*Cultural Diversity in Healthcare,* 1995). For companies to recruit and retain workers, industry will want to encourage organizational change and adopt attitudes that embrace this diverse workforce of the future. Along with these groups will come disadvantaged workers who bring needed skills but require workplace adaptations. Progressive industries will want the workforce to see that they hire to reflect the community where they operate (UCLA Institute of Industrial Relations, 1995).

IMPLICATIONS FOR NURSING PRACTICE

Health care is changing while the American population changes. Globalization is second nature to many businesses. Both nurses and patients come from across the world, bringing both strengths and challenges to health care. Because human resources are key to any business and to health care specifically, nurses must address several issues as the workforce and population become more diverse. Concepts such as communication, tolerance, and teamwork will lead this change if nurses are to be successful in embracing diversity. Each person must bring skills and uniqueness to professional practice and channel them in a positive way so both the client and the profession will benefit. Nurses must work collaboratively in teams without losing individuality. It is through diversity that differences can strengthen and bring new ideas to nursing practice, creating a synergy that is greater than any one person's idea alone.

Cultural Dimensions in Diversity

In a film produced by the American Journal of Nursing Company entitled, *Cultural Diversity in Healthcare* (1995), Dr. Joyce Newman Giger discusses six cultural dimensions in diversity. These are communication, spatial needs, social organization, time considerations, environmental control, and biological variation.

Communication

The first cultural dimension in diversity is **communication,** perhaps the most important. This involves understanding how diverse groups learn to communicate with others. For instance, the white-European culture tends to value direct eye contact, whereas this is less important to the African-American culture (*Cultural Diversity in Healthcare,* 1995). Body language is another form of communication; some groups gesture more than others when they talk. The key is to assess communication differences and translate them appropriately as nurses work together and care for patients.

Spatial Needs

Another dimension for consideration is **spatial needs.** This is a measure of acceptable personal space. Some cultures, such as Hispanics, value physical contact, whereas Europeans may be more distant or reserved (*Cultural Diversity in Healthcare,* 1995). Touching or being "in my face" may offend certain people and result in an uncomfortable work or patient care situation.

Social organization

Social organizations produce diversity. It is in social groups that each person learns behaviors that are acceptable there. These organizations could vary from our families and clans, to religious groups, to racial and ethnic or special interest groups. For example, Asians value the family above all else and will put a family member's health before their own (*Cultural Diversity in Healthcare,* 1995). What we learn and what we are taught are valued and are the norm from which each person functions in society. These variations are important as nurses work together and care for patients from varied social groups.

Time

Time considerations vary from culture to culture. People tend to function with time orientation of present, past, and future. For instance, Hispanics may not stick to a strict schedule as some other cultures may (*Cultural Diversity in Healthcare,* 1995). For the nurse with this orientation, being a few minutes late for a shift at work may only indicate a cultural value but may also put the nurse in conflict with a rigid schedule for the supervisor who values timeliness. Again, exploration of this issue is important as expectations are enforced.

Environmental control

Environmental control is another dimension of cultural importance. Actions may be the result of either an external or internal locus of control. For example, Italian persons may think there is little they can do to affect their future and rely more on the concept of fate, whereas white Europeans may function with the understanding that their present actions will directly affect an outcome (*Cultural Diversity in Healthcare,* 1995). This is an important concept for both the nurse and the patient receiving health care counseling and care.

Biological variation

The last area to consider is **biological variations.** People vary from culture to culture biologically, as well as socially. Body structure, skin color, and susceptibility to disease may vary among cultures. For example, hypertension is prevalent in 35% of African Americans over the age of 40, diabetes and tuberculosis are often seen in Native Americans, and diabetes is common in Hispanics (*Cultural Diversity in Healthcare,* 1995). These considerations are very important as nurses take proactive efforts to screen for health problems early to prevent premature onset in patients, as well as in themselves.

It is important for professional nurses to avoid stereotyping. When looking at general characteristics among cultures, one must remember that these are generalizations and do not always apply. In fact, stereotyping can build new barriers and produce conflicts.

IMPLICATIONS FOR RESOURCE MANAGEMENT

As health care reform continues, nurses are asked to do more with less and faster. A key to this is proactive assessment of the health care customer. Certain practices may be efficacious, or beneficial to the patient, and should be encouraged. Others may be neutral, or create no harm, and at best provide a psychological benefit. These should be accepted as important to the customer or patient. However, if the behavior is dysfunctional, such as eating harmful foods, nurses can take the opportunity to educate patients to more healthful behaviors, mindful of the cultural influence their existing behavior has for them (*Cultural Diversity in Healthcare,* 1995).

To provide cost-efficient, customer-focused care, a cultural assessment must be provided by each nurse on patient contact. This assessment includes cultural/racial/ethnic identity, language/communication barriers, religious beliefs and practices, illness and wellness behaviors, and healing beliefs and practices. Other important areas of assessment include family system functioning and values, nutritional behaviors, dietary needs and preferences, lifestyle and habits, and work and daily routines (*Cultural Diversity in Healthcare,* 1995). Effort up front with a thorough assessment and individualized planning of care can save wasted health care dollars and produce a happier patient/client.

Summary

As diversity continues and becomes a major change for the workforce of 2000, practicing nurses will meet new challenges of collaboration and team efforts. Nurses will come from various cultures and will bring strengths and new ideas to health care delivery. Care will be provided for patients or clients from various cultures. The challenge to the professional nurse is to recognize the importance of diversity, identify diversity, eliminate barriers, and collaborate to design the best health care practices possible. Nurse educators must accept the challenge of preparing students for "culturally competent practice." This includes teaching a deliberate practice of "respectful behaviors and interactions." (Lenburg, 1995) Because culture and ethnicity can influence health and illness, health care professionals must anticipate and resolve conflicts and manage bias for the good of the population as a whole and to improve the quality of care. This is of utmost importance as health care resources are procured and allocated in a changing environment.

At the Greater Victoria Hospital Society, promoting multiculturalism has been accomplished on a zero budget. Staff there launched a multicultural interest group in 1992. Anyone interested in joining was invited. The goal was to educate staff on multiculturalism, focusing on issues related to patient care. A valuable part of this process was an attitude survey, since being open to differences is necessary to embrace diversity. The success has been in the message carried by this group (Grewal and Butler, 1996):

> We instill confidence in the healthcare professional by training him or her to recognize the individual patient beyond the ethnic face, what is culturally meaningful and unique to that patient, while encouraging openness and respect for the complexity of cultural differences. Culture is not a strange unknown disease.

For more information on diversity and professional nursing practice, contact the American Nurses Association's Ethnic and Minority Program at (202) 651-7245 (NSNA, 1996).

Discussion Questions

1. What are the diversity trends occurring today as related to workforce demographics?
2. What are the nursing implications for increased diversity in the United States?
3. What impact do cultural differences have on patients? Nurses? Health care?

4. Why are recognition and understanding of diversity in the United States critical to resource management?

REFERENCES

Cejka S: The changing healthcare workforce: A call for managing diversity, *Healthcare Exec*, p 20, March/April 1993.

Cultural diversity in healthcare, Washington, DC, 1995, American Journal of Nursing Company (film).

Grewal S, Butler V: Promoting multiculturalism on a zero budget, *Leadership Health Serv* 5:5, 1996.

Keen CD: Emerging issues in human resources: Looking at the workplace of tomorrow today, Alexandria, Va, 1994, Society for Human Resource Management.

Lenburg C: *Promoting cultural competence in and through nursing education: A critical review and comprehensive plan for action,* monograph by American Academy of Nursing, Washington, DC, 1995.

National Student Nurses' Association (NSNA): Breakthrough to nursing (BTN) transcultural resource listing, New York, 1996.

UCLA Institute of Industrial Relations: *Human resources forecast,* supplement to *HR Magazine,* 1994.

chapter **twenty-one**

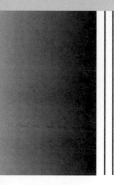

Continuous Quality Improvement: Practical Applications and Challenges

Marylane Wade Koch

Learning Objectives

- Discuss the key concepts from the Pew Health Professions Commission report "Healthy America: Practitioners for 2005" and relate them to quality improvement and resource management.
- Identify practical applications of continuous quality improvement.
- Describe future challenges of continuous quality improvement and relate these to resource management.

The future brings many challenges as customers such as consumers and payors demand high-quality health care services and outcomes at reasonable and affordable costs. Nurses and other health care professionals must find new ways to provide services and products to meet these customer requirements. A culture that supports the concepts and practice of **continuous quality improvement** in every step of delivering health care services will be necessary to continue to participate in the future marketplace. Key to this is recognizing environmental trends and identifying implications for improvement in customer service. Professionals who are proactive in identifying and implementing opportunities for improvement will be valued in independent practice or within the agency or organization where they work.

HEALTH CARE TRENDS

In October 1991 the Pew Health Professions Commission issued a report entitled, "Healthy America: Practitioners for 2005." The purpose of the report was to assist various schools that educate health care professionals in meeting the changing health care needs of America. The Pew Commission believes that if the recommendations presented are implemented, over time more efficient practice will result, as well as professionals' being more satisfied with their work. The goal is outcomes management that encourages more effective and efficient health care at less cost. The president of the Pew Charitable Trust, Dr. Thomas W. Langfitt, suggests that two paths must be followed to achieve necessary health care reform: (1) reorganization and (2) refinance of the present system to allow access and contain costs (Pew Health Professions Commission, 1991).

There are five broad trends identified in this report (Pew Health Professions Commission, 1991). These forces will vary in implication among professionals in various parts of the country, as well as within different sociocultural groups. However, the underlying issues remain the same.

Efficiency and Effectiveness through Coordinated Care

The emphasis to contain health care costs is a major force in the United States today. Coordinated care is one way to manage costs. To do this, a major priority has been established with most providers: improvement in costs, quality, and management. Coordinated care will come through integrated delivery systems with a change in focus from the health needs of the individual to the health needs of the community at large. New systems will diversify as the goal of cost-effective, appropriate care continues. This will result in a move from strictly curative care to preventive care. The U.S. population will receive more care in ambulatory care or community settings than in those of traditional hospital acute care. The coordinated care systems will measure outcomes, improve quality, increase practitioner accountability, and encourage standardized practice patterns. Practitioner value will come from both clinical and care management ability (Pew Health Professions Commission, 1991).

Diversity and Aging in the Population

The U.S. population is aging rapidly, with increasing numbers of persons living well beyond age 65. In fact, the average life expectancy is 77 years, with women's life expectancy being beyond 80; the fastest growing population segment is persons 85 years of age or older (Deets, 1995). The effect of this trend is an increase in health care resource consumption by older adults. Already, adults over age 65 spend 21% of their income on health care (excluding long-term care), whereas those under 65 spend only 8% of their income on the same (Deets, 1995).

This shift in demographics will also mean a shift in focus from acute to chronic disease care. To manage this situation cost effectively, health care practitioners must delay chronic disease onset through education and prevention. The United States will struggle with the dynamics of paying for these expanded services needed for an aging population as the older population grows faster than the younger population. This also results in fewer available persons to fill the roles of health care professionals.

The U.S. population is also becoming more diverse ethnically and racially. In fact, the number of persons from minorities is growing at a rate double that of whites (Pew Health Professions Commission, 1991). New cultural practices, economics, and disease patterns will result. More people from minorities will become health care practitioners as well. Diversity brings the need for understanding and relating to special needs of this segment of the population.

Tensions in the Expansion of Science and Technology

The trend toward new technology for diagnostic and therapeutic practice is under scrutiny. Although the U.S. population continues to embrace new treatments brought about by technology, the health care system must balance improvements with costs. Some issues to be considered are quality of life, access to care, individual choice, risk-benefit decisions, and integrity of life (Pew Health Professions Commission, 1991). Though valued, technology can further depersonalize and fragment care given by technically trained, specialized professionals.

Biotechnology will bring new dimensions to genetically based treatments, dictating changes in the delivery of health care. This brings both fear and hope to people in the United States while they adapt to change. Practitioners will lead this transition and establish new practice parameters.

Information technology will expand rapidly. Practitioners will be pressured to learn and use these tools in health promotion and disease prevention, as well as diagnosis and treatment. With the ability to gather and analyze group data, more opportunity exists to improve community population health. Biomedical research will be more specialized and utilized in practice more rapidly (Pew Health Professions Commission, 1991).

Consumer Empowerment

The relationship between the consumer and the provider is in transition. Among the issues at hand are informed consent, litigiousness, quality improvement, and cost containment (Pew Health Professions Commission, 1991). Mutual expectations and obligations between consumer and provider will require definition as focus shifts to health promotion and cost sharing by the consumer. Materials for health promotion must be written so all may understand and participate in health care decisions and accountability regardless of educational level.

Wellness emphasis has shifted care decisions to persons who pursue self-diagnostic, self-treatment methodologies. These consumers will not accept a passive role in their health care but demand information and assistance to improve and maintain their health. Consumers will have to share more accountability for health care costs as well as they select providers who are customer focused and cost-efficient.

Values That Shape Health Care

The aforementioned trends create a struggle between the rights of all humans to quality health care services and the implications for the common good of society itself. Issues such as quality of life, extension of life, and use of scarce health care resources surface. Many Americans are without health insurance or coverage for basic health care needs. Rural Americans live with less availability to care. Many die with preventable illnesses. Still costs continue to soar while government leaders discuss rationing of resources even further.

In the recent past the goal of health care has been cure with all measures taken to extend life. More and more the appropriateness of these practices is being challenged. This leads to discussion of patients' rights and choices for quality of life, extension of life, and the right to die comfortably. Hospices have grown in number across the United States, as have concerns about assisted suicide.

All of these trends are directly related to and support the need for continuous quality improvement. Coordinated and integrated care must produce the highest levels of positive clinical outcomes in a customer-friendly way at affordable costs. A change in U.S. demographics supports a shift from cure to care and acute to chronic disease management with understanding of and planning for cultural differences and health care practices. Again, professionals must use continuous quality improvement principles to actualize change in delivery of care with goals of improved outcomes and decreased costs. Technology offers improvements that result in increased longevity with expanded diagnostic and treatment modalities. The charge here is to continue improvements at affordable costs.

Consumers know more and want more control over health care decision making. Health care professionals must improve educational materials and methods to address consumer accountability and care cost sharing. Values will be diverse and have implications for quality-of-life and death-choice issues. The consumer must be informed to make the best individual decision.

PRACTICAL APPLICATIONS OF CONTINUOUS IMPROVEMENT

Many studies support the savings in health care costs, as well as improved quality and resource consumption, through continuous quality improvement. The following examples are but a few of the practical ways continuous quality improvement is benefiting health care in the current environment.

Continuous Improvement through Inventory Management

Rush-Presbyterian-St. Luke's Medical Center implemented an **inventory management** program that decreased supply utilization by $330,000 in 2 years. An automated system was installed in 1993, which reduced costs, reduced total supply usage by 20% per patient day, and improved supply usage based on actual need, rather than perceived need, by health care professionals ("Case in Point," 1996).

Continuous Improvement through Patient Documentation

Cincinnati Children's Hospital Medical Center implemented an automated **patient documentation** process that allows occupational, speech, and physical therapists to have detailed records that are electronically signed. When complete, these can be faxed directly to insurance companies or physicians. The records are downloaded each night. Before this automation 40% of the therapists' time was spent on administrative tasks; now therapists can spend more time with patients and are more productive. Start-up costs were recovered in 90 days, and the medical center is expecting an annual revenue increase of $1.2 million ("Case in Point," 1996).

Continuous Improvement through Variance Analysis

A St. Louis hospital, St. Mary's Health Center, uses a continuous quality improvement process called **"variance analysis"** to improve quality care. Care paths are used to plan treatments and for patient education and discharge planning. Any variance is examined to determine if there is an implementation problem or if the care path needs revision. An example is the care path for pneumonia. Two areas of concern surfaced when this care path was put in place. It was noted that patients were not receiving their antibiotics within the 4 hours specified and often were not getting the correct drug specified by the American Thoracic Society. Through continuous quality improvement processes of analysis of variances, the directive was clear: give the right antibiotic at the right time. The pathway was changed to reflect these initiatives. The results were (1) a decrease in mortality rate for pneumonia patients from 10.4% to 3.4%, (2) a decrease in average length of stay from 7.6 to 6.3 days, and (3) a decrease in average length of time between admission and administration of antibiotics from 5.3 to 3.5 hours ("News Digest," 1996).

Continuous Improvement through Cost Management

Castaneda-Mendez and Bernstein (1997) report the use and benefit of value-based **cost management** to integrate measures of activity-based costing, value-added analysis, and cost of quality. They wanted to measure the customer's perspective of value of services provided, the provider's perspective of being the customer's fiduciary, and the business side of achieving net income. The study focused on financial measures and looked at process measures of effectiveness, efficiency, and adaptability. The project studied the process of triage of patients with chest pain and the relationship to laboratory services. Cost-of-quality data linked effectiveness to prevention costs, processing costs, appraisal costs, failure costs, and outcome measures as value-added and activity-based costing. Implications for laboratory practice include offering more or different diagnostic information to clinicians using an improved process. The additional costs associated with this are prevention costs, which are recaptured as return on investment. Better results occur at the patient level, not just at the test result level. Using this approach to continuous quality improvement, laboratory professionals become collaborative team members in patient-focused care.

Continuous Improvement in Community Health

Another practical application of continuous quality improvement in **community health** is in the area of health research. For example, research related to the environmental effects on health by exposure to chemicals is important for prevention of illness and chronic disease. A study was funded by the National Institute of Nursing Research and the Center for Research on Occupational and Environmental Toxicology at Oregon Health Sciences University. The focus was on identifying the exposures of environmental agents associated with Parkinson's disease. The controlled study sampled persons who were diagnosed with Parkinson's before age 50.

A detailed survey was sent to address exposure at work, home, hobby, and travel to metals and chemicals. Several findings came to light from the 63 people who participated. There was a higher occurrence of Parkinson's disease in (1) persons who self-reported exposure to pesticides and (2) persons who live and work in agricultural communities. Specifically, persons who reported exposure to insecticides more than 10 times a year had a five times higher risk of Parkinson's disease. A planned study is to look at environmentally related cancer (Butterfield, 1996). The Parkinson's disease study is but one of many examples of research-based nursing studies that can improve the quality of life and patient care outcomes for more effective use of limited resources and dollars for treatment.

Another study looked at antibiotics and other drugs for the common cold. Using 1993-1994 data from Kentucky Medicaid programs, the study reviewed medical records for either outpatient or emergency department visits. This study grew from the concern that drug-resistant bacteria are more and more prevalent as a result of antibiotic overuse. Often antibiotics are prescribed for the common cold even though colds are caused by viruses and antibiotics are not effective in treatment. The number of persons reviewed was 1439 individuals, mostly children, with 2171 visits. Some 60% got an antibiotic. Investigators estimate the cost of prescribing antibiotics for the common cold to be at least $37.5 million per year in health care expenditures. This study resulted in the recommendation for improvement in practice by guidelines that prevent unnecessary prescribing and limit development of drug-resistant bacteria ("Advances," 1996).

FACING NEW CHALLENGES

Although continuous quality improvement offers many solutions to health care challenges, it cannot be viewed as a panacea. Many organizations become disillusioned with continuous improvement when results do not quickly bolster the bottom line. To directly link continuous improvement to the financial welfare of an organization, the leaders must tie efforts directly to business goals and operational plans. Quality leaders must integrate continuous improvement efforts with business management (Godfrey, 1997).

Sibbald (1996) writes about a project led by Pat Armstrong in which researchers interviewed 25 groups of employees at 10 hospitals, a total of 96 people, to get their opinion of continuous quality improvement as a management philosophy. The study showed that workers became disillusioned with continuous improvement because it seemed that the focus was always on cost cutting rather than the delivery of quality care. Workers expressed a concern that continuous improvement was used for a short-term cost saving and cuts were often directed at those delivering the services. Armstrong believes that management can lose support for continuous quality improvement when they focus on the cost of human resources instead of seeing the people as valued for the savings in their ideas. The study does support the importance of quality improvement but warns management to look at its message if it wants to keep employees producing quality improvement ideas.

LEGAL ISSUES IN CONTINUOUS QUALITY IMPROVEMENT

There are often legal implications affecting the practice of continuous quality improvement. In the past persons looked to the community standard to establish acceptable practice standards. Now more national standards of practice have been established to determine if a health care defendant is competent and was prudent in delivery of care. In fact, the federal government is now establishing clinical practice standards through the Agency for Health Care Policy and Research (AHCPR). This agency was established in 1989 by Congress to develop and disseminate national guidelines to support clinical health care professionals (Cross and Schmele, 1996).

Peer review laws are more common because many states and the federal government have enacted laws to improve the quality of health care in this country. The Health Care Quality Improvement Act of 1986 (HCQIA) requires physicians and facilities to report payments made on malpractice and peer review activities to a national data bank. It also requires reporting of any adverse actions taken concerning either a license or clinical privilege. Reporting requirements are mandated for hospitals, boards of medical examiners, any health care agency, professional societies, and insurance companies who work with physicians, dentists, and other licensed health care professionals (Cross and Schmele, 1996).

Self-directed work teams and employee empowerment are key to keeping any business financially healthy. Most managers will tell you that their most important resources are the human resources at the organization. More and more businesses are recognizing that quick, friendly response to customers is as important as a good service or product. The people customers care about are those who answer their calls or help them get the service or product they desire. This means that employees must be given the information needed to take action to help the customer. Managers will be most successful with continuous quality improvement when they empower employees by sharing information (Blanchard, 1996).

Leaders of the future will view the total organization and identify systems and processes that are supporting or constraining forces for organizational performance improvement. Resource management will focus on strategic mission and find ways to improve organizational processes for enhanced performance (Castaneda-Mendez, 1997). Leadership is key to success, and continuous quality improvement is key to leadership success.

Summary

The future is full of challenges for health care professionals. Continuous quality improvement is one current philosophy that holds promise to both improve the quality of health care in this country and manage costs for health care products and services. Nursing must embrace the concept of resource management as a way to secure better health care provided by the professional nurse.

Dieter (1996) writes about the implications of continuous quality improvement for clinical nurse specialists, although his comments are applicable to all areas of practice. He challenges that quality nursing care and cost-effectiveness can coexist in a culture of continuous improvement. He further asserts that nurses in the twenty-first century must be aware of the bottom line when designing new plans, using current research, or requesting more equipment or staffing changes. Nurses must be comfortable demonstrating cost-effectiveness and proper resource management. Educators must incorporate basic principles of accounting and economics into professional nurse curricula so nurses have some understanding of business. Using continuous quality improvement, nurses can show good stewardship of health care resources and continue to be key players in today's evolving health care system.

Discussion Questions

1. As nurses prepare for professional practice in the coming decades, what are the health care trends that may affect that practice? Why are skills and knowledge in continuous quality improvement important to professional nursing practice in the future?
2. What are some practical applications of continuous quality improvement in the hospital, community, or outpatient settings? What are common beneficial outcomes, and how do they affect nursing practice?
3. Is continuous quality improvement the answer to providing cost-efficient, quality health care in the future? What role does leadership play in ensuring that organizational success is achieved for improved quality care?

REFERENCES

Advances: Research note, *Q Newsletter Robert Wood Johnson Foundation* 4:6, 1996.

Blanchard K: Sharing information is key, *Qual Digest* 16(6):19, 1996.

Butterfield PG: Seeking clues to Parkinson's disease, *Reflections* 22(3):14, 1996.

Case in point, *J Healthcare Res Manage* 15(10):24, 1996.

Castaneda-Mendez K: Value-based cost management: The foundation of a balanced performance measurement system, *J Healthcare Qual* 19(4):6, 1997.

Castaneda-Mendez K, Bernstein L: Linking costs and quality improvement to clinical outcomes through added value, *J Healthcare Qual* 19(2):11, 1997.

Cross LL: Legal implications of quality management. In Schmele JA, editor: *Quality management in nursing and health care,* Albany, NY, 1996, Delmar.

Deets H: Home care in the 21st century, *Caring Magazine* 14(9):50, 1995.

Dieter DC: Cost effectiveness and quality nursing care, *Clin Nurse Specialist* 10(3):153, 1996.

Godfrey B: The bottom line, *Qual Digest* 17(2):17, 1997.

News digest: Variance analysis improves health care, *Qual Digest* 16(6):10, 1996.

Pew Health Professions Commission: Healthy America: Practitioners for 2005, Durham, NC, 1991, Duke University Medical Center.

Sibbald BJ: The painful price of TQM, *Can Nurse* 92(7):6, 1996.

Index

Page numbers in italics indicate illustrations,
boxes, and tables.